Environmental Health in the 21st Century

Environmental Health in the 21st Century

From Air Pollution to Zoonotic Diseases

Volume 2: L–Z

RICHARD CRUME, EDITOR

GREENWOOD™

An Imprint of ABC-CLIO, LLC
Santa Barbara, California • Denver, Colorado

Library of Congress Cataloging-in-Publication Data

Names: Crume, Richard V., editor.
Title: Environmental health in the 21st century : from air pollution to zoonotic diseases / Richard Crume, editor.
Description: Santa Barbara, California : Greenwood, [2018] | Includes bibliographical references and index.
Identifiers: LCCN 2017037595 (print) | LCCN 2017039061 (ebook) | ISBN 9781440843655 (ebook) | ISBN 9781440843648 (set : alk. paper) | ISBN 9781440848728 (vol.1 : alk. paper) | ISBN 9781440848735 (vol. 2 : alk. paper)
Subjects: | MESH: Environmental Pollution | Environmental Illness | Environmental Exposure | Environmental Health—history | Encyclopedias
Classification: LCC RA566 (ebook) | LCC RA566 (print) | NLM WA 13 | DDC 363.73—dc23
LC record available at https://lccn.loc.gov/2017037595

ISBN: 978-1-4408-4364-8 (set)
978-1-4408-4872-8 (vol. 1)
978-1-4408-4873-5 (vol. 2)
978-1-4408-4365-5 (ebook)

22 21 20 19 18 1 2 3 4 5

This book is also available as an eBook.

Greenwood
An Imprint of ABC-CLIO, LLC

ABC-CLIO, LLC
130 Cremona Drive, P.O. Box 1911
Santa Barbara, California 93116-1911
www.abc-clio.com

This book is printed on acid-free paper ∞

Manufactured in the United States of America

Dedicated to the civil servants of the U.S. Environmental Protection Agency, who have devoted their careers to solving the most challenging environmental health issues while providing global leadership and making the world a better place for future generations. Their hard work, professionalism, and commitment to public service often go underappreciated.

Contents

Alphabetical List of Entries

Topical List of Entries

Environmental Pollution

Health Sciences

Energy and Climate

Waste Management

Built Environment

L

LABORATORY QUALITY ASSURANCE

Analyses of environmental pollutants are usually conducted in laboratories, where trained scientists and technicians apply standard operating procedures to achieve consistent and reproducible results. To ensure that the correct processes and procedures are followed, including appropriate instrumentation and calibration protocols, a quality assurance (QA) evaluation is often performed by someone independent of the laboratory. QA is important to establish that environmental contaminants are correctly identified so that appropriate measures can be taken to protect public health.

To be confident that a laboratory provides accurate results, a QA plan is created that (1) describes their polices, objectives, principles, organizational authority, responsibilities, accountability, and implementation plans and (2) provides the framework for planning, implementing, and assessing their work. QA plans are often required by organizations like the federal government before the organization will do business with the laboratory. Independent auditors ordinarily carry out QA evaluations to ensure that the QA results are unbiased.

Often a QA plan is developed that is specific to a particular project, for example, analyzing a large quantity of samples from a contaminated stream or industrial smokestack. This plan is commonly referred to as a quality assurance project plan (QAPP). QAPPs integrate all technical and quality aspects of the project, including planning, implementation, and assessment. The purpose of the QAPP is to document the analytical approach and to provide a project-specific "blueprint" for obtaining the type and quality of environmental data needed for a specific purpose.

Once the QAPP is finalized and approved, each person associated with requirements of the QAPP must be provided a copy, and system must be in place to track revisions and document distributions. Additionally, training is required for anyone

What Are Standard Operating Procedures?

An important laboratory QA requirement is that all routine processes and procedures used in the laboratory must be documented as standard operating procedures (SOPs). These SOPs must be detailed enough to ensure that a scientist or technician knows exactly how to follow the processes and procedures to achieve accurate and reproducible results. Well-written SOPs are essential for an effective QA program.

implementing any part of the QAPP, and this training must be documented. Any controls or standards used to perform and validate the analyses, including equipment calibrations, must be checked and verified to ensure they meet any certification requirements.

Before beginning any measurement and data collection activity, it is imperative to understand the monitoring objectives and to document them in the QAPP. All collected data inherently have some degree of uncertainty, and it is important to establish the acceptable level of uncertainty before beginning the measurement and data collection activity. A systematic approach to establishing the acceptable degree of uncertainty involves developing data quality objectives (DQOs). These can be viewed as quantitative and qualitative objectives for measuring data in terms of precision, accuracy, representativeness, comparability, and completeness, and they are frequently cited as the level of uncertainty acceptable to a decision maker. Ideally, the DQO process leads to efficient and effective expenditure of resources; consensus on the type, quality, and quantity of data needed to meet the project goals; and the full documentation of actions taken during the development of the project.

Joe Elkins and Richard Crume

See Also: Ames Test; Environmental Auditing

Further Reading

Hibbert, D. B. *Quality Assurance for the Analytical Chemistry Laboratory.* New York: Oxford University Press, 2007.

Konieczka, Piotr, and Jacek Namieśnik. *Quality Assurance and Quality Control in the Analytical Chemical Laboratory: A Practical Approach.* Boca Raton, FL: CRC Press, 2009.

U.S. Environmental Protection Agency. *How EPA Manages the Quality of Its Environmental Data.* http://www.epa.gov/quality (accessed December 31, 2015).

World Health Organization. *Quality Assurance.* http://www.who.int/diagnostics_laboratory/quality/en/ (accessed December 31, 2015).

LAND DISPOSAL OF WASTE MATERIALS

What are waste materials? Garbage is so pervasive in our society that we know what it is intuitively, but often the exact definition eludes us. The U.S. Environmental Protection Agency (EPA) considers solid waste as "any garbage or refuse, sludge from a wastewater treatment plant, water supply treatment plant, or air pollution control facility and other discarded material, resulting from industrial, commercial, mining, and agricultural operations, and from community activities." Just about everything we do leaves behind some type of waste material. Note that the definition of solid waste includes wastes that are liquid, semisolid, or contained gases. In the United States, wastes amount to about 260 million tons (236 million metric tons) per year, or around 4.4 pounds (2.0 kilograms) per person per day.

The four most common components of municipal solid waste in the United States are paper, food, yard trimmings, and plastics (see Table 9). Additionally, there

Table 9. Municipal solid waste components in the United States.

Municipal Solid Waste Material	Percentage of Total Solid Waste (By Weight, before Recycling)
Paper	26.6
Food	14.9
Yard trimmings	13.3
Plastics	12.9
Rubber, leather, textiles	9.5
Metals	9.0
Wood	6.2
Glass	4.4
Other	3.2

are other types of wastes that are sometimes more difficult to account for, including sewage, radioactive and other hazardous waste materials, petroleum refining by-products, and electronic wastes.

Efforts over the past few decades by the EPA and other government agencies to deal with waste and its associated problems, including public health issues and environmental degradation, have yielded mixed results. Recycling rates have risen, but so has the total amount of solid waste generated, such that the quantity of waste being disposed of today is still slightly more than it was in 1980. Recycling rates in the United States lag behind many other developed nations. For example, some northern European countries (e.g., Sweden and the Netherlands) recycle over half of their wastes and incinerate the remainder. Relying on recycling and incineration, Germany landfills are less than 1 percent of overall waste, and Japan has a very extensive recycling program where very little goes to waste.

There are three main paths for waste materials once they are ready for disposal: they can be recycled, incinerated, or placed in a landfill. In the past, some wastes were simply left out to rot in open dumps, often at sites near waterways. This practice created a number of environmental hazards, including water contamination, toxic gas releases, fire hazards, and infestations. At the turn of the 20th century, the United States imported incinerator technology from England, and around the time of World War II, the concept of landfilling became attractive for large American cities.

Today, waste materials that are landfilled must be disposed of in a capped and carefully controlled landfill environment. Between 1984 and 1988, new regulations and enforcement of the Resource Conservation and Recovery Act required safety standards at disposal sites, including rejecting certain hazardous materials, which required processing in special facilities. Beginning in 1991, federal regulations began requiring landfills to have waterproof plastic liners to keep liquefied garbage (leachate) from leaking into the surrounding soil. Landfills must now also

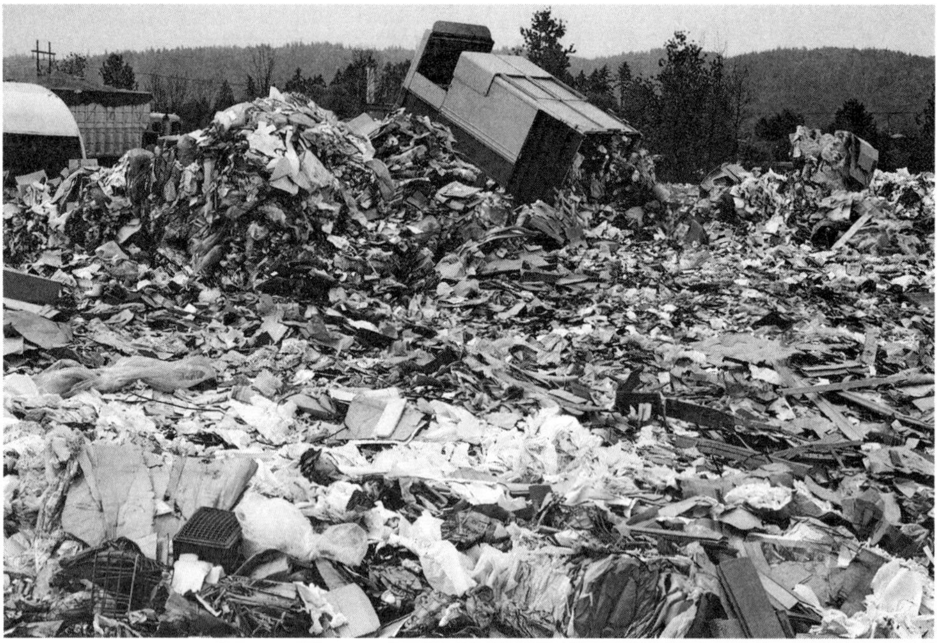

Large piles of garbage at a landfill. Many municipal landfills are reaching full capacity, causing cities to find alternatives to the land disposal of wastes, including waste reuse, reduction, and recycling programs. (PhotoDisc, Inc.)

monitor leachate and methane gas collection. At many modern landfills, the controlled release of gases through pipes is allowed, or the gases are captured and burned to produce energy.

Landfill space is becoming a major issue in the United States as older sites become filled and citizens reject new sites in close proximity to their communities. In 1970, there were over 16,000 authorized waste disposal landfill sites in the United States, but that number had fallen to 1,200 by 2011 (although many of the remaining sites are far larger than their predecessors). As new landfills are created farther away from the cities where the wastes originate, this creates secondary impacts on the environment, such as air pollution emissions from garbage trucks. Although many landfills have closed over the past few decades, there is still plenty of space available for new landfills outside of urban areas. As of 2015, 22 states reported having landfill space available into the next decade, and it has been estimated that current landfills can meet U.S. trash disposal needs for years to come.

Modern landfills are often considered preferable to waste incinerators from a public health perspective because incineration creates toxic air pollution emissions, including dioxin compounds, that are hazardous to health and may be carcinogenic. Incinerators also cause gaseous and particulate matter pollution, although emission controls today are effective in reducing (but not eliminating) these pollutants.

Incinerator technology, which is now used mainly for waste-to-energy purposes (i.e., incinerators that produce useful heat or electricity), can be less expensive than a comprehensive recycling program when energy recovery is taken into account.

Aaron Dorman

See Also: Bioremediation for Waste Treatment; Dioxin Pollution; Electronic Waste Disposal; Environmental Protection Agency; Landfill Gas Pollution; Municipal Solid Waste Management; Ocean Dumping and the Pacific Garbage Patch; Particulate Matter and Bioaerosols Pollution; Recycling; Resource Conservation and Recovery Act; Three Rs of Waste Management; Waste Incineration

Further Reading

Advancing Sustainable Materials Management: 2014 Fact Sheet. Washington, DC: U.S. Environmental Protection Agency, 2016.

Humes, Edward. *Garbology: Our Dirty Love Affair with Trash.* New York: Avery, 2013.

Lacy, Peter, and Jakob Rutqvist. *Waste to Wealth: The Circular Economy Advantage.* New York: Palgrave Macmillan, 2015.

Pichtel, John. *Waste Management Practices: Municipal, Hazardous, and Industrial.* Boca Raton, FL: CRC Press, 2014.

U.S. Environmental Protection Agency. *Clean Air Act Guidelines and Standards for Waste Management.* https://www.epa.gov/stationary-sources-air-pollution/clean-air-act-guidelines-and-standards-waste-management (accessed September 21, 2016).

U.S. Environmental Protection Agency. *Controlling Air Pollution from Boilers and Process Heaters.* https://www.epa.gov/boilers (accessed December 21, 2016).

U.S. Environmental Protection Agency. *Criteria for the Definition of Solid Waste and Solid and Hazardous Waste Exclusions.* https://www.epa.gov/hw/criteria-definition-solid-waste-and-solid-and-hazardous-waste-exclusions (accessed December 21, 2016).

Van Haaren, Rob, Nickolas Themelis, and Nora Goldstein. "The State of Garbage in America." *BioCycle*, vol. 51, no. 10 (October 2010): 16.

Williams, Timothy. "Garbage Incinerators Make Comeback, Kindling Both Garbage and Debate." *New York Times*, January 10, 2015, https://www.nytimes.com/2015/01/11/us/garbage-incinerators-make-comeback-kindling-both-garbage-and-debate.html?.

LANDFILL GAS POLLUTION

In the United States and many other nations, much of the municipal garbage is deposited in landfills (also called sanitary landfills), which are specially designed facilities for burying wastes (e.g., kitchen garbage, yard wastes, used packing materials, and sometimes commercial wastes and other nonhazardous waste materials). Landfills may also be designed to receive construction and demolition debris and hazardous wastes. Over time, microorganisms begin to break down and decompose landfill wastes, resulting in the release of gases, including methane, a highly flammable and potent greenhouse gas. These gases can be harmful to human health and contribute to climate change.

Fighting Climate Change by Recycling

How much trash does the average American create every day? Would you believe over 4 pounds (1.8 kilograms)? For all Americans, that adds up to over 250 million tons (227 million metric tons) of trash each year! About 35 percent of these waste materials are recycled or composted, which has prevented the release of over 200 million tons (181 million metric tons) of carbon dioxide (CO_2) per year from landfills and incinerators, the equivalent of taking nearly 40 million cars of the road. Reducing CO_2 emissions is important because the increasing concentrations of CO_2 in the atmosphere, mainly due to human activities beginning with the industrial revolution, are the primary cause of climate change.

Kitchen garbage and other wastes contain many organic compounds that microorganisms feed on, forming methane and other gases. These gases migrate upward through the landfill, eventually being released to the surrounding air. Typically, about half of landfill gases consists of methane, and most of the remainder is carbon dioxide. While both methane and carbon dioxide contribute to global warming, methane is a much more potent greenhouse gas. (In the United States, nearly 20 percent of methane associated with human activities comes from landfills.) The remaining landfill gases are composed of hundreds of different compounds, including complex organic molecules and hydrogen sulfide. The makeup of landfill gases varies greatly from site to site, depending on factors such as the type of waste and the climate.

Landfill gases often contain certain organic compounds that are considered hazardous air pollutants (also called air toxics) and are known or suspected to cause cancer and other adverse health effects in humans. Toluene, benzene, xylenes, vinyl chloride, and ethyl benzene are examples of these types of air pollutants. Although typically present at very low concentrations relative to methane and carbon dioxide, these toxic pollutants can still represent a significant health risk to the surrounding population.

Another problem with landfill gases is odor. Well-designed and well-operated facilities typically do not have odor problems. But under certain weather conditions (e.g., during an atmospheric inversion when pollutants tend to be trapped near the ground), nearby residents may be able to smell the landfill. One common component of landfill gases, hydrogen sulfide, smells like rotten eggs and can easily be detected by the human nose, even at concentrations as low as 0.5 to 1 part per billion. The ammonia present in landfill gases also has a distinctively pungent odor. When exposed to landfill gas odors, some people may experience headaches or nausea, although medical attention is seldom required. Families living close to landfills may find the odors disruptive to their daily lives.

Landfill gases can be collected using a system of wells, trenches, piping, and fans (or other gas-moving equipment). After being collected, the gases may enter a combustion device (e.g., a boiler, engine, turbine, or flare), which destroys the methane and many of the organic and odorous compounds. Because methane can be used as a fuel, combusting it in a boiler, engine, or turbine to generate power (e.g., electricity or heat) is an attractive benefit of collecting landfill gases. (Roughly a quarter of U.S. landfills collect gases for power production, mostly electricity.) Landfill gas emissions can also be reduced by producing less waste to begin with, by recycling waste materials instead of sending them to the landfill, and by finding other uses for wastes, such as composting.

Due to concern about landfill gases, the U.S. Environmental Protection Agency has issued rules requiring owners of large landfills to capture and control gases emitted from their facilities. Owners have the option of burning the gas in a combustion device (e.g., a boiler, engine, or turbine) to generate energy, collecting and treating the gas for sale or other beneficial use, or destroying it in a flare. These rules are part of the nation's climate strategy to reduce methane emissions. Additionally, the rules reduce emissions of other organic compounds, including some hazardous air pollutants, and pollutants causing odors.

Richard Crume

See Also: Bioremediation for Waste Treatment; Carbon Dioxide and the Carbon Cycle; Climate Change and Human Health; Environmental Protection Agency; Hazardous Air Pollutants; Hazardous Waste Disposal; Land Disposal of Waste Materials; Municipal Solid Waste Management; Odor Pollution; Open Burning of Waste; Recycling; Three Rs of Waste Management; Waste Incineration

Further Reading

Emerging Technologies for the Management and Utilization of Landfill Gas. Washington, DC: U.S. Environmental Protection Agency, 2013.

Landfill Gas: Creating Green Energy in Your Community (Landfill Methane Outreach Program). Washington, DC: U.S. Environmental Protection Agency, 2008.

Pawlowska, Malgorzata. *Mitigation of Landfill Gas Emissions*. London: CRC Press, 2014.

Townsend, Timothy G., et al. *Sustainable Practices for Landfill Design and Operation*. New York: Springer, 2015.

U.S. Environmental Protection Agency. *Landfill Methane Outreach Program*. https://www.epa.gov/lmop (accessed August 15, 2016).

U.S. Environmental Protection Agency. Municipal Solid Waste Landfills. https://www.epa.gov/landfills/municipal-solid-waste-landfills#regs (accessed September 8, 2017).

LAPPÉ, FRANCES MOORE

Frances Moore Lappé (1944–), author of the 1971 best seller *Diet for a Small Planet*, which has sold 3 million copies worldwide, grew up in a Fort Worth, Texas, household where meat and white bread were the centerpieces of what was then considered to be a healthy family meal. But her life led her on a path to redefining what healthy eating should be and exploring how individuals can make a difference in their own lives and the lives of others by changing their eating habits. The impact Lappé has had on world hunger and health is extensive and multifaceted. She has written 18 books, is a world-renowned spokesperson on the topic of solving world hunger, and has founded and contributed to a wide variety of organizations focusing on food, hunger, and the environment.

Solving Our Biggest Global Challenges

Thinking like an ecosystem, we see that, since we are all connected, we are all implicated in every social outcome.

An Interview with Frances Moore Lappé

Best-selling author, public speaker, and activist

Frances Moore Lappé is the author or coauthor of 18 books, including the groundbreaking best seller Diet for a Small Planet, *which began a revolution over 30 years ago in how America and the world think about food and hunger. (J. M. Hirsch of the Associated Press calls* Diet for a Small Planet *"the blueprint for eating with a small carbon footprint since long before the term was coined.") She has received 18 honorary doctorates and a large number of awards, including the James Beard Foundation Humanitarian of the Year Award for her lifelong impact on the way people all over the world think about food, nutrition, and agriculture. She is also a member of the World Future Council and the International Commission on the Future of Food and Agriculture. With her daughter, Anna Lappé, Frances Moore Lappé cofounded the Small Planet Institute. Her most recent work is* World Hunger: 10 Myths *(coauthored with Joseph Collins).*

Recently you have written that to address our biggest global challenges, whether hunger, environmental pollution, or climate change, we need to rid ourselves of what you term the scarcity-mind. Can you elaborate on this concept and why it is important to you?

Much of humanity is now trapped in a truly dangerous mental map, a worldview that fails to protect life because it is perversely aligned with nature, including with human nature. I say perversely because its assumptions elicit the worst in us while stifling the best, and they defy the laws of wider nature as well, thus bringing both human and environmental destruction. From this profound malalignment, humans end up creating together a world that few, if any, of us would individually choose. I believe the core assumptions of this deadly mental map are *separateness* (we each exist apart from one another and from nature), *stasis* (reality is best understood as fixed and finished), and *scarcity* (there is not enough of anything). These assumptions make up what I call *scarcity-mind*. Through it, we see ourselves in perpetual competition with other selfish creatures over scarce goods. The conditions flowing from scarcity-mind—concentrated power, lack of transparency, and a culture of blame—are precisely those proven repeatedly to bring forth the worst in our species. The Holocaust, after all, was not the work of only a few mad men. And extreme chronic undernourishment harms 795 million people today, even as food production per person has increased over 65 percent since the 1960s, now supplying nearly 2,900 calories for each of us daily.

Let me now introduce another concept: *eco-mind*. This evidence-based way of seeing is emerging worldwide and draws on ancient wisdom and disciplines from anthropology to neuroscience, and I believe it can free us from the self-reinforcing destructiveness of scarcity-mind. For some time, science has confirmed what great seers have told us for eons, that the true nature of reality is *connection* (all exists in relationship with all else), *continuous change* (change is the one constant we can count on), and *co-creation* (if connection and change are both givens, then all is both shaped by and shaping all that emerges in ongoing co-creation). This evidence-based view of reality, the eco-mind, suggests thinking like an ecosystem. Its most obvious and helpful lesson is that we humans are like every other organism in the ecosystem: what we express is largely shaped by our context and the stimuli around us. With this realization, we can form a hypothesis about human nature—identifying what useful human traits are there to be tapped by our social environment for meeting the goal of planetary transition to life-serving cultures, and what tendencies need to be minimized by social rules and conditions, if we are to thrive.

And finally, there is the concept of *living democracy*. Through this lens, we can envision a more functional social ecology—rules and norms we create that are positively aligned both with our nature and the laws of wider nature. I mean that we can perceive mechanisms for making choices together—governance, formal and informal—that align positively with our nature, and we can understand why they are essential to wider, ecological health. In other words, we are thinking like an ecosystem and applying it to our social reality. The term living democracy suggests democracy as both a lived experience and an evolving, organic reality itself, "easily lost but never finally won," in the words of the first African-American federal appellate judge, William Hastie.

Thinking like an ecosystem, we see that because we are all connected, we are all implicated in every social outcome. We can, therefore, forego preaching and pleading, as we realize that much of the terrible dysfunction evident today—from random violence to environmental destruction to persistent, massive hunger—is the result of social systems created by us and perversely aligned with our nature.

Lappé's consciousness about world hunger was raised during the 1960s at the University of California, Berkeley, where she first started to realize that a plant-centered diet was best for everyone. She also began researching why there was such a huge hunger problem in a world with an abundance of food available. She has demonstrated that the world's food availability is economically driven by the extreme inequalities around the globe, pointing out in her many publications and presentations that millions of people are too poor to buy food at marketplace prices. As a result, grain that could feed hungry people instead feeds meat sources (e.g., beef cattle), which are unnecessary for a healthy diet. She emphasizes that if only diets around the world would focus on plant-based foods, our worldwide hunger problems would disappear.

In 1975, she and Joseph Collins founded the Institute for Food and Development Policy (also known as Food First), which focuses on educating Americans about the political and economic causes of and solutions to the global hunger problem. The institute's first book, *Food First: Beyond the Myth of Scarcity*, coauthored by Lappé and Collins, explains that scarcity and overpopulation are not the causes of world hunger and describes how grassroots organizations can help the poor improve their health through democratic processes.

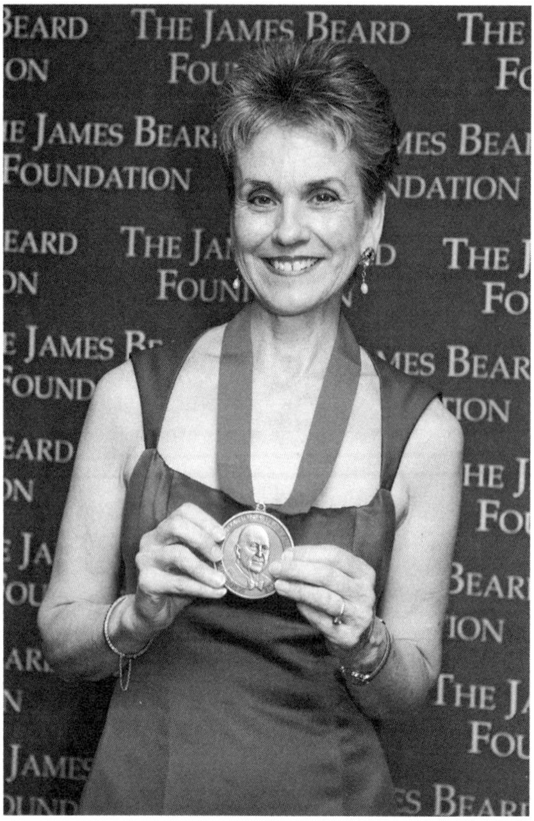

Frances Moore Lappé, author and world hunger activist. Lappé's 1971 best seller *Diet for a Small Planet* demonstrated how people can make a difference in their own lives and the lives of others by changing their eating habits. (AP Photo/Diane Bondareff)

Lappé calls her solution to the world's hunger crisis "living democracy," meaning that by making wise food choices on a day-to-day basis, individuals are not only contributing to their own well-being but to the good health of the entire world as well. In 1990, Lappé and her husband, Paul Martin Du Bois, founded the Center for Living Democracy. Their 1994 book, *The Quickening of America: Rebuilding Our Nation, Remaking Our Lives*, shows how ordinary people can solve the world's hunger problems by participating in this living democracy. In 2002, Lappé and her daughter, Anna Lappé, created the Small Planet Institute, a collaborative network that promotes the living democracy tenets through education and research. She and her daughter also founded the Small Planet Fund to connect resources to global efforts supporting the living democracy concept.

Lappé has received countless awards and 17 honorary degrees from universities all over the world. In 1987, she was only the fourth American to ever receive the Right Livelihood Award in Sweden, and in 2003, she was honored by the National Nutritional Foods Association with the prestigious Rachel Carson Award. In 2008, Lappé received the James Beard Foundation's Humanitarian of the Year Award.

Susan J. Montgomery

See Also: Environmentalism; Food Supply, Environmental Threats to; Organic Agriculture; Pesticides and Herbicides

Further Reading

Frances Moore Lappé: Delicious Food Is Not an Indulgence—It's a Way to Solve Our Ecological Crises. Yes! Magazine (November, 2013). http://www.yesmagazine.org/issues/how-to-eat-like-our-lives-depend-on-it/choosing-deliciousness (accessed March 18, 2016).

Grassroots International. *Frances Moore Lappé Biography*. http://grassrootsinternational.org/frances-moore-lappé-biography (accessed March 18, 2016).
Public Broadcasting Service. *Now, Frances Moore Lappé*. http://www.pbs.org/now/politics/lappe.html (accessed March 18, 2016).
Right Livelihood Award Foundation. *The Right Livelihood Award for Outstanding Vision and Work on Behalf of Our Planet and Its People*. http://www.rightlivelihood.org/moore_lappe.html (accessed March 18, 2016).
Shareable. *Dignity, Democracy and Food: An Interview with Frances Moore Lappè*. http://www.shareable.net/blog/dignity-democracy-and-food-an-interview-with-frances-moore-lappè (accessed March 18, 2016).

LEAD POISONING PREVENTION

Lead, one of the earth's natural elements, is a bluish-white, lustrous metal that is extracted from various underground ore deposits. Lead is extremely dense, corrosion resistant, and malleable, and it has a low melting point, making it an important component in batteries, X-ray shields, ammunition, electronics, and industrial paints. Historical records indicate humans began mining lead over 6,000 years ago due to its unique properties, and the toxic effects of lead exposure have been known for 2,500 years. In ancient times, the Romans used lead to glaze pottery, construct water pipes and aqueducts, make cosmetics, and sweeten wine as a flavoring additive. Due to its prolific use, many individuals were exposed to lead, and lead poisoning symptoms were described throughout ancient history as lead colic, paralysis, palsy, and lead madness.

Lead Exposure: A Problem of the Past?

Lead poisoning has been perceived by some as a problem of the past, given that lead paint is no longer used and lead gasoline is no longer sold at the gas pumps. In addition, blood lead levels in children have dropped significantly since the late 1970s due to various laws and programs that eliminate the use of lead in certain products, thereby preventing future exposures. Nevertheless, lead exposure, especially for children, remains a concern, a problem highlighted by research showing that there is no safe level of lead in the bloodstream.

Recently, public water supplies have come under investigation for lead contamination. For example, the water supply of Flint, Michigan, became contaminated with lead in 2014 after the city tapped into the Flint River as a backup water source while constructing a new pipeline to Lake Huron. The corrosive Flint River water, which had not been treated with an anticorrosion agent (in violation of federal law), caused lead in aging water service lines to leach into the residential water supply, resulting in unacceptably high lead concentrations. Various complaints, criminal charges, and lawsuits were filed, including felony charges against four officials for mishandling funds. President Barack Obama visited Flint in 2016 to meet with residents and discuss federal assistance.

Lead in Drinking Water

While exposure to lead in paint and soil is well understood, less is known about lead in drinking water, especially at low concentrations.

An Interview with Jennifer Chavez

Staff Attorney, Earthjustice

Jennifer Chavez is a staff attorney with Earthjustice, a nonprofit environmental law advocacy organization, where she is involved with a number of cases related to protecting water resources in the Washington, D.C., and Chesapeake Bay regions and to stopping mountaintop removal mining in the Appalachian coalfields. Chavez previously worked for a Chicago-area law firm representing municipal governments.

We have known about the hazards of lead exposure for a long time, but problems with lead in drinking water continue to surface. Why hasn't more been done to address an obviously serious problem?

Lead in drinking water is invisible to the ordinary person, and the factors that cause lead contamination of water are outside of the ordinary person's control, so most of the public has remained in the dark and powerless to do anything about the problem. The U.S. Environmental Protection Agency (EPA) has been regulating lead in drinking water for a long time, but the permissible levels are not low enough to prevent lead exposure problems. Furthermore, the EPA rules have too many loopholes that allow drinking water utilities to comply with the law while still exposing water consumers to dangerous levels of lead in water.

It was recently discovered that the drinking water supply of Flint, Michigan, has high levels of lead contamination. Yet, little was done to address this problem until outspoken residents and environmental activists got involved. Is this an example of an environmental justice situation, where low income and minority people often bear the brunt of environmental contamination and exposure? (Flint is 56 percent African American, and the median household income is below $30,000 per year.)

In a sense, environmental justice is embedded in the nation's drinking water supply system in that lead and other contaminants often occur in older homes and inner city locations where low income and minority people tend to live. Thus, it is reasonable to ask whether the response to the Flint crisis would have been different if a community with a different composition were involved. Ultimately, as long as there are some cities and neighborhoods that get their water through drinking water pipes and fixtures that contain lead, even in wealthy neighborhoods, people will be at risk of drinking lead. The only way to fully remediate the problem is to remove all of the lead from our drinking water systems.

Evidence is building that even low doses of lead can be harmful, especially in children. Is there a safe level below which we need not be concerned?

I am an attorney, not a health scientist, but there is a consensus building that low levels of lead contamination in drinking water can be harmful and that there may not be a threshold level below which adverse health effects will not appear.

For most people lead in drinking water is not their main source of exposure, but it can be a significant source in addition to paint and air pollution. For some people, including pregnant women and fetuses, lead in water can be the primary source of lead exposure at a time when they are highly susceptible to lifelong harm. While public health departments know a lot about lead in paint and soil, they are less knowledgeable about lead in water. If lead paint is discovered in an old home and the children show symptoms of exposure, the drinking water should also be tested, but this is seldom done.

What is a good career path for a recent college or university graduate who is interested in addressing urban environmental problems such as lead exposure among inner city children?

There is a disconnect between scientists and advocacy groups, and closer coordination between these groups is needed. Whatever career recent graduates select, they should look for opportunities to merge science and advocacy so that clear and unambiguous messages about environmental pollution are conveyed to the public.

In the modern era, three major uses for lead resulted in millions of people, primarily children, getting lead poisoned. Beginning in the late 1800s, lead was used as a performance additive in household paint and gasoline. In paint, lead provided durability, flexibility, and a glossy appearance, and it repelled mold and mildew. Tetraethyl lead was added in gasoline to improve performance and curb engine knocking. Lead was also used to make water pipes and as a solder to seal pipe joints. Due to these long-standing uses, lead poisoning often occurred from ingesting or inhaling lead paint chips and dust, inhaling automobile exhaust, and drinking contaminated water. The risks of exposure were higher in children due to their smaller stature and greater likelihood of touching contaminated surfaces, licking fingers, and inhaling contaminated air collecting closer to the ground.

Exposure to lead causes a variety of adverse health effects. Lead poisoning can impact nearly all organs in the body but primarily affects the blood system, brain, and central nervous system, leading to anemia, behavioral and learning problems, reduced IQ, delayed growth, kidney problems, and even death. These health effects are more pronounced in children, who have a faster metabolism, higher absorption and lower excretion rate, and greater risk of toxic effects on developing organs and the central nervous system.

Throughout the nineteenth and twentieth centuries, physicians and scientists documented illnesses and deaths in children and workers associated with lead exposure, and the Centers for Disease Control and Prevention (CDC) established blood lead health standards. These concerns resulted in two major U.S. laws that banned lead in residential paint in 1978 and phased out lead in gasoline through 1986. These two regulatory actions resulted in significant reductions in lead exposure, preventing millions of future lead poisoning cases.

The primary cause of lead poisoning today is from older homes (built before 1978) that were painted with lead paint. The CDC estimates there are 24 million homes in the United States that have deteriorating lead paint and high levels of lead dust, with approximately 4 million of these homes inhabited by children. State public health programs report blood lead results to the CDC, and based on this information, it is estimated that over a half-million U.S. children ages 1 to 5 have blood lead levels of 5 microgram/deciliter or greater, with significant disparities between African American and Caucasian children. When a child's blood lead level exceeds this reference level, family lead prevention education, removing the sources of lead exposure, and medical case management are recommended.

Preventing lead poisoning is the primary goal of public health programs. Beginning with the laws that banned lead paint and leaded gasoline, public health agencies have worked hard to get additional laws passed to prevent new lead poisoning cases. In 1986, the Environmental Protection Agency (EPA) banned lead for use in plumbing, and in 1992, the EPA required landlords and sellers of property built before 1978 to notify tenants and homebuyers of potential lead hazards. In 1995, the U.S. Food and Drug Administration banned the use of lead solder in food cans, and in 1999, the U.S. Department of Housing and Urban Development enacted a lead safe housing rule that targeted homes federally owned or receiving federal housing assistance. The EPA established lead dust and soil hazard standards in 2001 that are used by public health officials when investigating lead exposure associated with housing and taking enforcement actions. Additionally, the EPA established rules that all home renovators must follow to ensure safe work practices where lead is present.

In addition to these prevention laws, public health agencies promote prevention through case surveillance, education, lead testing of children, mandatory blood lead reporting, inspections, and housing regulation enforcement. Public health agencies work closely with geographers to develop risk maps that target older neighborhoods, and they partner with the U.S. Department of Housing and Urban Development to rehabilitate older homes, making them lead safe and preventing future exposures. These types of prevention programs, along with collaboration among government agencies, have resulted in blood lead levels dropping significantly since 1978. However, lead poisoning prevention remains a concern because there is no safe blood lead level, and exposure continues in millions of homes with deteriorating lead paint.

R. Christopher Rustin

See Also: Automobile and Truck Emissions and Controls; Centers for Disease Control and Prevention; Children's Environmental Health; Environmental Protection Agency; Flint, Michigan, Contaminated Drinking Water in; Heavy Metal Pollution

Further Reading

Hernberg, Sven. "Lead Poisoning in a Historical Perspective." *American Journal of Industrial Medicine*, vol. 38, no. 3 (September 2000): 244–254.

Segarra, Marielle. *Lead Poisoning: A Doctor's Lifelong Crusade to Save Children from It*. National Public Radio (Weekend Edition Sunday), Washington, DC, 2016. http://www.npr.org/2016/06/05/480595028/lead-poisoning-a-doctors-lifelong-crusade-to-save-children-from-it.

U.S. Agency for Toxic Substance and Disease Registry. *Toxicological Profile for Lead.* https://www.atsdr.cdc.gov/toxprofiles/tp.asp?id=96&tid=22 (accessed January 31, 2017).
U.S. Centers for Disease Control and Prevention. *Lead.* https://www.cdc.gov/nceh/lead/ (accessed January 31, 2017).
U.S. Department of Housing and Urban Development. *The Lead-Safe Housing Rule.* https://portal.hud.gov/hudportal/HUD?src=/program_offices/healthy_homes/enforcement/lshr (accessed January 26, 2017).
U.S. Environmental Protection Agency. *Integrated Risk Information System, Lead and Compounds (Inorganic).* https://cfpub.epa.gov/ncea/iris2/chemicalLanding.cfm?substance_nmbr=277 (accessed January 31, 2017).
U.S. Environmental Protection Agency. *Lead.* https://www.epa.gov/lead (accessed January 31, 2017).

LEADERSHIP IN ENERGY AND ENVIRONMENTAL DESIGN

Leadership in Energy and Environmental Design (LEED) is a certification program for buildings and communities that promotes sustainability through building design, construction, operation, and maintenance. Projects receiving LEED certification must meet certain prerequisites to become certified at the silver (least rigorous), gold, and platinum (most rigorous) levels. The LEED program is important for environmental health because it leads to building and communities that use less energy, thereby helping to reduce greenhouse gases and other environmental pollutants. Additionally, LEED-certified buildings cost less to operate.

How Green Buildings Benefit Society

Green buildings are buildings where steps have been taken to reduce the amount of energy consumed over the life cycle of the building. Additionally, green buildings reduce impacts on human health and the environment by efficiently using water, reducing wastes, incorporating sustainable materials, and creating a healthy indoor environment. Residential and commercial buildings account for about 40 percent of total U.S. energy consumption, and much of this energy comes from electric power plants that burn fossil fuels—coal, oil, and natural gas. Green buildings help fight climate change by using less electricity, which results in fossil fuel power plants emitting less carbon dioxide, the most widespread greenhouse gas in the United States. Using less electricity also results in power plants emitting lesser amounts of other air pollutants, such as particulate matter and sulfur dioxide, that directly affect human health. Additionally, green buildings typically have lower operating expenses (e.g., lower electric and water utility bills) than other buildings, which helps make green buildings more affordable in the long run. The U.S. Green Building Council's LEED program is one of the most widely used systems for rating green buildings, both in the United States and globally. Additionally, Energy Star, a program run jointly by the U.S. Environmental Protection Agency and the U.S. Department of Energy, qualifies newly built or renovated buildings as being energy-efficient, awarding them the Energy Star label.

The LEED program is sponsored by the U.S. Green Building Council (USGBC), headquartered in Washington, D.C. The USGBC was established in 1993 to "promote sustainability-focused practices in the building and construction industry." Initially, the USGBC comprised a coalition of architects and building industry representatives having the common goal of creating a green building rating system for buildings that achieve environmental and sustainability standards. The result of this collaboration was the creation of the LEED certification program in 2000.

LEED certification applies to all types of buildings, including office buildings, commercial space, factories, warehouses, data centers, hospitals, schools, historical buildings, and homes. Unique standards and rating criteria have been established for each of the following categories:

- Building Design and Construction: buildings that are being newly constructed or going through major renovation
- Interior Design and Construction: projects that are a complete interior fit-out, including commercial interiors, retail, and hospitality
- Building Operation and Maintenance: existing buildings that are undergoing improvement work or little to no construction
- Neighborhood Development: new land development projects or redevelopment projects containing residential uses, nonresidential uses, or a mix
- Homes: single family homes, low-rise multifamily units (one to three stories), or midrise multifamily units (four to six stories)

The LEED certification program is used around the world, with about 1.85 million square feet (172,000 square meters) certified daily.

In addition to running the LEED program, the USGBC advocates for green building policies and programs, establishes strategic partnerships with government and industry leaders, and campaigns for standards, programs, and regulations that promote green buildings and communities. According to the USGBC, its advocacy priorities include government leadership by example, private-sector market transformation, raising the bar on codes and regulations, and community-wide sustainability. Additionally, USGBC presents national awards to individuals and organizations and, in collaboration with Bank of America, provides funding and educational materials to developers interested in constructing LEED-certified affording housing.

Richard Crume

See Also: Climate Change and Human Health; Electric Power Generation, Health Implications of; Energy Star; Environmental Protection Agency; Greenhouse Effect and Global Warming; Renewable Energy, Health Implications of; Sustainable Development and Health

Further Reading

Ching, Frank, and Ian M. Shapiro. *Green Building Illustrated*. Hoboken, NJ: John Wiley and Sons, 2014.

Kibert, Charles J. *Sustainable Construction: Green Building Design and Delivery*. Toronto, Canada: John Wiley and Sons Canada, 2016.
Kubba, Sam. *Handbook of Green Building Design and Construction: LEED, BREEAM, and Green Globes*. Amsterdam, the Netherlands: Elsevier/Butterworth-Heinemann, 2017.
U.S. Green Building Council. *Green Building Information Gateway*. http://www.gbig.org (accessed September 19, 2016).
U.S. Green Building Council. *Home Page*. http://www.usgbc.org (accessed September 19, 2016).

LEAL, JOHN

John Leal (1858–1914) was a physician and water expert who earned the moniker "father of chlorine" for leading the first large-scale water chlorination project in the United States. Chlorination kills bacteria that cause waterborne diseases. Its use has saved millions of lives, provided untold economic benefits, and transformed water-related leisure activities. Furthermore, chlorination can be done quickly and inexpensively. However, waterborne disease continues to be a major cause of death in areas of the world where chlorination systems are inadequate.

Born in Andes, New York, on May 5, 1858, Leal moved with his family to Paterson, New Jersey, when he was still a child. He attended Princeton University and then obtained his medical education at Columbia College of Physicians and Surgeons, graduating in 1883. Leal then returned to Paterson to practice medicine. As a city health officer, he became a public health expert and later took advisory positions with private water companies, including the Jersey City Water Supply Company. Working to make the water supply safer was a good fit for Leal. The emerging field of bacteriology had long captured his interest. Additionally, while serving in the Civil War, his own father had become ill from drinking contaminated water, dying after almost two decades of suffering.

The Jersey City Water Supply Company was contracted by Jersey City, New Jersey, to improve the city's poor water quality. The expensive project involved damming the Rockaway River and creating Boonton Reservoir, which began delivering water in 1904. Using the results of new bacteriological tests to argue that the water quality was still problematic, the city took the company to court, claiming it had violated the contract. In a 1908 ruling, the court found that the city's water quality was improved but that bacteria rates spiked several times a year after high water and flooding. As a remedy, the city wanted expensive sewers built, but the court agreed to allow Leal's company 90 days to put another solution in place and prove its efficacy. To Leal, who had experimented with disinfection methods in the lab, that solution was chlorination.

The idea of putting chlorine, a potentially lethal chemical, into the water supply was radical at the time. Even though there were some cases of chlorine having limited success in European water supplies, chemical disinfection of water was not a popular idea with many scientists or the public. Leal lacked specific permission to add chlorine to the water supply, so his project was an especially bold and risky move.

Leal enlisted MIT-educated sanitation engineer and filtration expert George Warren Fuller to quickly design a chlorine delivery system that could meet the challenge of treating 40 million gallons (151 million liters) of water daily. Chlorination plant operations were initially directed by George A. Johnson, who had recently used chloride of lime (the same chemical originally used in Jersey City) as a successful disinfection agent for the much smaller Chicago stockyard water supply. Leal took over plant operations a few months after the plant opened.

Jersey City's water treatment plant opened on September 26, 1908, with great success. Infant mortality, cholera, and typhoid fever rates fell dramatically, and water utilities around the country moved quickly to chlorinate. Meanwhile, a second lengthy court case required that Leal defend the project.

Leal died from complications of diabetes on March 13, 1914. For the next century, he remained a relatively obscure name in public health history, with credit for chlorination largely going to Johnson. For unknown reasons, perhaps family tensions, his grave in a Paterson cemetery remained unmarked for a century. Leal was finally commemorated on the 155th anniversary of his birth with the installation of a grave marker heralding him as a "Hero of Public Health."

Kathy Stolley

See Also: Cholera; Drinking Water Quality and Regulation; Environmental Health Profession; Sewage Treatment and Disposal; Waterborne Diseases

Further Reading

American Chemistry Council. *A Public Health Giant Step: Chlorination of U.S. Drinking Water*. http://www.waterandhealth.org/drinkingwater/chlorination_history.html (accessed February 18, 2017).

Johnson, Steven. *How We Got to Now: Six Innovations That Made the Modern World*. New York: Riverhead Books, 2015.

McGuire, Michael J. *The Chlorine Revolution: Water Disinfection and the Fight to Save Lives*. Denver, CO: American Water Works Association, 2013.

Public Broadcasting System. *How We Got to Now: How One Man Poisoned a City's Water Supply (and Saved Millions of Children's Lives in the Process)*. http://www.pbs.org/how-we-got-to-now/blogs/howwegottonext/how-one-man-poisoned-a-citys-water-supply-and-saved-millions-of-childrens-lives-in-the-process (accessed September 8, 2017).

LEGIONNAIRES' DISEASE

Legionnaires' disease is a serious, potentially fatal pneumonia caused by gram-negative bacteria from the *Legionella* genus. The bacterial pneumonia affects 10,000 to 15,000 people per year in the United States and more than 7,000 people per year across the European Union, although these estimates are generally thought to be significantly underreported. In hospitalized patients, Legionnaires' disease can have up to a 39 percent fatality rate, with a typical fatality rate of about 10 to 15 percent seen globally.

The disease was discovered in 1976, when participants of the American Legion's annual convention in Philadelphia developed a strange pneumonia, and 29 subsequently died. The causative agent was later determined to be *Legionella pneumophila*, a previously unrecognized freshwater bacterium. There are currently 60 different species of *Legionella*, and most are considered pathogenic. (Most cases of the disease are caused by *Legionella pneumophila* serogroup 1.)

Legionella bacteria are found naturally in freshwater sources worldwide in concentrations that rarely, if ever, cause human disease. Legionnaires' disease is largely a problem created by humans. The bacteria thrive in created aquatic environments, such as the plumbing of large and complex water supply systems, cooling towers of large air-conditioning units, decorative fountains, hot tubs, humidifiers, and aquariums. In these environments, *Legionella* can become aerosolized in water droplets and inhaled, causing infection.

Hotels, resorts, and cruise ships are frequent outbreak locations for *Legionella* due to their large water systems and other aerosol-generating sources (e.g., a shower head or mist-generating water cooling tower). This is also true for hospitals and long-term care facilities, whose inhabitants may be more susceptible to infection due to illness or age. Risk factors for developing Legionnaires' disease include preexisting renal or hepatic failure, diabetes, chronic lung disease, systemic malignancy, smoking (current or past), immune system disorders, and being age 50 and older.

Symptoms of infection are indistinguishable from other causes of pneumonia. Patients with Legionnaires' disease usually experience fever, loss of appetite, mild cough, headache, malaise, and lethargy. Some people also experience myalgias, rigors, dyspnea, and diarrhea. Those who survive the infection occasionally suffer from long-term health effects, including restrictive lung disease, weakness, poor memory, fatigue, retrograde amnesia, or cerebellar symptoms.

Proper diagnosis of Legionnaires' disease is crucial to appropriate patient management as well as accurate reporting to health departments. Diagnostic tests begin with a general chest x-ray. From there, the gold standard for diagnosis is both a culture of lower respiratory secretions and the *Legionella* urinary antigen test. Treatment centers on antibiotic therapy and supportive respiratory care. Typical antibiotic therapy consists of a combination of potent antipneumococcal beta-lactam and either a macrolide or fluoroquinolone.

Because there is currently no vaccine for *Legionella*, prevention, infection control, and outbreak investigation are key environmental and public health priorities. There are numerous standards and guidelines for preventing *Legionella* in specific environments, such as the Centers for Disease Control and Prevention's (CDC) Guideline for Prevention of Nosocomial Pneumonia, New York State Department of Health recommendations for hospitals and nursing homes, and the Veterans Health Administration's Directive 2008–010, Prevention of Legionella Disease for Healthcare. The CDC has a vessel sanitation program for cruise ships and heating, ventilation, and air-conditioning systems. Additionally, the American Society of Heating, Refrigerating, and Air-Conditioning Engineers has published

Guideline 12–2000, Minimizing the Risk of Legionellosis Associated with Building Water Systems.

Timothy J. Sutton

See Also: Indoor Environment; Infectious Diseases; Respiratory Disease and Air Pollution

Further Reading

Centers for Disease Control and Prevention. *Legionella (Legionnaires' Disease and Pontiac Fever): About the Disease*. https://www.cdc.gov/legionella/about (accessed February 1, 2017).

Che, D., et al. "Sporadic Cases of Community Acquired Legionnaires' Disease: An Ecological Study to Identify New Sources of Contamination." *Journal of Epidemiology and Community Health*, vol. 57, no. 6 (June 2003): 466–469.

Fields, Barry S., Robert F. Benson, and Richard E. Besser. "Legionella and Legionnaires' Disease: 25 years of Investigation." *Clinical Microbiology Reviews*, vol. 15, no. 3 (July 2002): 506–526.

Hilbi, Hubert, et al. "Update on Legionnaires' Disease: Pathogenesis, Epidemiology, Detection, and Control." *Molecular Microbiology*, vol. 76, no. 1 (April 2010): 1–11.

Phin, Nick, et al. "Epidemiology and Clinical Management of Legionnaires' Disease." *The Lancet Infectious Diseases*, vol. 14, no. 10 (October 2014): 1011–1021.

Sabrià, Miguel, and Magda Campins. "Legionnaires' Disease: Update on Epidemiology and Management Options." *American Journal of Respiratory Medicine*, vol. 2, no. 3 (February 2003): 235–243.

Shelton, Brian G., et al. "Review of Legionnaires' Disease." *American Industrial Hygiene Association Journal*, vol. 61, no. 5 (September–October 2000): 738–742.

Vergis, Emanuel N., Efsun Akbas, and Victor L. Yu. "Legionella as a Cause of Severe Pneumonia." *Seminars in Respiratory and Critical Care Medicine*, vol. 21, no. 4 (July–August 2000): 295–304.

LEUKEMIA AND ENVIRONMENTAL EXPOSURE

Leukemia is a type of cancer affecting the bone marrow, lymphatic system, and other tissues involved with blood formation. The disease typically causes the formation of white blood cells that are abnormal and function improperly. Because these abnormal cells tend to grow and divide faster and live longer than healthy cells, they can overwhelm the supply of blood cells, resulting in a diminished numbers of healthy white blood cells, red blood cells, and platelets. A combination of genetic and environmental factors appears to cause leukemia, although as with most cancers, the exact mechanism is not well understood.

Cases of leukemia are classified according to how quickly the disease progresses and the types of cells involved. Although often considered a children's disease, most leukemia cases occur in older adults, usually over 65 years of age. Symptoms vary but commonly include fever, fatigue, frequent or severe infections, weight loss, loss of appetite, nosebleeds, enlarged liver or spleen, swollen lymph nodes, swollen or bleeding gums, easy bleeding or bruising, sweating at night, bone or joint pain, anemia, and petechiae (small red or purple spots on the skin). These symptoms are also associated with other often less serious conditions, and diagnosis by a healthcare professional is essential.

In both children and adults, exposure to ionizing radiation (e.g., from cancer radiation therapy) is the most firmly established environmental risk factor for leukemia. (Japanese atomic bomb survivors who were exposed to high radiation levels were also found to have a higher incidence of leukemia.) Additionally, an elevated risk of developing the disease is linked to benzene (e.g., a chemical used in the chemical industry and found in gasoline), agricultural exposure (e.g., pesticides), and smoking. For children, the parent's exposure to pesticides and other chemicals may also increase risk. Other risk factors for leukemia include previous cancer treatments, genetic disorders, and a family history of leukemia. Exposure to certain rare viruses may also be a factor.

Benzene exposure is of particular interest from an environmental health perspective because it is an environmental pollutant that is regulated by the U.S. Environmental Protection Agency (EPA), and the association between benzene exposure and leukemia has been well documented in the agency's Integrated Risk Information System database. The EPA has determined that benzene is a "known" human carcinogen for all routes of exposure, based on "convincing human evidence as well as supporting evidence from animal studies." Cancer-causing substances are designated as "known" when there is sufficient evidence from epidemiological studies to establish a causal relationship between exposure and the formation of cancer.

The type of treatment selected for leukemia depends on several factors, including the patient's age, white blood cell count, the cancer genetics, if there was a preleukemic condition, and whether the patient was previously treated for cancer. The usual treatment is chemotherapy, sometimes in combination with bone marrow transplants, radiation therapy, interferon therapy, and surgical removal of the spleen. According to the Leukemia and Lymphoma Society, the overall five-year relative survival rate for leukemia over the period 2005 to 2011 was about 62 percent. (Survival rates for specific types of leukemia may differ from this overall figure.) With the treatments available today, leukemia can be managed and even cured in many cases.

While medical science does not yet know how to prevent leukemia, the most significant avoidable risk factor for adults is smoking, and avoiding benzene exposure may also lower the risk of developing the disease. The risk of leukemia is higher for people previously receiving radiation and chemotherapy treatments for other cancer types, taking immune suppressing drugs, and having certain genetic conditions like Down's syndrome.

Richard Crume

See Also: Automobile and Truck Emissions and Controls; Cancer Clusters; Cancer Risk from Environmental Exposure; Children's Environmental Health; Environmental Protection Agency; Integrated Risk Information System; Pesticides and Herbicides; Radiation, Ionizing and Nonionizing

Further Reading

American Cancer Society. *Leukemia*. http://www.cancer.org/cancer/leukemia (accessed October 24, 2016).

DeVita, Vincent T., Theodore S. Lawrence, and Steven A. Rosenberg. *Lymphomas and Leukemias: Cancer—Principles and Practice of Oncology*. Philadelphia, PA: Wolters Kluwer, 2016.

Leukemia and Lymphoma Society. *Facts and Statistics*. http://www.lls.org/http%3A/llsorg.prod.acquia-sites.com/facts-and-statistics/facts-and-statistics-overview/facts-and-statistics (accessed October 24, 2016).

Mayo Clinic. *Diseases and Conditions: Leukemia*. http://www.mayoclinic.org/diseases-conditions/leukemia/basics/definition/con-20024914 (accessed October 24, 2016).

National Cancer Institute, National Institutes of Health. *Leukemia—Patient Version*. https://www.cancer.gov/types/leukemia (accessed October 24, 2016).

U.S. Environmental Protection Agency. *Integrated Risk Information System: Benzene*. https://cfpub.epa.gov/ncea/iris2/chemicalLanding.cfm?substance_nmbr=276 (accessed October 24, 2016).

LIFE CYCLE ASSESSMENT

Life cycle assessment (LCA) is a method of evaluating the potential environmental impacts associated with all stages of a product or process. LCAs may be either attributional (the most common type) or consequential. Attributional LCAs are based on known past environmental impacts, while consequential LCAs seek to identify the future environmental consequences of a proposed decision. The product or process stages examined include raw material extraction, manufacturing, distribution, use or reuse, and disposal. LCAs are an important tool for both corporate and government decision makers to limit environmental impacts and avoid unnecessary risks to human health.

The purpose of an LCA is to make comparisons between competing products or processes based on known data. The results may then be used to identify ways to modify a product or process to reduce adverse environmental impacts. LCAs are used primarily within industries to design and develop products. However, LCAs may also be used to help policymakers decide which plans to implement, and they may be helpful to consumers in making informed decisions when purchasing products.

Whereas a traditional cost-benefit analysis focuses on financial considerations, the primary benefit of an LCA is the ability to evaluate environmental impacts. For instance, a company might choose to use LCA if they want to model the environmental implications of changing various steps of their production process. However, the downside of an LCA is that it can be quite time-consuming and expensive.

The LCA process has been established by the International Organization for Standardization under two standards:

- ISO 14040:2006, Environmental Management—Life Cycle Assessment—Principles and Framework: overview of the practice, applications, and limitations of LCA

- ISO 14044:2006, Environmental Management—Life Cycle Assessment—Requirements and Guidelines: guidance on preparing, conducting, and reviewing LCAs, including assessing impact, interpreting results, and evaluating the nature and quality of data collected

A typical LCA assessment involves three phases: (1) defining the goal and scope of the project; (2) compiling an inventory of inputs and outputs; and (3) evaluating potential impacts and making a recommendation. These phases are described next.

Defining Goals and Scope. The first LCA phase is to establish the goal and scope of a given LCA. This begins with defining the processing steps, or "gates," which may range from (1) extracting raw materials to disposing of goods (called cradle-to-grave); (2) extracting raw materials to finishing the production of goods (called cradle-to-gate); or (3) one processing stage to another (called gate-to-gate). Additionally, discrete environmental impact categories must be identified, for example, toxicity to humans, depletion of abiotic resources, emissions of greenhouse gases, stratospheric ozone depletion, toxicity to aquatic or terrestrial organisms, and eutrophication. A final step in identifying the goals and scope of an LCA is to define the functional unit to be compared across products. For example, to compare energy required by compact fluorescent lamps (CFL) versus incandescent light bulbs, the functional unit might be defined as "450 lumens of light for 5,000 hours," and the LCA might demonstrate that the energy used by one 9-watt CFL is comparable to that of five 40-watt incandescent light bulbs.

Compiling an Inventory. The second phase of LCA involves quantifying all the inputs and outputs of materials as well as evaluating how these materials may affect the environment. The inventory is based on either national data (known as environmental input-output data) or on a survey of the actual process or product (known as unit process data). The resulting life cycle inventory is usually illustrated with a flowchart or process tree. Given the technical nature and the volume of data usually involved, LCA inventories are often performed using computer models, for example, Argonne National Laboratory's Greenhouse Gases, Regulated Emissions, and Energy Use in Transportation (GREET) model.

Evaluating Potential Impacts. The third phase involves evaluating the significance of potential environmental impacts. For example, an industry might use LCA to develop a plan that is less damaging to the environment than other possible plans. In the impact assessment process, various outputs are converted to equivalent measures. As an illustration, because both atmospheric carbon dioxide and methane contribute to climate change, methane would be converted to equivalent units of carbon dioxide for the purpose of evaluating the global warming potential of competing processes.

One well-known example of the usefulness of LCA is the evaluation of environmental impacts related to the "eat local" movement in the United States. By calculating miles traveled per item of food, researchers found that conventional food distribution networks use more fuel and emit more carbon dioxide than locally sourced food. Thus, proponents of eating locally held that buying food produced within 100 to 250 miles (161 to 402 kilometers) of their homes would have less environmental impact. Yet, the initial research overlooked several factors, including the resources needed to grow the food and the method of transportation. For example, if local tomatoes are grown in greenhouses while imported tomatoes are grown in sun-warmed fields, then the local tomatoes may have a greater environmental impact. In another example, potatoes shipped via train for 1,000 miles (1,609 kilometers) may emit the same amount of carbon dioxide as potatoes trucked for 100 miles (161 kilometers) because freight cars are less resource-intensive than trucks. If every step of the process in food production is equal—from growing conditions to transportation methods—then "eating local" does indeed have less impact on the environment, but in most cases, the circumstances of local and imported food products are not the same. Therefore, LCA helps people make decisions based on holistic data.

Alisha K. Newton

See Also: Environmental Auditing; Environmental Impact Assessment; Laboratory Quality Assurance; Recycling

Further Reading

Argonne National Laboratory. *GREET Model*. https://greet.es.anl.gov (accessed February 21, 2017).

Crawford, Robert H. *Life Cycle Assessment in the Built Environment*. London: Taylor and Francis, 2011.

DeWeerdt, Sarah. "Is Local Food Better?" *World Watch Magazine*, vol. 22, no. 3 (May/June 2009).

ISO 14040:2006, Environmental Management—Life Cycle Assessment—Principles and Framework. Geneva, Switzerland: International Organization for Standardization, 2006.

ISO 14044:2006, Environmental Management—Life Cycle Assessment—Requirements and Guidelines. Geneva, Switzerland: International Organization for Standardization, 2006.

Jolliet, Olivier, et al. *Environmental Life Cycle Assessment*. Boca Raton, FL: CRC Press, 2015.

LIGHT POLLUTION

It is difficult to imagine a world without lighting. We depend on artificial lighting (light created by humans) for a wide range of activities that would otherwise be difficult if not impossible. However, sometimes lighting can become a nuisance when it disturbs sleep or interferes with stargazing. When this happens, we refer to the lighting as light pollution.

Light pollution is usually caused by outdoor lighting, for example, a security light on a house that shines through a bedroom window next door, keeping the neighbor awake at night. And a flashing neon sign on a local business might also interfere with sleep patterns for people living nearby. When this happens, light pollution becomes a health issue that needs to be addressed. However, unless one's property is large or in a remote area, it can be difficult to prevent outdoor lighting from spreading onto neighboring properties and becoming a nuisance.

Astronomers also struggle with light pollution when they attempt to view celestial objects from an urban location. The light from buildings, motor vehicles, and streetlights can fill the evening sky, making astronomical observations difficult with even the most powerful telescopes. This is why observatories are often located on mountaintops or in secluded areas, far away from the city lights.

Furthermore, light pollution can be a hazard to certain wildlife species that depend on light for navigation and biological cues. City lights can easily disorient birds that migrate at night and navigate by the moon and stars. And female sea turtles may not lay eggs if the lighting from beachfront homes and businesses causes the turtles to confuse day and night. Sometimes a bright light at night will act like a magnet, attracting moths and other insects, which, in turn, can entice hundreds of bats looking for a meal.

The behavior of animals, including feeding and migration patterns, can also be altered when nighttime lighting disrupts their circadian rhythms. In plants, the closing of flowers and changes in leaf position at night can be thrown off rhythm if artificial lighting disturbs the evening darkness. Humans need darkness too: to regulate our internal clockwork, sleep well at night, and wake up in the morning feeling refreshed.

Issues surrounding light pollution can be complicated. For example, homeowners may feel it is their right to protect their property with a security light, whereas neighbors may contend that the light interferes with their right to privacy and a good night's rest. In most cases, these issues can be resolved through friendly conversations. But sometimes to resolve the matter, a local conflict resolution service is needed, or a city or state light ordinance must be invoked.

Several steps can be taken to reduce light pollution. One effective approach is to locate outdoor lighting far from neighboring properties or to direct the light away from the properties. Another approach is to put the lighting on a timer switch that turns the light off later at night when neighbors are trying to sleep. Of course, outdoor lights should always be switched off when not needed, which saves energy too. Using low-wattage, energy-efficient light bulbs also reduces energy consumption and, depending on the type of bulb, may reduce light intensity. In a high-rise building, closing the curtains at night can prevent birds from crashing into windows while improving visibility of the moon and stars for others.

Security lighting is often located over an entry door or in a dark corner of a property to discourage intruders. Reducing light pollution from security lighting can be especially challenging because it is not always possible to locate security lights where they are not visible from a neighbor's bedroom window. However, if the light fixture is equipped with a motion detection switch, the light stays off unless an intruder is in the vicinity. Another option is to fit the light fixture with a shield that blocks light from the neighbor's view. A spot light, which focuses more narrowly than other types of lighting, can also be helpful.

Specific concerns about light-emitting diode (LED) street lighting have been raised by the American Medical Association (AMA), which has issued community guidance for reducing the harmful human and environmental effects of roadway lighting systems using LEDs. This type of lighting consumes less energy than conventional lighting, resulting in a lower reliance on fossil fuels to generate electricity, and about 10 percent of existing street lighting in the United

States has already been converted to LED technology. However, according to the AMA, LED lighting emits large amounts of blue light that appears white to the naked eye and can cause a hazardous nighttime glare for drivers. Furthermore, the blue LED light suppresses melatonin at night, resulting in a five times greater impact on circadian sleep rhythms compared with conventional street lighting. This can result in reduced sleep time, diminished sleep quality, impaired daytime functioning, and even obesity. Outdoor LED lighting can also disorient birds, insects, turtles, and fish. The AMA guidelines recommend that communities use the lowest intensity lighting possible to minimize blue-rich light, properly shield the lights to minimize glare, and consider dimming the lighting during off-peak periods.

Richard Crume

See Also: Energy Star; Leadership in Energy and Environmental Design

Further Reading

AMA Adopts Community Guidance to Reduce the Harmful Human and Environmental Effects of High Intensity Street Lighting. American Medical Association, Chicago, IL, 2016. http://www.ama-assn.org/ama/pub/news/news/2016/2016-06-14-community-guidance-street-lighting.page.

Anderson, Jay, ed. *Environmental Impact of Light Pollution and Its Abatement*. Toronto, Canada: Royal Astronomical Society of Canada, 2012.

Bogard, Paul. *The End of Night: Searching for Natural Darkness in an Age of Artificial Light*. New York: Back Bay Books, 2014.

Fighting Light Pollution: Smart Lighting Solutions for Individuals and Communities. Mechanicsburg, PA: Stackpole Books, 2012.

International Dark Sky Association. *Home Page*. http://darksky.org (accessed June 3, 2017).

Meier, Josiane, et al., eds. *Urban Lighting, Light Pollution, and Society*. New York: Routledge, 2015.

Mizon, Bob. *Light Pollution: Responses and Remedies*. New York: Springer, 2012.

Scriber, Brad. "Light Pollution, Ecological Light Pollution, Got Milky Way, Getting Back in the Black, Nightlight Savings Time, Lights and Safety." *National Geographic GeoPedia* (October 2008). http://ngm.nationalgeographic.com/geopedia/Light_Pollution.

LONDON SMOG DISASTER

In early December 1952, a blanket of deadly smog lay over the city of London for about four days, killing around 4,000 people. The smog spanned roughly 1,000 square miles (2,590 square kilometers), but the public was not too alarmed at the time. Due to London's developing industrial sector and geographic location, residents were used to a heavy fog.

Power plants in London burned large amounts of bituminous coal, which the city heavily relied on. Also, industrial plants constantly emitted a smoky soot full of hydrocarbons, a by-product of burning coal containing high amounts of sulfur and nitrogen. In the early 20th century, 76,000 tons (68,900 metric tons) of soot were emitted in London each year, about 650 tons (590 metric tons) for every square mile. But the industrial companies were not to blame for the majority of this soot.

Londoners were very fond of their domestic open-fire kitchens. While other European countries had transitioned to stoves and ovens, London was less interested in these new cooking technologies. Roughly two-thirds of London's soot was a result of these domestic fires. During World War II, the British government even encouraged residents to burn these fires in their homes, thinking the soot would serve as camouflage from enemy air bombings.

On December 4, 1952, the soot mixed with fog to create a thick, lethal smog. The particular toxicity of this fog was caused, in large part, by a temperature inversion that tended to prevent the smog from dispersing, holding it in place. (London is susceptible to this type of meteorological phenomenon because of its topography, surrounded by low hills that allow air to stagnate above the bustling streets.) That morning in December, a cool, high-pressure system encroached upon London, trapping the fog beneath and preventing the pollution from dissipating. In addition, house fires during the evening were created to warm the houses from the cold air, in turn emitting large amounts of sulfur dioxide and other noxious gases into the stagnant air. Soot and smoke from industrial plants added to the mix.

The smog was at times nearly black and at other times yellow, and some reports say it turned green. The visibility that morning was only 70 to 80 yards (64 to 73 meters), and street lamps were lit during the daytime. The port of London on the Thames River had to be closed because of the limited visibility, shutting in over 100 ships and excluding another 200 waiting to enter, and the poor visibility also resulted in an uptick in burglaries around the city. Londoners coughed up soot, felt pain in their throats and lungs, and experienced difficulty breathing, especially babies and the elderly. By the third day of the smog, the insides of London homes were covered in soot.

A few weeks after the incident, reports of nearly 1,000 deaths surfaced, but the health minister subsequently reported the number to be closer to 3,000, and later studies estimated 7,000 to 12,000 deaths. The devastation the city felt after so many illnesses and deaths eventually caused momentum to build for the passage of the British Clean Air Act of 1956. The act required Londoners to burn smokeless fuel in their homes or switch to gas or electricity. Since then, London has only had one other dangerous fog, this one occurring in 1962.

Mallory L. Daily

See Also: Air Pollution; Electric Power Generation, Health Implications of; Hazardous Air Pollutants; Ozone and Smog in the Urban Environment; Particulate Matter and Bioaerosols Pollution; Polycyclic Aromatic Hydrocarbons; Regional Haze Pollution; Respiratory Disease and Air Pollution

Further Reading

Corton, Christine L. *London Fog: The Biography*. Cambridge, MA: Belknap Press, 2015.

Corton, Christine L. "The Return of London's Fog." *New York Times*, November 6, 2015, https://www.nytimes.com/2015/11/08/opinion/sunday/the-return-of-londons-fog.html?.

50 Years On: The Struggle for Air Quality in London since the Great Smog of December 1952. London: Greater London Authority, 2002.

Hernan, Robert Emmet. *This Borrowed Earth: Lessons from the Fifteen Worst Environmental Disasters around the World.* New York: St. Martin's Press, 2010.

Stoddrad, Katy. "Fog Brings London to a Standstill, December 1952." *Guardian*, November 2, 2015, https://www.theguardian.com/uk-news/from-the-archive-blog/2015/nov/02/fog-great-smog-london-1952.

Tracton, Steve. "The Killer London Smog Event of December, 1952: A Reminder of Deadly Smog Events in U.S." *Washington Post*, December 20, 2012, https://www.washingtonpost.com/blogs/capital-weather-gang/post/the-killer-london-smog-event-of-december-1952-a-reminder-of-deadly-smog-events-in-us/2012/12/19/452c66bc-498e-11e2-b6f0-e851e741d196_blog.html.

LOVE CANAL INCIDENT

The Love Canal incident is perhaps one of the best known examples of the serious adverse health effects resulting from the indiscriminant dumping of toxic wastes. Love Canal is officially defined as a 36-square-block area in Niagara Falls, New York, where refuse was dumped for decades, including 22,000 tons (19,960 metric tons) of toxic waste buried by the Hooker Chemical Company.

Lessons from Love Canal

After all these years, the scars still remain with the former residents of Love Canal.

An Interview with Luella Kenny

Former Love Canal resident

Luella Kenny, a former resident of Love Canal, helped lead the fight to clean up the Love Canal hazardous waste dump site and address the adverse health conditions, including cancer, experienced by many residents. Kenny has remained active in community and environmental organizations, including serving on the boards of the Center for Health, Environment, and Justice and the Love Canal Medical Fund, and she has participated in panels sponsored by the New York Department of Health and the U.S. Environmental Protection Agency. Kenny has spoken about hazardous waste to many high school and university students and to various grassroots community groups. Her passion lies in educating young people about the dangers of exposure to toxic chemicals.

The Love Canal incident is recognized as one of the great environmental disasters of the twentieth century in the United States, leading to creation of the Comprehensive Environmental Response, Compensation, and Liability Act (also known as Superfund) in 1980. Having lived through the Love Canal tragedy, can you comment on the challenges that were faced by residents of

the area, both physical and emotional? After all these years, have families recovered or are there lingering effects?

The Love Canal period was a time of great stress and chaos for the residents of Love Canal. Because the danger was not immediately evident to the residents, it caused conflict within families. This was not like a hurricane or tornado, where residents seek shelter because they know it is coming. There were times when chemicals permeated the air or barrels surfaced. But most of the residents grew up in Niagara Falls, whose primary industry was the chemical plants, and the chemical odors were familiar. Husbands and wives were always arguing, usually because the wife wanted to leave and protect her family, whereas the male of the time felt duty bound to provide shelter for his family. As children and family members became ill, it was difficult to be told you had to remain in your contaminated house until the government finally purchased your residence. Enormous stress was caused by the lack of support from government and health officials, family illnesses, burglaries, mothers forced to spend time away from home to fight for their rights, and the uncertain future.

After all these years, the scars still remain with the former residents of Love Canal. Children whose childhood was disrupted were the most vulnerable, and many are still unable to talk about this period of their lives. There are two types of former residents: the ones who want no identity with the Love Canal disaster and those who feel it is important to educate people about the dangers of toxic waste exposure. Certainly, the lives of residents were permanently changed.

Many concerned citizens fought to clean up Love Canal and hold responsible those who caused the physical and financial distress experienced by so many local residents. What were the most important lessons learned, and in retrospect, are there any other actions you wish you had taken?

It was important that the concerned residents be at the forefront of the fight for relocation. Certainly, support from high profile individuals was welcomed and encouraged, but the affected residents were the driving force. Politics was an important dynamic that needed to be gauged and used to the residents' advantage. Regretfully, greater initiative was needed to prevent rehabitation of the area. The dump still contains 20,000 tons (18,144 metric tons) of chemicals that are supposedly contained, but there are signs of leakage, and several current residents are ill with diseases that can reasonably be associated with exposure to Love Canal chemicals.

There may be hundreds of other sites like Love Canal across the United States that have not yet even been discovered. What advice do you have for community groups concerned with hazardous waste dump sites in their neighborhoods?

Communities faced with a hazardous waste problem need to unite and educate themselves about the problem. Take advantage of the leadership training and technical assistance offered by many environmental groups. Persevere until you reach your goal. Government officials may try to get you to settle for less, but you must remain firm until you reach your goal. There can be no compromise when your family's life is at stake.

What would be a good career path for a recent college or university graduate wanting to help communities find solutions to local environmental problems?

There are many avenues open to students who are interested in preserving the environment. Obviously, many branches of science and engineering will further their knowledge of how toxic chemicals affect humans and how the toxic effects can be mitigated. Lawyers and politicians who will make and protect the laws that will protect the environment are needed, as are teachers who will mold young minds to realize the importance of the environment. Leaders in all walks of life are important because we are all responsible for protecting the environment. Together we can make a difference!

In the late 1890s, William T. Love conceived of a plan to dig a canal connecting the Niagara River to Lake Ontario, thereby avoiding Niagara Falls. Before Love ran out of funding, only about a mile (1.6 kilometers) long, 50 feet (15 meters) wide, and 10 to 40 feet (3 to 12 meters) deep section of the canal was excavated. The abandoned canal was used as a municipal dump for the city of Niagara Falls in the 1920s. By 1942, Hooker Electrochemical Company (later becoming Hooker Chemical Company) was given permission to dispose of wastes in the canal. They first drained the canal and lined it with a thick clay, which was supposed to prevent leakage. Then they began placing 55-gallon (208-liter) barrels into the pit. The city of Niagara Falls and the U.S. Army also continued to dispose of refuse there. The dump site remained in operation until 1953, when it was covered over with soil, allowing vegetation to grow on it. On April 28, 1953, Hooker Chemical Company sold the site for $1 to the Niagara Falls City School District, with a written agreement that clearly disclosed the unsuitability of the site for development. Nevertheless, in 1955, the school board completed construction of the 99th Street School beside the site, and soon thereafter, they built the 93rd Street School, located six blocks away. The remaining land was then sold to private developers who built single-family residences and low-income housing. In 1957, sewer lines, which breached the protective clay walls, were installed, and the protective clay cap was partially removed by the city. This allowed the dangerous chemicals buried there to migrate away from the canal bed.

From the 1960s onward, residents of the area complained about the appearance of strong "chemical" odors, foul substances, and puddles of strange oily and odd-colored liquids in their basements and yards. By the mid- to late 1970s, residents, with support from local journalists, began discussing unusually high incidences of birth defects and other abnormalities. Also, children who played in the vicinity of the dump site talked about playing with "hot rocks," which were conglomerations of chemicals that had oozed out and, when smashed, would sometimes release sparks and smoke. Children would sometimes return home with chemical burns on their hands and feet from playing in the area.

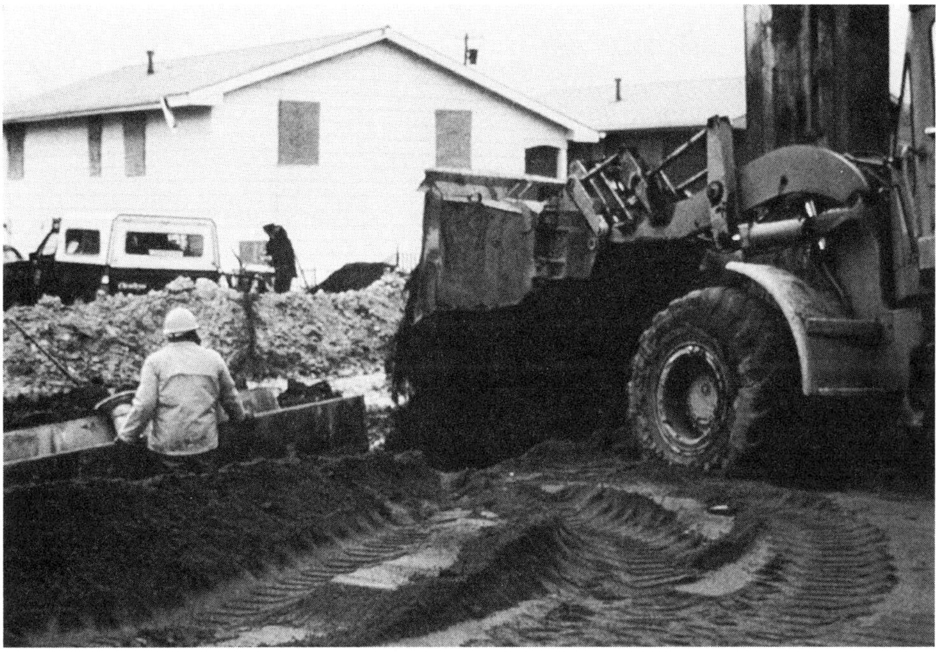

Cleanup of the Love Canal waste dump in Niagara Falls, New York, where industrial wastes were dumped for decades. When waste materials began to surface and an abnormal number of illnesses were reported, President Carter declared an environmental emergency for the site. (Centers for Disease Control and Prevention)

The New York State Health Department found an abnormally high rate of miscarriages, and on August 2, 1978, when a state of emergency was declared for the dump site, homeowners began to organize. (When Lois Gibbs was elected president of the Love Canal Homeowners' Association, her son was experiencing an array of health problems, including asthma, epilepsy, low white blood cell counts, and urinary tract infections. She was later to become a well-known environmental activist.) Efforts were mounted to collect evidence indicating the buried toxic waste was responsible for the health problems experienced by residents. It became nearly impossible for houses to be sold, and some families simply abandoned their homes. Over 800 families were eventually relocated and reimbursed for their homes. All of the residences to the west and most of those to the east of the site were demolished. Subsequently, the Comprehensive Environmental Response Compensation and Liability Act (known as Superfund) was passed to help fund remediation of toxic waste sites located in residential areas.

Unfortunately, Love Canal is not a unique environmental catastrophe. In fact, Love Canal is only one of thousands of industrial waste sites around the country that evolved through collaboration between local governments and corporate entities. Many of these sites continue being a threat to the health and safety of the public living near them.

Victor B. Stolberg

See Also: Asthma; Children's Environmental Health; Environmentalism; Hazardous Waste Disposal; Land Disposal of Waste Materials; Superfund Act

Further Reading

Blum, Elizabeth D. *Love Canal Revisited: Race, Class, and Gender in Environmental Activism*. Lawrence: University Press of Kansas, 2008.

Gibbs, Lois Marie. *Love Canal and the Birth of the Environmental Health Movement*. Washington, DC: Island Press, 2010.

Levine, Adeline Gordon. *Love Canal: Science, Politics, and People*. Lexington, MA: D.C. Heath and Company, 1982.

Paigen, Beverly, et al. "Growth of Children Living Near the Hazardous Waste Site, Love Canal." *Human Biology*, vol. 59, no. 3 (June 1987): 489–508.

LYME DISEASE

Lyme disease, caused by the bacteria *Borrelia burgdorferi sensu lato* and transmitted by black-legged ticks, is the most common vector-borne disease in the United States. Following a tick bite, bacteria are able to establish a skin infection, resulting in a "bull's-eye" skin rash and then spreading to different organs. This can lead to the severe inflammation of heart and joints and neurological abnormalities. Even after two to four weeks of treatment with antibiotics, some patients still suffer from fatigue, pain, or joint aches, a condition known as posttreatment Lyme disease syndrome.

The number of the Lyme disease cases has surged since the disease was first identified in 1975, and each year about 30,000 cases (mostly in northern, eastern, and midwestern areas of the United States) are reported by state health departments and the District of Columbia. Despite the large number of cases, no human

Avoiding Lyme Disease

If you want to avoid getting Lyme disease, the Mayo Clinic advises staying away from areas that attract deer ticks. This includes wooded and bushy areas with long grass. Other approaches include the following:

- Wear clothes that cover your skin (e.g., long-sleeved shirts and long pants) when walking in wooded or grassy areas. (Do not let dogs run free.)
- Use insect repellents, being careful to follow directions.
- If you have a yard, clear away brush and leaves where ticks can live.
- Check yourself, children, and pets for ticks after visiting wooded or grassy areas. (Taking a shower can help remove ticks too.)

Because deer ticks are often no larger than the head of a pin, they are hard to identify and remove. If you find a tick, remove it with tweezers, pulling carefully and steadily to avoid crushing it.

vaccine against Lyme disease is currently available, although considerable vaccine research is underway.

Vaccination against pathogens has been considered as the most effective way to control an infectious disease such as Lyme disease. (Pathogen proteins are vaccinated into humans to induce antibodies that destroy pathogens during infection.) However, unlike other pathogens, Lyme disease-causing bacteria are transmitted from reservoir animals in the environment (in the United States mostly from white-footed mice) to humans via ticks. Consequently, the work on developing a vaccine against Lyme disease has focused on interrupting bacterial transmission. Researchers believe this can be achieved by immunizing humans or reservoir animals with bacterial proteins or bacteria with reduced virulence.

The only transmission blocking vaccine (LYMErix) approved by the U.S. Food and Drug Administration targets the surface protein OspA from the Lyme disease-causing bacteria. This protein is produced when the bacteria are in ticks and is reduced when the bacteria enter animals. Thus, when humans are immunized with the OspA protein, the OspA antibody is induced to eliminate bacteria during tick feeding. However, a few patients have developed arthritis after immunization, likely because of the autoimmune response triggered by the OspA protein, and this has led to withdrawal of the vaccine from the market. The current research focus is to develop the OspA protein as a reservoir animal-based vaccine by immunizing the white-footed mice as opposed to humans, thereby blocking mouse-tick-human transmission. Another option under investigation is to evaluate other proteins from Lyme disease-causing bacteria as vaccine candidates.

An alternative to human- or reservoir animal-based vaccines is a vector-targeted vaccine. These vaccines would target the tick proteins that facilitate feeding or bacterial survival in ticks or transmission to animals. Therefore, the antibodies targeting on these proteins would be expected to block tick feeding, eventually preventing bacterial transmission. One example is a tick saliva protein (Salp15) that helps the bacteria to escape from the immune response of humans and animals, resulting in efficient transmission. Vaccinating Salp15 protein has been demonstrated to prevent Lyme disease infection in mice, making this protein a vaccine candidate.

The conventional strategy in developing human- or animal-based vaccines for the prevention of Lyme disease is challenging. However, multiple bacterial or tick proteins being tested for their abilities to prevent diseases will likely produce next-generation vaccines against Lyme disease, resulting in improved public health by preventing new Lyme disease cases.

Yi-Pin Lin

See Also: Infectious Diseases; Zoonotic Diseases

Further Reading

Centers for Disease Control and Prevention. *Lyme Disease*. https://www.cdc.gov/lyme (accessed November 29, 2016).

Dai, Jianfeng, et al. "Antibodies against a Tick Protein, Salp15, Protect Mice from the Lyme Disease Agent." *Cell Host and Microbe*, vol. 6, no. 5 (November 2009): 482–492.

Embers, Monica E., and Sukanya Narasimhan. "Vaccination against Lyme Disease: Past, Present, and Future." *Frontiers in Cellular and Infection Microbiology*, vol. 3, no. 6 (February 2013): 1–15.

Gomes-Solecki, Maria. "Blocking Pathogen Transmission at the Source: Reservoir Targeted OspA-Based Vaccines against *Borrelia Bburgdorferi*." *Proceedings of the National Academy of Sciences*, vol. 112, no. 38 (September 2015): 11752–11753.

Mayo Clinic. *Lyme Disease*. http://www.mayoclinic.org/diseases-conditions/lyme-disease/basics/prevention/con-20019701 (accessed November 29, 2016).

LYMPHATIC FILARIASIS

Lymphatic filariasis is an infection that causes elephantiasis, an irreversible enlarging and hardening of the limbs. The disease is found in tropical and subtropical regions, and it is caused by microscopic filarial worms that are transmitted to humans by mosquito bites. By blocking the lymphatic system, these worms cause fluids to collect in tissues, resulting in swelling and bacterial infections. It is estimated that around 120 million people are infected with the disease, and in the hardest hit communities, up to 10 percent of men and women exhibit swollen limbs critical enough to severely affect their quality of life. Many victims of this disease experience pain and physical disability and must contend with the social stigma associated with their physical appearance.

Infection usually occurs during childhood, but the effects are typically not apparent until later in life, when the condition can become debilitating. There is no cure for lymphatic filariasis, but medicines are available to control the spread of the disease and to limit further disability among patients. Additionally, the severity and progression of the disease can be reduced with simple hygiene and skin

The Carter Center's Fight against Lymphatic Filariasis

The Carter Center has been working with countries in Africa and Hispaniola to stop the spread of lymphatic filariasis by distributing medicines that prevent mosquitoes from transmitting the parasite. And to protect pregnant women and children who cannot take the medicines, the center distributes long-lasting insecticidal bed nets, which have the added benefit of protecting against other mosquito-borne diseases like malaria. In Nigeria, a country especially hard-hit by the disease, the center has delivered millions of medicinal treatments and bed nets and assisted with educational programs, with the result that by 2012 transmission of the disease had been stopped. The Carter Center was created in 1982 by former U.S. president Jimmy Carter to find solutions to the global problems of protecting human rights and alleviating human suffering. It is located near the Jimmy Carter Presidential Library and Museum in Atlanta, Georgia.

care, with exercise, and by elevating affected limbs. And in some cases, tissue swelling can be alleviated with surgery. People living in mosquito-infested areas should avoid mosquito bites by using insect repellents on exposed skin, wearing long-sleeve shirts and trousers, and sleeping under insecticide-treated nets. Indoor mosquito sprays can also be effective.

Lymphatic filariasis infections can be asymptomatic, acute, or chronic. Most cases are asymptomatic, where there are no external signs of the disease, but damage to the lymphatic and immune systems and kidneys can still occur. Acute infections involving inflammation of the skin, lymph nodes, and lymphatic vessels may occur, and these infections often accompany chronic cases of lymphoedema (tissue swelling) or elephantiasis (skin/tissue thickening) involving the limbs, breasts, and genital organs.

Because many lymphatic filariasis patients have difficulty making a living, eradication of the disease would contribute to reducing worldwide poverty. Eradication may be possible on a global scale if the spread of the disease can eventually be stopped, although close monitoring would be required to ensure the disease does not reemerge, and many patients already infected would need continuing care for a lifetime. Although lymphatic filariasis has not been reported in the United States since the early 20th century, nearly 1 billion people in 54 countries are at risk of infection.

Richard Crume

See Also: Carter Center; Communicable Diseases; Infectious Diseases; World Health Organization; Zoonotic Diseases

Further Reading

The Carter Center. *Lymphatic Filariasis Elimination Pro*gram. https://www.cartercenter.org/health/lf (accessed November 6, 2017).

Centers for Disease Control and Prevention. *Parasites—Lymphatic Filariasis*. https://www.cdc.gov/parasites/lymphaticfilariasis (accessed November 6, 2017).

Devaney, Eileen. *Lymphatic Filariasis*. Oxford, UK: Blackwell Science, 2001.

Goel, Trilok Chandra. *Lymphatic Filariasis*. Singapore: Springer, 2017.

Lymphatic Filariasis, Fact Sheet. World Health Organization, Geneva, Switzerland, 2016. http://www.who.int/mediacentre/factsheets/fs102/en.

Nutman, Thomas B. *Lymphatic Filariasis*. London: Imperial College Press, 2000.

M

MALARIA

Named for the Italian for "bad air," malaria has afflicted the human race for over 4,000 years of recorded history. First described in ancient Chinese medical texts, malaria epidemics may have contributed to the downfall of both the Greek city-states and the Roman Empire. Today, over 200 million cases of malaria worldwide occur every year. While over 800,000 deaths were attributed to this disease in 2000, this number has dropped to just under 500,000 in 2015. This improvement in mortality rates has been attributed to better therapeutics and malaria prevention efforts targeting the vector (carrier of disease).

Malaria is caused by members of the *Plasmodium* genus, a group of eukaryotic single-celled parasites. The life cycle of these organisms is complex, involving both the human host and the mosquito vector. In humans, the parasites grow and multiply in human liver cells before invading the red blood cells. In the case of *Plasmodium vivax* and *Plasmodium ovale* infections, dormant cells can remain in the liver and reactivate after months or years without symptoms. In the red blood cells, the parasites continue to reproduce until the cell bursts, resulting in the release of waste products and merozoites (daughter *Plasmodium* cells) that continue the cycle by invading more red blood cells. Eventually, the parasite is transmitted to a mosquito when the infected individual is bitten. There, the parasite undergoes further different rounds of growth and development until it reaches the mosquito's salivary glands and can be transmitted to another human host. A variety of genetic defenses against this disease have arisen in humans, including sickle-cell anemia, thalassemia, and glucose-6-phosphate dehydrogenase deficiency, all of which make the red blood cells less hospitable for the parasite.

There is an incubation period of 7 to 30 days between infection with *Plasmodium* and the onset of malaria symptoms that correlates with the period the parasites incubate in the liver before expanding to the blood. The exact length of this incubation period varies based on the exact species. If travelers take antimalarial drugs to prevent the disease, this can delay the onset of symptoms, sometimes for months. The classical presentation of malaria involves a cold stage with shivering, followed by fever with vomiting and headache, and then a final "sweating" stage in which the patient returns to normal temperature. This pattern can repeat every two or three days depending on the strain of parasite. However, this presentation is infrequent, and most patients experience a combination of flu-like symptoms, including fever, chills, body aches, nausea, and vomiting. In severe cases, seizures, brain damage, liver disease, coma, and death can occur. A variety of treatments for malaria are currently available, and it is recommended that treatment is initiated as quickly as possible after diagnosis of the disease.

Malaria can only be transmitted by mosquitos in the genus *Anopheles*. There are over 400 identified species in this genus, but only 30 to 40 commonly transmit the *Plasmodium* parasites. *Anopheles gambiae* is particularly well known because it plays a predominant role in the transmission of *Plasmodium falciparum*, which causes the deadliest form of malaria. The mosquito life span and eating habits play a large role in malaria transmission rates, and transmission occurs more frequently in regions where the mosquitos live longer and prefer to bite humans rather than animals. Climate also plays a large role in malaria transmission, as humidity, temperature, and rainfall regulate both the mosquito life cycle and the length of time the parasite must incubate in the mosquito before it can pass to a human host. Because the mosquito plays such a large role in disease transmission, prevention and eradication efforts often focus on preventing mosquito bites and eliminating the vector entirely when possible. In areas where malaria is endemic, the World Health Organization recommends mosquito netting around beds as well as the treatment of indoor surfaces with insecticide.

Repeated exposure to the parasite can cause partial immunity, which reduces the risk of severe disease. Because of this, most malaria deaths in Africa (where the disease is endemic and transmission rates are high) occur in young children who have not previously been exposed to the disease. In areas where people are not as exposed to malaria, and thus cannot benefit from this partial immunity, all age groups are potentially at risk. In 2015, 212 million new cases of malaria and 429,000 deaths due to malaria were reported. Children under the age of five in sub-Saharan Africa accounted for the vast majority of these deaths. While malaria is no longer endemic in the United States, approximately 1,500 cases occur annually among U.S. citizens, primarily among travelers to countries in which malaria is still pervasive.

To date, the most effective methods to prevent malaria target the mosquitos that transmit the disease. Malaria was endemic in the southeastern United States until 1951, when the disease was eradicated by the combined efforts of the Centers for Disease Control and Prevention (CDC) and state and local health agencies. This success prompted the formation of a global program to eradicate malaria. However, along with drainage and removal of mosquito breeding sites, one of the primary mechanisms of eradication was the liberal use of dichlorodiphenyltrichloroethane (DDT). This insecticide has since been linked to adverse reproductive effects and may cause cancer. DDT is capable of traveling long distances in the atmosphere, accumulates in fatty tissue, and is extremely persistent in the environment. Due to controversy surrounding the use of DDT as well as logistical difficulties and challenges, the global effort to eradicate malaria was halted in 1969. However, new advances in drug and vaccine development, as well as a better understanding of the socioeconomic effects of malaria, have recently brought global eradication back into discussion. Various governing and private organizations are actively pursuing this goal.

Marilyn Holt

See Also: Centers for Disease Control and Prevention; DDT Exposure; Infectious Diseases; Insect-Borne Diseases; World Health Organization

Further Reading

Centers for Disease Control and Prevention. *Malaria*. https://www.cdc.gov/malaria (accessed April 30, 2017).

Webb, James L. A. *Long Struggle against Malaria in Tropical Africa*. Cambridge, UK: Cambridge University Press, 2016.

White, N. J., et al. "Malaria." *The Lancet*, vol. 383, no. 9918 (February 2014): 723–735.

World Health Organization. *Malaria*. http://www.who.int/mediacentre/factsheets/fs094/en (accessed April 30, 2017).

MARINE POLLUTION, INTERNATIONAL TREATIES TO PREVENT

The 1972 Convention on the Prevention of Marine Pollution by Dumping of Wastes and Other Matter, otherwise known as the London Convention, is an international treaty for protecting the marine environment from human activities. It was developed and administered by the International Maritime Organization, a UN agency responsible for regulating international shipping. The London Convention took effect in 1975, and its primary objective is to control all sources of marine pollution, including waste dumping. There are currently 87 signatory states that are parties to this convention. The London Convention was modernized by the 1996 London Protocol. There are currently 48 parties to the London Protocol, which will eventually replace the London Convention.

The United States has signed but not ratified the London Protocol, which means that the United States is not bound by this treaty. However, the United States actively participates in the annual Consultative Meeting of Contracting Parties to the London Convention and London Protocol and supports the treaty through, for example, compliance and monitoring support, capacity building, and scientific and technical guideline development. The U.S. Environmental Protection Agency, supported by the U.S. State Department, participates in annual joint meetings of the London Convention Scientific Group and London Protocol Scientific Group. These groups of scientists are responsible for advising the Consultative Meeting with the best scientific and technical advice on marine ecology and pollution.

Under the London Protocol, which took effect in March 2006, parties are prohibited from all ocean dumping, except for the wastes explicitly listed in the protocol's Annex 1. Wastes that may be considered for dumping include the following:

- Dredged material
- Sewage sludge

- Fish wastes or material resulting from industrial fish processing operations
- Vessels and platforms or other man-made structures at sea
- Inert, inorganic geological material
- Organic material of natural origin
- Bulky items primarily comprising iron, steel, concrete, and similarly unharmful materials for which the concern is physical impact, and limited to those circumstances where such wastes are generated at locations with no land-based alternatives
- Carbon dioxide streams from carbon dioxide capture processes for sequestration in sub-seabed geological formations

Furthermore, the London Protocol restricts commercial-level ocean fertilization as a greenhouse gas mitigation technique but allows for scientific research on the technique and, in future meetings, for revisiting the topic and developing guidelines. The London Protocol is a critical international treaty to protect and preserve international waters, ocean wildlife, and marine ecosystems. This is particularly so in the context of climate change, which will not only create new challenges for the oceans but exacerbate existing ones as well.

Ans Irfan

See Also: Biosphere, Environmental Threats to; Carbon Capture and Sequestration; Climate Change and Human Health; Environmental Protection Agency; Ocean Dumping and the Pacific Garbage Patch

Further Reading

International Maritime Organization. *Convention on the Prevention of Marine Pollution by Dumping of Wastes and Other Matter*. http://www.imo.org/en/OurWork/Environment/LCLP/Pages/default.aspx (accessed January 3, 2017).

1996 Protocol to the Convention on the Prevention of Marine Pollution by Dumping of Wastes and Other Matter, 1972 (as Amended in 2006). London: International Maritime Organization, 2006.

U.S. Environmental Protection Agency. *Ocean Dumping: International Treaties*. https://www.epa.gov/ocean-dumping/ocean-dumping-international-treaties (accessed January 3, 2017).

MARINE VESSELS, POLLUTION FROM

At any given point in time, there are tens of thousands of ships sailing between our ports and the oceans. Most of this traffic comprises shipping vessels, as over 90 percent of global trade occurs through sea lanes. Also, there has been a global increase in cruise ships over the past few decades, and there are thousands of naval vessels at sea. Those ships generate a large amount of pollution for both the oceans and atmosphere. Marine pollution can be divided between direct sources, such as emissions and waste discharge, and incidental problems, like oil spills or inadvertent transport of invasive species in cargo or on ship hulls.

Exhaust pollution from ships typically includes sulfur oxides, nitrogen oxides, and particulate matter. Not only is this a problem while at sea, but ships can also contribute heavily to local smog while docked, which can lead to respiratory disease and other adverse health issues. Some research indicates that the emissions from marine vessels contribute to a number of premature deaths in port cities every year.

The living organisms that travel on the bottom of a ship's hull or in the ballast water, disrupting destination ecosystems as invasive species, are another form of pollution. Traditionally, people tried to counter this by using antifouling agents like paint. But some of the toxins contained in these agents exacerbated the problem by poisoning the waters the ships sailed through. Today, antifouling paints are regulated by the International Maritime Organization (IMO) to prevent toxic accumulation in the oceans. There are also alternatives to paints, such as ultrasonic waves or electrochlorination.

Some of the worst forms of marine pollution come from accidents at sea, such as oil spills. However, these incidents have declined 85 percent since 1985 as a result of regulation and changes to ship design, including the monitoring of oily water discharges and a requirement that oil tankers have double hulls. Pollution from marine vessels is surprisingly only 10 percent of total oceanic pollution because the majority originates from land. Shipping only accounts for 2.2 percent of global carbon emissions, although these emissions are expected to increase over 200 percent by the year 2050. Nevertheless, shipping is much more energy efficient than land-based transportation.

Much of international marine pollution is regulated through the IMO. Global standards were instituted in 2005 under a treaty that limits emissions of sulfur and nitrogen oxides from engine exhaust. Illegal dumping of toxic materials was addressed in the London Protocol, which went into effect in 2006. Engines installed on U.S. vessels must adhere to fuel standards promulgated under the Clean Air Act. Finally, the U.S. Environmental Protection Agency bans ocean dumping for a variety of hazardous materials, including radioactive waste and other forms of toxic garbage.

Aaron Dorman

See Also: Air Pollution; Clean Air Act; Climate Change and Human Health; Ecosystems, Importance of; Environmental Protection Agency; Invasive Species and Human Health; Particulate Matter and Bioaerosols Pollution; Respiratory Disease and Air Pollution

Further Reading

International Maritime Organization. *Marine Environment*. http://www.imo.org/en/OurWork/environment (accessed May 7, 2017).

Karim, Md Saiful. *Prevention of Pollution of the Marine Environment from Vessels*. Basil, Switzerland: Springer, 2014.

U.S. Environmental Protection Agency. *EPA Collaboration on International Air Pollution Standards for Marine Vessels*. https://www.epa.gov/regulations-emissions-vehicles-and-engines/epa-collaboration-international-air-pollution-standards (accessed May 7, 2017).

U.S. Environmental Protection Agency. *Learn about Ocean Dumping*. https://www.epa.gov/ocean-dumping/learn-about-ocean-dumping (accessed May 7, 2017).

MAUNA LOA OBSERVATORY, CARBON MEASUREMENTS AT

The Mauna Loa Observatory is the site of the longest continuous measurement of carbon dioxide (CO_2) in the atmosphere. Measurements of CO_2 are important because CO_2 is considered the primary cause of climate change, which has the potential to seriously disrupt natural systems and compromise human health.

The observatory is located at an elevation of 3,397 meters (11,145 feet) on the northern flank of the Mauna Loa volcano on the island of Hawaii. This is considered an ideal location because of the elevation and pristine environment. Since measurements began in 1958, there has been a steady increase in CO_2 concentrations in the atmosphere, and the amount of increase has been growing from year to year. For example, in 2015, the increase in CO_2 concentrations over the previous year was 3.05 parts per million, which is the largest year-to-year increase ever recorded at the observatory.

The main cause of increasing CO_2 concentrations in the atmosphere is electric power generation at power plants that are fueled with coal, oil, or natural gas. These power plants emit vast quantities of CO_2, and while some CO_2 is taken in by vegetation or absorbed by ocean waters, enough remains in the atmosphere to

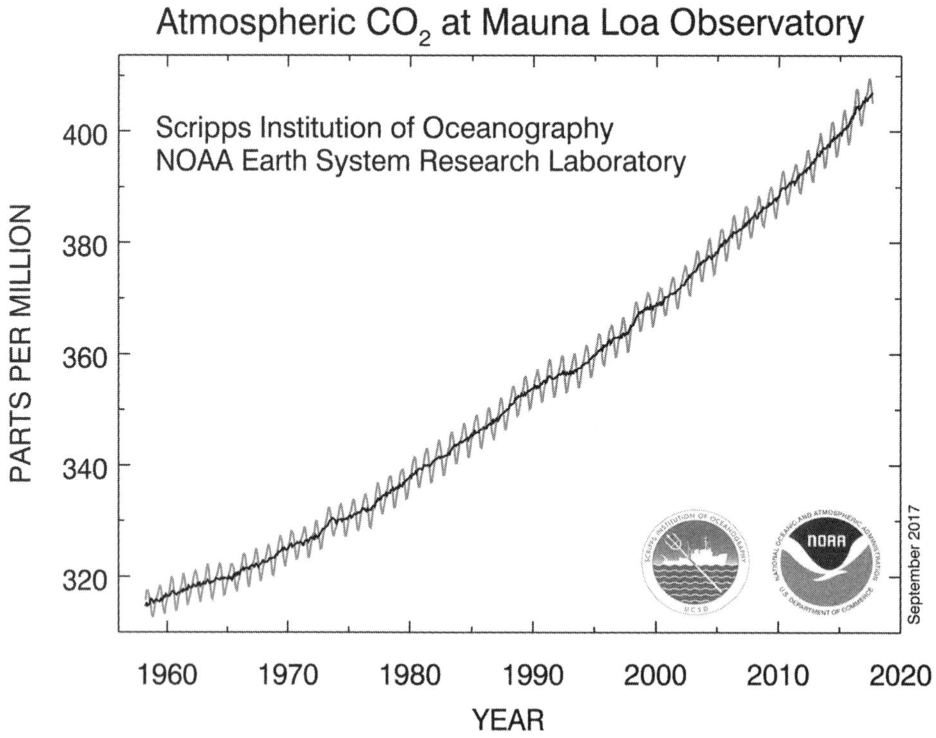

Monthly mean atmospheric carbon dioxide concentrations at the Mauna Loa Observatory, 1958–2016. The darker curve represents seasonally corrected data. (National Oceanic and Atmospheric Administration, https://www.esrl.noaa.gov/gmd/ccgg/trends/full.html)

alter the earth's climate. Measurements at Mauna Loa and other observatories help environmental scientists estimate how much power plants and other CO_2 sources contribute to climate change and predict how much the earth may warm in the future.

Measurements of CO_2 are made using an instrument called CO_2 analyzer, which passes infrared light through a small cell containing a sample of air. An infrared light detector is located at the end of the cell opposite the light source, and because CO_2 absorbs infrared light, the instrument can estimate the amount of CO_2 in the air by the amount of light absorbed. Atmospheric scientists believe that the measurements made at the Mauna Loa observatory accurately represent actual atmospheric concentrations because the analyzer is calibrated frequently and rigorously, and independent measurements using other instruments confirm the accuracy of the analyzer.

Richard Crume

See Also: Biosphere, Environmental Threats to; Carbon Dioxide and the Carbon Cycle; Climate Change and Human Health; Electric Power Generation, Health Implications of; Greenhouse Effect and Global Warming

Further Reading

Cerling, Thure E., M. Denise Dearing, and James R. Ehleringer. *A History of Atmospheric CO2 and Its Effects on Plants, Animals, and Ecosystems*. New York: Springer Science+Business Media, 2005.

Mims, Forrest M. *Hawaii's Mauna Loa Observatory: Fifty Years of Monitoring the Atmosphere*. Honolulu: University of Hawaii Press, 2012.

National Oceanic and Atmospheric Administration. *Trends in Atmospheric Carbon Dioxide*. http://www.esrl.noaa.gov/gmd/ccgg/trends/full.html (accessed August 10, 2016).

National Oceanic and Atmospheric Administration. *Welcome to Mauna Loa Observatory!* http://www.esrl.noaa.gov/gmd/obop/mlo (accessed August 10, 2016).

Volk, Tyler. *CO2 Rising: The World's Greatest Environmental Challenge*. Cambridge, MA: MIT Press, 2010.

MEDICAL AND INFECTIOUS WASTE MANAGEMENT

Public pressure to regulate medical waste began in the late 1980s when needles and other medical waste washed ashore on beaches in New Jersey during the summer—the height of beach season. The medical waste found on these popular beaches was tracked back to a barge that disposed of hospital waste materials by dumping them into the ocean. Not only was the waste unsightly, but there was much concern about sanitation and safety as well.

In response to the public outcry, the U.S. Congress enacted the Medical Waste Tracking Act (MWTA) of 1988 as an amendment to the Resource Conservation and Recovery Act. The MWTA required the U.S. Environmental Protection Agency (EPA) to promulgate regulations governing medical waste management. The EPA published its final medical waste tracking regulations in 1989, and the rules went into effect as a two-year pilot program in four states (New York, New Jersey, Connecticut, and Rhode Island). Following completion of the pilot program, the EPA determined that medical waste can be safely regulated by the states without the need for federal oversight.

As a result of the two-year pilot program, the EPA found that medical waste is most hazardous at the point of generation (e.g., hospitals, nursing homes, and home-health settings), and the greatest disease-causing potential of medical waste was to healthcare workers. The Centers for Disease Control and Prevention estimates there are approximately 385,000 needlesticks and other sharp-related injuries to hospital workers each year, an estimate that does not take into account needlesticks at healthcare setting outside the hospital, for example, doctor offices and home healthcare settings.

In addition to concerns over the health and safety of hospital and healthcare workers, improper disposal of needles and other sharp items poses a health risk to waste disposal workers. For example, janitors, housekeepers, and sanitation workers could be stuck by needles or other sharps while collecting trash and transporting garbage bags. Sticks from used needles can result in infection or exposure to blood-borne illnesses, such as hepatitis B or C or HIV/AIDS.

In 1991, the U.S. Occupational Safety and Health Administration (OSHA) developed regulations designed to protect workers from blood-borne pathogens. These regulations required employers to evaluate whether their operations could expose workers to needles and sharps, and if so, to create exposure control plans that would reduce exposure and protect employees. The OSHA program relied heavily on educating employees on the health dangers of medical sharps and training employees to use proper disposal techniques and containers when dealing with medical wastes that contain blood or other body fluids. The program also mandated that medical wastes be clearly labeled and placed in bright red-orange containers so that all workers will know to take caution when handling.

The U.S. Department of Transportation (DOT) also developed guidelines requiring those who ship medical waste to take precautions to prevent workers and the general public from exposure to pathogens. Similar to the OSHA regulations, the DOT regulations focus on training workers to properly identify, label, and package medical wastes so that people are warned of the potential for exposure and protected from an accidental stick. In addition to the OSHA and DOT regulations, many states provide additional rules and guidelines for employers to help protect workers from the health risks associated with blood-borne pathogens and other medical wastes.

Prior to 1997, most medical waste in the United States was incinerated. However, public health studies showed that waste incineration contributed to smog and other harmful air pollution, and in 1997, the EPA published regulations reducing emissions from medical waste incinerators. Even with these regulations, medical waste incineration continued to be the third leading source of dioxin emissions and the fourth leading source of mercury emissions in the United States.

The EPA continued to revise its medical waste incineration regulations in response to public health concerns, with the most recent revisions promulgated in 2013.

Elizabeth Ann Glass Geltman

See Also: Centers for Disease Control and Prevention; Dioxin Pollution; Environmental Protection Agency; Hazardous Waste Disposal; Mercury Pollution; Occupational Safety and Health; Occupational Safety and Health Administration; Resource Conservation and Recovery Act; Waste Incineration

Further Reading

Crouch, James. *Hazardous Waste in Healthcare: A Guide to Regulatory Compliance*. Middleton, MA: HCPro, 2016.

U.S. Centers for Disease Control and Prevention. *Sharps Safety for Healthcare Settings*. https://www.cdc.gov/sharpssafety (accessed March 8, 2017).

U.S. Environmental Protection Agency. *Medical Waste*. https://www.epa.gov/rcra/medical-waste (accessed March 8, 2017).

Windfeld, Elliott Steen, and Marianne Su-Ling Brooks. "Medical Waste Management—A Review." *Journal of Environmental Management*, vol. 163 (November 2015): 98–108.

MERCURY POLLUTION

Mercury is a dense element that occurs naturally throughout the world, either in elemental form or in chemical compounds. In its elemental form, it is the only metal that occurs as a liquid. It has been known since antiquity for a variety of uses, such as making mirrors (due to its reflective properties), extracting gold, and a component in medicines. It is most commonly known for its use in thermometers. Mercury can be highly toxic.

Mercury can enter the environment in several ways. It can be released naturally during volcanic activity and by the weathering and erosion of rocks containing mercury and mercury compounds. Additionally, it is present in many (particularly older) manufactured products and can be released when those products are disposed of. Mercury can also be a by-product of industrial processes, including the burning of coal in electric power plants.

Mercury can be very toxic in the environment, and human exposure should be avoided. In aquatic environments, microorganisms can transform mercury into methylmercury, which is a more bioavailable form. Methylmercury is a persistent, bioaccumulating, and toxic substance, which means it persists and magnifies in the food chain and can build up to concentrations high enough in fish and shellfish to be toxic to humans.

Exposure to mercury appears to be predominately via inhalation, while exposure to methylmercury tends to be through diet. There are a wide variety of health effects to humans from mercury and methylmercury, including fetal damage, impacts to childhood development and learning, and various forms of toxicity to adults, including damage to the nervous system. Some symptoms of acute or prolonged exposure include tremors, emotional changes, headaches, and poor performance on tests of mental function. In animals, mercury exposure can cause reduced reproduction, slower growth and development, and abnormal behavior.

One of the most recognized cases of mercury poisoning occurred in Japan and came to be known as Minamata disease. Mercury discharged into Minamata Bay from an industrial source was taken up by the fish and shellfish, which were then eaten by people living along the bay. The first case was noted in 1956, with more cases identified throughout the 1960s. The observed health effects included paralysis and death. Another case occurred in 1965 at a different location in Japan, which was also linked to mercury contamination from an industrial source. The health effects among the Japanese remained long after exposure ended.

Mercury fish consumption advisories remain in place throughout the Great Lakes region of the United States and Canada. Numerous actions to reduce mercury pollution have been underway for a number of years, ranging across local, state/provincial, federal, and binational levels. Work at the federal level has included rules on incineration sources (e.g., municipal and medical waste), rules pertaining to certain industrial sources (e.g., chlor-alkali plants), and more recently, rules addressing mercury and other toxic chemicals from coal-fired power plants. Federal and state laws and rules have restricted mercury use in many products over the past three decades, including paints and batteries, and other programs (e.g., environmentally preferable purchasing) have led to reduced use of mercury-containing products in health care and other fields. Ongoing research, monitoring, assessment, and outreach work around mercury have been carried out through various initiatives over the past decade, including the U.S. Great Lakes Restoration Initiative, and additional work is being carried out under the amended Great Lakes Water Quality Agreement, including an assessment for the International Joint Commission highlighting the continued importance of atmospheric deposition of mercury in the Great Lakes and the need to address mercury sources, both near and far.

Thomas B. Lawrence

See Also: Electric Power Generation, Health Implications of; Fish Consumption Advisories; Great Lakes Pollution; Heavy Metal Pollution; Minamata Disease; Persistent, Bioaccumulating, and Toxic Chemicals

Further Reading

Agency for Toxic Substances and Disease Registry. *Public Health Statement for Mercury*. https://www.atsdr.cdc.gov/phs/phs.asp?id=112&tid=24 (accessed April 30, 2017).

Alloway, Brian J. *Heavy Metals in Soils: Trace Metals and Metalloids in Soils and Their Bioavailability*. New York: Springer Verlag, 2014.

Bank, Michael S. *Mercury in the Environment: Pattern and Process*. Berkeley: University of California Press, 2012.

The Economic and Environmental Impact of Great Lakes Manufacturing: Snapshot of Emissions, Pollution Prevention Practices, and Economic Impact Using Public Data. Champaign, IL: Great Lakes Regional Pollution Prevention Roundtable, 2016.

George, Timothy S., Masazumi Harada, and Sachie Tsushima. *Minamata Disease (English)*. Kumamoto, Japan: Kumamoto Nichinichi Shinbun Culture and Information Center, 2004.
U.S. Environmental Protection Agency. *International Actions for Reducing Mercury Emissions and Use*. https://www.epa.gov/international-cooperation/international-actions-reducing-mercury-emissions-and-use (accessed April 30, 2017).
U.S. Environmental Protection Agency. *Mercury in Your Environment*. https://www.epa.gov/mercury (accessed April 30, 2017).
Wuana, Raymond A., and Felix E. Okieimen. "Heavy Metals in Contaminated Soils: A Review of Sources, Chemistry, Risks, and Best Available Strategies for Remediation." *International Scholarly Research Notices*, vol. 2011, article 402647 (August 2011).
Zuber, Sharon L., and Michael C. Newman. *Mercury Pollution: A Transdisciplinary Treatment*. Boca Raton, FL: CRC Press, 2012.

MINAMATA DISEASE

Minamata disease is a form of poisoning that causes severe damage to the central nervous system among people exposed to methylmercury by eating contaminated fish and shellfish. The contamination occurred when methylmercury in wastewater was released into the environment from industrial facilities and accumulated in marine life. The first outbreak of Minamata disease was reported in 1956 in the town of Minamata in southern Japan, followed by a separate outbreak (known as Niigata Minamata disease) nine years later in the northern Japan town of Niigata.

Methylmercury is a highly potent neurotoxin. The symptoms of poisoning include numbness in hands and feet, ataxia (inability to control muscles in arms and legs), loss of peripheral vision, damage to hearing and speech, excruciating pain, paralysis, coma, and even death. Methylmercury is known to be passed from pregnant mothers to unborn babies, causing congenital Minamata disease, a condition resembling cerebral palsy. There is no cure for Minamata disease, and the treatment options are limited to symptom management and functional rehabilitation. The total number of Minamata disease victims is estimated between 20,000 and 30,000.

The best known pollution source of Minamata disease was the Minamata Plant of Chisso Corporation, which had regularly discharged industrial wastewater contaminated with methylmercury from its acetaldehyde production line into Minamata Bay and the Minamata River over a period of 36 years, between 1932 and 1968. The beginnings of this environmental pollution and its health consequences were insidious, but gradually, people started noticing worrisome indications: sightings of dead fish and the general disappearance of fish and shellfish from the bay, reports of cats and dogs acting strangely and unexpectedly dying, and rumors of people afflicted with a strange disease. Cats were especially susceptible, and the term "dancing cat fever" was coined by local citizens to describe the agonizing jerky movements of cats that had eaten contaminated seafood. Despite increasing suspicion and accusations, Chisso Corporation initially denied any link between the wastewater from its plant and these incidents.

The first cases of Minamata disease in humans were officially recognized in 1956 when Dr. Hajime Hosokawa (1901–1970), the Chisso hospital director, reported an epidemic of an unknown central nervous system disease to the local public health office. Even when its own internal toxicology data conclusively linked their wastewater to methylmercury poisoning, the Chisso Corporation chose to hide this information from the public. Chisso Corporation operated their facility for another 12 years before discontinuing the operation in 1968 when acetaldehyde production was no longer profitable. In that same year, the Japanese government belatedly announced its official determination linking the methylmercury contamination from the Chisso Minamata plant with Minamata disease.

At the center of the controversy surrounding Minamata disease, continuing even today, is the victim certification program. The program started in 1959 and was formalized in 1969 under Japan's Law Concerning Special Measures for the Relief of Pollution-Related Health Damage. When certified, victims become eligible for free medical care, pensions, and lump-sum compensation payments. However, critics point out that the program, in spite of numerous revisions, has been too restrictive, and the burden of proof is too high for many victims in need of assistance. The Japanese Supreme Court agreed with the critics in 2014, ordering the government to be less restrictive in compensating victims. Even so, the total number of certified victims to date remains less than 3,000.

Efforts to control contaminated seafood started in the mid-1950s, including bans on the sale of contaminated seafood, self-imposed fishing restrictions by the fishing industry, a Chisso Corporation buyback program to purchase contaminated fish, and the installation of nets to block contaminated fish from leaving Minamata Bay. These efforts were fueled by economic interests of the local fishing industry along with local health concerns. However, with 77 to 165 tons (70 to 150 metric tons) of mercury remaining in the sedimentary sludge at the bottom of Minamata Bay and surrounding waters, the control efforts were only partially effective. In some areas, the contaminated sludge reached 13 or more feet (4 or more meters) deep. In a 1977 survey, the concentration of mercury in some sludges approached an extremely high level (7,700 parts per million [ppm]).

The environmental restoration of the Minamata Bay and surrounding waters, mainly by dredging the bottom to remove contaminated sludge, started in 1977. In heavily contaminated areas, the contaminants were contained by covering the area with heavy metal sheets. When the restoration project was finished in 1988, the highest concentration of mercury detected in the sludge was 14.7 ppm, which was below the 25 ppm level established by Japanese environmental officials as the restoration goal.

The programs to assist and compensate the Minamata disease victims, as well as various pollution prevention and environmental restoration programs, have been financed jointly by the polluters (Chisso in Minamata and Showa-Denko in Niigata), city and prefectural governments, and the Japanese government. Additionally, the prefectural and national governments created the National Institute for Minamata Disease in 1977 as the hub for medical research focusing on Minamata disease and public education. The institute is designated a World Health Organization cooperative research center for studying the health effects of organic mercury.

Yoko S. Crume

See Also: Environmental Toxicology; Fish Consumption Advisories; Mercury Pollution; Neurotoxicants; Water Pollution; World Health Organization

Further Reading

Harada, Masazumi (Translated by Sachie Tsushima and Timothy S. George). *Minamata Disease*. Kumamoto, Japan: Kumamoto Nichinichi Shinbun Culture and Information Center, 2004.

Ishimure, Michiko (Translated by Livia Monnet). *Paradise in the Sea of Sorrow: Our Minamata Disease*. Ann Arbor: University of Michigan Center for Japanese Studies, 2003.

Minamata Disease: Its History and Lessons. Minamata, Japan: Minamata City Planning Division, 2007.

Sato, Hisashi. *Niigata Minamata Disease: Methyl Mercury Poisoning in Niigata, Japan*. Niigata, Japan: Niigata Nippo Jigyosha, 2009.

MOLD AND DAMPNESS

Mold is a naturally occurring substance that can be found almost anywhere and cause a variety of adverse health effects, depending on the sensitivity of the exposed individual. Mold concentrated inside a building, particularly in damp areas, can increase exposure and worsen adverse health effects. Common human reactions to mold exposure include an itchy throat or ears, hives, sneezing, runny or stuffy nose, and eyes that are swollen, itchy, or watery. Highly sensitive individuals can develop atopic conditions, such as eczema, allergies, and asthma.

A variety of mold species can trigger allergic symptoms, including rhinitis, wheezing, chest tightness, and difficulty breathing. Rhinitis, the inflammation of mucous membranes inside the nose, is a common nonspecific symptom of mold exposure. Adverse health effects can occur from both chronic and acute exposures to mold. Populations at particular risk are those that have experienced recent flood damage in their homes or workplaces, and children in general, who are more susceptible to the effects of mold than adults.

Exposure to a variety of mold species, including *Cladosporium, Penicillium, Mucor, Aspergillus*, and *Alternaria*, has been associated with the exacerbation of asthma. (When asthma worsens due to mold exposure, the reaction may be called a mold allergy.)

The likeliness of mold causing an asthmatic episode varies with location. For example, spending time in a damp, mold-infested room, such as a basement or an attic with a leaky roof, leads to increased risk of mold-induced asthma attacks. In addition to exacerbating asthma, mold can sometimes lead to the initial onset of asthma, particularly in damp, indoor environments. Populations exposed to mold are twice as likely to develop asthma as those not exposed.

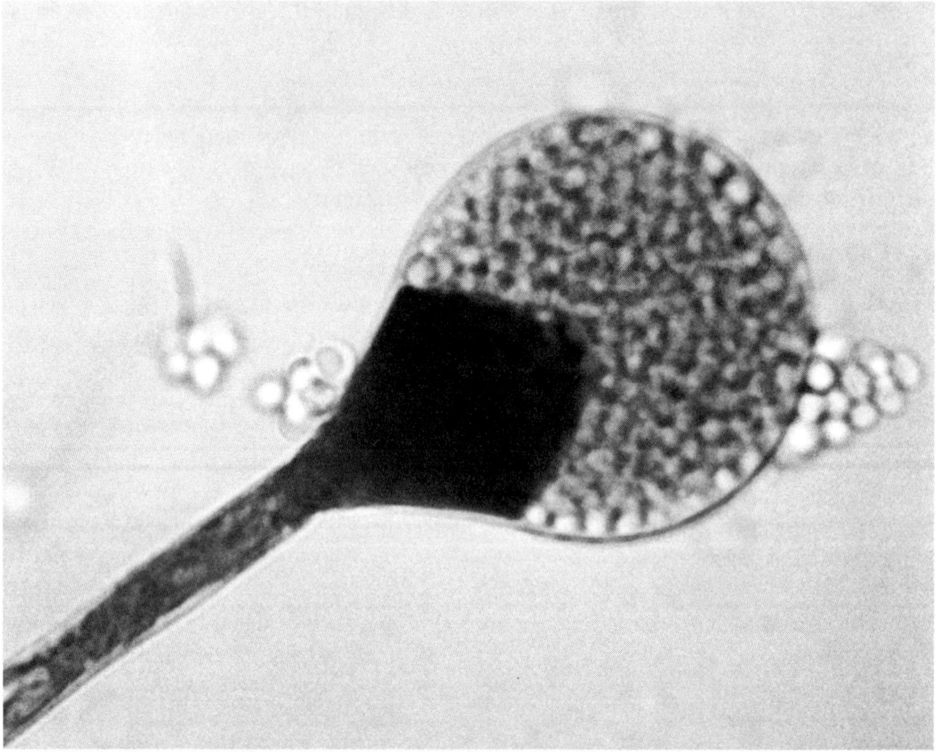

Magnified view of a mold spore. Indoor molds can cause a variety of respiratory and skin infections. (Centers for Disease Control and Prevention/Lucille K. Georg)

Other serious health conditions triggered by mold exposure include allergic bronchopulmonary aspergillosis (a strong response of the immune system, causing dilation of the airways) and hypersensitivity pneumonitis (an inflammation of the alveoli). Inhaling or ingesting mold can also lead to fungal infections that may be difficult to treat. And sometimes mold metabolized by the human body may form toxic compounds known as mycotoxins, which cause chronic effects that persist from months to years, depending on the severity of exposure.

Based on the extent of the mold contamination, there are several ways to remove mold and remediate buildings infested with mold. The two simplest ways to remove mold are damp wiping and wet vacuuming. Damp wiping is the best option for everyday mold and small areas where mold grows following a flood, leak, or plumbing problem. Damp wiping involves scrubbing a surface with water, detergent, or both. Once damp wiping is complete, the surface must be thoroughly dried to prevent mold from growing back. For surfaces with larger swaths of mold, wet vacuuming can be used in conjunction with damp wiping to remove basic mold contamination. (Wet vacuuming can only be used on surfaces that are still wet.) For severe mold contamination of building material (e.g., a wall or ceiling), the only option may be to completely remove and replace the material.

Disposal of mold-contaminated materials must follow environmental guidelines to protect workers doing the removal as well as those handling the garbage. Protections include (1) putting the mold-contaminated materials in large, thick garbage bags that can hold a large volume without breaking; (2) placing a warning label on the bag, indicating it contains hazardous material; and (3) notifying the removal company that they are handling a hazardous substance. Of course, specific disposal requirements can differ by locality.

Preventative measures should be taken whenever possible to avoid or minimize mold growth so that remediation is not necessary. Because mold grows in places with high humidity, keeping humidity levels low (below 50 percent) in homes, offices, and other buildings will reduce mold growth. Additionally, mold growth can be reduced or prevented by regular heating and air-conditioning equipment maintenance (including routine cleaning and filter replacement), repairing leaks as soon as they are found, cleaning damp or wet spots immediately following discovered leaks, and venting kitchens, bathrooms, and equipment like clothes dryers.

Mold represents a serious public health concern that should be addressed immediately. It is especially important as a preemptive measure to help those with asthma or allergies avoid having adverse episodes.

Elizabeth Ann Glass Geltman and Adam Hess

See Also: Allergens in the Environment; Asthma; Children's Environmental Health; Naturally Occurring Toxins

Further Reading

American Industrial Hygiene Association. *Facts about Mold*. https://www.aiha.org/publications-and-resources/TopicsofInterest/Hazards/Pages/Facts-About-Mold.aspx (accessed February 25, 2017).

Indoor Air Quality—Information about Mold (Fact Sheet). Troy: New York State Department of Health, 2011.

Lankarge, Vicki. *What Every Home Owner Needs to Know about Mold and What to Do about It*. New York: McGraw-Hill, 2003.

National Institute of Environmental Health Sciences. *Mold*. https://www.niehs.nih.gov/health/topics/agents/mold (accessed February 25, 2017).

Occupational Safety and Health Administration. *Mold Remediation*. https://www.osha.gov/SLTC/etools/hurricane/mold.html (accessed February 25, 2017).

U.S. Environmental Protection Agency. *Mold*. https://www.epa.gov/mold (accessed February 25, 2017).

MUNICIPAL SOLID WASTE MANAGEMENT

Municipal solid waste (MSW), otherwise known as garbage, is a mixture of a wide variety of household and commercial wastes. MSW in the United States, before any recycling, has the following average composition:

- Paper (26.6 percent of total)
- Food (14.9 percent of total)

- Yard trimmings (13.3 percent of total)
- Plastics (12.9 percent of total)
- Rubber, leather, and textiles (9.5 percent of total)
- Metals (9.0 percent of total)
- Wood (6.2 percent of total)
- Glass (4.4 percent of total)
- Other (3.2 percent of total)

Paper, food products, yard trimmings, and plastics make up almost 70 percent of MSW. If properly handled, MSW ordinarily does not present a significant health hazard. However, potential groundwater contamination and toxic air emissions at landfills remain concerns for people living in close proximity to these facilities, as do toxic air emissions at waste incinerators.

Around the time of World War II, American cities began switching from less healthy methods of garbage disposal (e.g., open burning in dumps and use as farm animal feed) to so-called sanitary landfills, where the garbage was capped (i.e., contained) under a layer of soil. At first, there was not much of a difference between a landfill and an open garbage dump other than the landfill's thin cap. However, various health issues associated with landfills have led to tighter regulatory practices over the past 50 years. Many older landfills became toxic Superfund sites by the 1980s, as the U.S. Environmental Protection Agency (EPA) began closing down hundreds of landfills and issuing more stringent standards to make landfills safer to nearby communities.

Today, most landfills are considered safe, although health concerns continue to arise in nearby communities from time to time. Complaints commonly include headaches, respiratory and gastrointestinal problems, objectionable odors, throat and eye irritation, and stress caused by living in close proximity to the facility. Some scientists and government agencies are also concerned about toxic air pollutants coming from landfills that could potentially cause more severe health problems, including cancer. When a garbage truck reaches a landfill, the wastes are sorted and screened for any toxic or hazardous materials, such as paints, cleaning chemicals, motor oil, batteries, and pesticides, which must be handled separately

Garbage Trucks Fueled with Garbage?

Landfill gas is already being used as a fuel to produce useful heat or electricity. What if landfill gas were converted to compressed natural gas and used to power garbage trucks? It is estimated that the average landfill could power a fleet of up to 40 natural gas-powered garbage trucks while reducing pollutants that would otherwise be emitted from diesel-powered trucks. Although the technology exists today, vehicle modifications and refueling infrastructure would be needed to realize such a goal.

and possibly taken elsewhere for processing. Some of these materials, like batteries, can be recycled.

What happens to MSW once it is placed in a landfill? The wastes begin to degrade, the rate and extent depending on the type of waste and landfill design. Some materials deteriorate quickly, while others may take decades or even centuries to break down. During this process, landfills create two major by-products: gas (mainly methane and carbon dioxide), which rises to the top, and a liquid called leachate, which sinks to the bottom.

The methane and carbon dioxide emitted from landfills are generally not a health concern, although they both contribute to climate change. Because methane is a combustible fuel, landfill gas can be converted to compressed natural gas or hydrogen or channeled to waste-to-energy plants, which are basically combustors that recover energy to produce useful steam or electricity. As of 2016, there were 648 sites converting landfill gas into energy, and the EPA estimates there are another 400 landfill sites that are good candidates for such purposes. Landfill gas may also contain small quantities of hydrogen sulfide (which smells like rotten eggs), ammonia (which smells like decaying fish), and various toxic compounds that have the potential to cause more serious, long-term health problems. The toxic leachate created by landfills can also present a health concern if it breaks through the liner and contaminates groundwater or gets into nearby surface water.

Although Americans are recycling more waste materials than ever before, progress has been slow. The EPA estimates that the United States recycles only about one-third of its MSW, and that number may be overstated due to inexact data collection methods. The recycling rates for lead-acid batteries (98.9 percent) and corrugated boxes (89.5 percent) are high, with tires (40.5 percent), glass containers (32.5 percent), and plastic bottles and jars (about 30 percent) at the other end of the spectrum. On average, about half of all aluminum beer and soda cans are recycled. Although recycling rates are improving, increases in population and consumption mean that the quantity of solid waste continues to increase.

MSW is increasingly used for composting. Specifically, organic waste material, such as food scraps and yard trimmings, can be processed and stored under conditions that cause it to decompose. Eventually, the compost can be used as a natural fertilizer. The composting of MSW may be more complicated than it first appears. For example, the waste materials vary widely in size, composition, and moisture and nutrient contents, and wastes unsuitable for composting (including some potentially toxic or hazardous materials) may also be mixed in. Sophisticated technology is required to separate out and process compostable materials that are safe for use in gardens and on agricultural lands.

Aaron Dorman

See Also: Carbon Dioxide and the Carbon Cycle; Composting, Health Benefits of; Environmental Protection Agency; Groundwater Pollution and Depletion; Hazardous Air Pollutants; Hazardous Waste Disposal; Odor Pollution; Open Burning of Waste; Recycling; Respiratory Disease and Air Pollution; Superfund Act; Waste Incineration

Further Reading

Advancing Sustainable Materials Management: 2014 Fact Sheet. Washington, DC: U.S. Environmental Protection Agency, 2016.

Humes, Edward. *Garbology: Our Dirty Love Affair with Trash.* New York: Avery, 2013.

Lacy, Peter, and Jakob Rutqvist. *Waste to Wealth: The Circular Economy Advantage.* New York: Palgrave Macmillan, 2015.

National Geographic. *Toxic Waste, Man's Poisonous Byproducts.* http://environment.nationalgeographic.com/environment/global-warming/toxic-waste-overview (accessed October 5, 2016).

Pichtel, John. *Waste Management Practices: Municipal, Hazardous, and Industrial.* Boca Raton, FL: CRC Press, 2014.

Rogers, Heather. *Gone Tomorrow: The Hidden Life of Garbage.* New York: New Press, 2006.

U.S. Environmental Protection Agency. *Municipal Solid Waste Landfills.* https://www.epa.gov/landfills/municipal-solid-waste-landfills (accessed December 21, 2016).

U.S. Environmental Protection Agency. *What if Garbage Fumes Powered More of Our Cars, Trucks, and Buses?* https://www.epa.gov/greenvehicles/what-if-garbage-fumes-powered-more-our-cars-trucks-and-buses-0 (accessed December 21, 2016).

Van Haaren, Rob, Nickolas Themelis, and Nora Goldstein. "The State of Garbage in America." *BioCycle,* vol. 51, no. 10 (October 2010): 16.

Vrijheid, M. "Health Effects of Residence Near Hazardous Waste Landfill Sites: A Review of Epidemiologic Literature." *Environmental Health Perspectives,* vol. 118, supplement 1 (March 2000): 101–112.

Williams, Timothy. "Garbage Incinerators Make Comeback, Kindling Both Garbage and Debate." *New York Times,* January 10, 2015.

N

NANOMATERIALS

Nanomaterials are defined by their size, requiring one dimension of the particle to be less than 100 nanometers. (A nanometer is equivalent to one-billionth of a meter.) Although there are many natural particles that fall within the definition of nanomaterials, the particles of concern are those engineered specifically on the nanoscale. These nanomaterials have unique properties that are different from the original bulk materials. For example, engineered nanomaterials can affect chemical reactivity, electrical properties (e.g., conductivity and fluorescence), magnetism, optical properties (e.g., color and transparency), and physical properties (e.g., hardness, strength, elasticity, and melting and boiling points). These engineered properties can be useful for different applications, but they can also introduce health issues.

One important characteristic of the small size of nanomaterials is increased relative surface area per unit of mass, which leads to greater reactivity that can be harnessed for medical and environmental applications, such as drug delivery, improved catalysts, and water purification. However, this greater reactivity can also result in harm to living cells. Other important nanomaterial characteristics are shape, type of material, surface charge, and surface coating, all of which can impact both the fate of the nanomaterials as well as their toxicity. The most common nanomaterials are composed of silver, zinc oxide, titanium dioxide, and carbon-based materials, including carbon nanotubes, fullerenes, and buckyballs. Many nanomaterials are coated to enhance their stability in the environment and to prevent aggregation with other nanomaterials or naturally occurring particles.

Engineered nanomaterials are currently being used in many consumer and industrial applications, which can result in direct and indirect releases to the environmental release. Unfortunately, there is not a full understanding of the implications of such releases. The antimicrobial behavior of nanomaterials is one of the main reasons for their use in consumer products and medical applications. These consumer products include personal care products as well as clothing, both of which likely result in nanomaterials being released into surface waters during normal use and disposal. (Researchers have documented the release of nanomaterials from socks during simulated washing.) Nanomaterials are also increasingly used for environmental cleanup of contaminants in soil and water, resulting in direct release to the environment. Weathering over time releases nanomaterials found in outdoor paints into surface waters. Additionally, accidental releases into the environment would be expected during manufacturing, use, and disposal of nanomaterials and products containing nanomaterials.

Once in the environment, many potential transformations of nanomaterials are likely to occur, including oxidation, reduction, photochemical reactions, dissolution, and aggregation. Nanomaterial fate and transport in the environment are also impacted by properties of the media (e.g., pH, temperature, humidity, ionic strength, and the presence of other particles). Dissolution of nanomaterials can result in the release of toxic-free metals into the environment. While increased aggregation will likely result in nanomaterial settling out of suspension, the smaller, more stable particles will remain suspended longer and travel farther in air and water.

Researchers have demonstrated nanomaterial uptake by aquatic organisms as well as terrestrial plants. Uptake into cells may occur through active mechanisms, such as phagocytosis, or by passive pathways, such as diffusion. In vitro laboratory studies with a range of mammalian and human cell lines indicate that exposure to nanomaterials can result in cell death, oxidative stress, cell dysfunction, DNA damage, increased immune response, and physical impairment. While oxidative stress appears to be the main route of toxicity, nanoparticles may also act as Trojan horses because their small size allows them to enter cells, release free ions, and deceptively cause other harmful reactions. In vivo experiments indicate the uptake and accumulation of nanomaterials, and other research demonstrates that trophic transfer is possible, resulting in nanomaterials accumulating up the food chain.

Humans may be exposed to nanomaterials via contaminated air inhalation and ingestion of contaminated water and food. Research is ongoing regarding the health effects of exposure to nanomaterials in humans and other organisms, particularly at the trace concentrations predicted in the environment. Additional studies are investigating the effects of mixtures of nanomaterials and the nanomaterial properties leading to the greatest toxicity.

Talia E. Abbott Chalew

See Also: Bioaccumulation of Environmental Contaminants; Heavy Metal Pollution; Particulate Matter and Bioaerosols Pollution; Personal Care Products, Health Issues with

Further Reading

Elsaesser, A., and C. V. Howard. "Toxicology of Nanoparticles." *Advanced Drug Delivery Reviews*, vol. 64, no. 2 (February 2012): 129–137.

Klaine, Stephen. J., et al. "Nanomaterials in the Environment: Behavior, Fate, Bioavailability, and Effects." *Environmental Toxicology and Chemistry*, vol. 27, no. 9 (September 2008): 1825–1851.

Schultz, C., et al. "Analytical Approaches to Support Current Understanding of Exposure, Uptake, and Distributions of Engineered Nanoparticles by Aquatic and Terrestrial Organisms." *Ecotoxicology*, vol. 24, no. 2 (March 2015): 239–261.

Sellers, K., et al. *Nanotechnology and the Environment*. Boca Raton, FL: CRC Press, 2008.

Shatkin, Jo A. *Nanotechnology: Health and Environmental Risks*. Boca Raton, FL: CRC Press, 2012.

U.S. Environmental Protection Agency. *Research on Nanomaterials*. https://www.epa.gov/chemical-research/research-nanomaterials (accessed December 29, 2016).

Weisner, Mark R., and Jean-Yves Bottero. *Environmental Nanotechnology: Applications and Impacts of Nanomaterials.* New York: McGraw Hill, 2007.
YouTube. *The Air You Breathe—Do Nanoparticles Pose a Health Risk?* https://www.youtube.com/watch?v=QvvatP5woLM.

NATIONAL AIR TOXICS ASSESSMENT

The National Air Toxics Assessment (NATA) is a program of the U.S. Environmental Protection Agency (EPA) to assess nationwide health risks from exposure to hazardous air pollutants, also known as toxic air pollutants, or simply, air toxics. Air toxics are air pollutants that may cause or contribute to cancer or other serious adverse health problems, including cardiovascular, immune system, kidney, liver, neurological, reproductive, and respiratory effects. Air toxics can also adversely affect ecology and the environment.

The goal of NATA is to identify the air toxics, emission sources, and source locations representing the greatest concern to public health. This information is then used by air pollution experts and agencies to focus resources on the populations at greatest risk for adverse health effects. Because resources (e.g., funds, agency experts, and field technicians) are often limited for air pollution research and control, NATA helps set priorities and direct air pollution professionals toward the emissions and sources presenting the greatest threat.

NATA allows the risk of cancer and other adverse health effects to be estimated, based on the amount of pollutants inhaled, duration of exposure, and toxicity of the pollutants. Because of uncertainties inherent in determining exposure and toxicity, NATA risk estimates are just that—estimates. These risk estimates are not exact, and for this reason, NATA analyses are usually designed to err on the side of safety. This means that NATA is more likely to overestimate health risk than to underestimate it.

Three examples of the types of air pollutants found in NATA assessments are benzene (present in gasoline), tetrachloroethylene (a solvent sometimes used in dry cleaning), and methylene chloride (an industrial solvent and paint stripper). A total of 187 air toxics are identified in the Clean Air Act, and these are emitted from electric power plants, various industrial and commercial operations, and mobile sources (e.g., cars and trucks). When the EPA uses NATA to estimate risk associated with these pollutants, the results are ordinarily reported at the census tract level.

There are some important limitations to keep in mind when using NATA data. NATA provides information on exposure and risk across broad geographical areas, and it cannot be used to estimate exposure and risk for specific individuals or small regions, such as specific census blocks or areas immediately surrounding a particular industry. Furthermore, the assessments generally use emission data averaged over a year and thus do not estimate short-term risks and acute exposure scenarios. Not all possible air toxics are included in NATA assessments, and the effects of mixtures of air toxics are difficult to evaluate. There are also limitations in the accuracy of computer models, exposure assumptions, and emission inventory data, and episodic emissions are not considered (e.g., higher emissions from certain industrial equipment during periods of startup, shutdown, and malfunction). Finally, NATA does not consider exposure occurring indoors or from ingestion or dermal contact.

Although there are a number of limitations to the use of NATA assessments, they are still very useful for several purposes, including:

- prioritizing pollutants and emission sources for further investigation and control;
- identifying geographical locations for further investigations;
- providing a starting point for more detailed local investigations;
- helping with the placement of air pollution–monitoring equipment; and
- empowering citizens and local governments to make decisions concerning pollution sources and health threats.

When the EPA conducts a NATA assessment, the first step is to create an inventory of emission sources. With this information, sophisticated computer models are used to estimate air toxic concentrations in the ambient air and the population exposed to these concentrations. This work is done on a nationwide basis so that estimates can be made for all regions of the United States. The final step is to characterize the potential inhalation health risks for these regions. NATA assessments are published every few years, with the intervening years needed to analyze data. Thus, the NATA assessment for 2011 was not released to the public until 2015. Other assessments are available for the years 1996, 1999, 2002, and 2005, and the EPA is currently compiling data for future assessments.

When characterizing the possibility that someone in a population might develop cancer due to exposure to air toxics, the EPA often uses a probability calculation. For example, a cancer risk of 1-in-1-million indicates the possibility that one person would develop cancer out of every 1 million people exposed to the same concentration of the same pollutant over the same timeframe. This is generally considered an upper-bound estimate because it assumes a constant exposure, 24-hour per day, over 70 years, whereas people actually move around during the day and often relocate their homes to other neighborhoods or cities. Thus, this approach may be overly protective based on the level and duration of exposure. On the other hand, the estimate does not take into account exposure to other air toxics that may be present or whether a person is more vulnerable to exposure due to factors such as age or preexisting conditions.

The question of what level of cancer risk is acceptable or unacceptable is controversial, although the EPA has made case-specific determinations for some regulatory programs. For health risk other than for cancer, case-specific determinations are also made. Factors considered include confidence in the underlying health and dose-response data, uncertainties inherent in calculations and modeling, the level and duration of exposure, and the hazard quotient (the ratio of the actual exposure level to the level where no adverse health effects are expected).

The 2011 NATA assessment indicates that millions of Americans live in areas where air toxics may present potential health concerns and that, on average, about 1 of every 25,000 Americans (i.e., 40-in-1-million) could develop cancer associated with air toxics if exposed over 70 years. The assessment found that formaldehyde, benzene, and acetaldehyde contribute the most to nationwide cancer risk, and acrolein, diesel particulate matter, and chlorine contribute the most to nationwide health risk other than cancer. (The cancer risk assessment did not evaluate the contribution of diesel particulate matter.) However, for the reasons described earlier, there are considerable uncertainties in the NATA assessments, and caution should be exercised in applying the results and drawing conclusions.

Richard Crume

See Also: Air Pollution; Cancer Risk from Environmental Exposure; Clean Air Act; Dose-Response Assessment; Environmental Protection Agency; Hazardous Air Pollutants; Integrated Risk Information System

Further Reading

Guidelines for Carcinogen Risk Assessment (EPA/630/P-03/001F). Washington, DC: U.S. Environmental Protection Agency, 2005.

U.S. Environmental Protection Agency. *National Air Toxics Assessment*. https://www.epa.gov/national-air-toxics-assessment (accessed March 25, 2017).

U.S. Environmental Protection Agency. *2011 NATA: Assessment Results*. https://www.epa.gov/national-air-toxics-assessment/2011-nata-assessment-results (accessed March 25, 2017).

Zhou, Y., et al. "Carcinogenic Air Toxics Exposure and Their Cancer-Related Health Impacts in the United States." *PloS One*, vol. 10, no. 10 (October 2015).

NATIONAL CENTER FOR ENVIRONMENTAL ASSESSMENT

The National Center for Environmental Assessment (NCEA) is one of seven research centers and laboratories making up the Office of Research and Development at the U.S. Environmental Protection Agency (EPA). The NCEA's aim is to inform researchers, regulators, and members of the public about the potential effects that common pollutants and other stressors can have on human health and the environment. Through the integration of research and risk assessments, the NCEA provides technical reporting leading to a better understanding of the impact of exposure to environmental pollutants.

The NCEA is divided into four divisions and an Immediate Office (IO). The IO, located in Arlington, Virginia, manages all assessment programs in NCEA, including the Human Health Risk Assessment (HHRA) and Global Change programs. The HHRA program is largely responsible for providing peer-reviewed human health assessments related to chemicals that are already present in the environment. The Global Change program uses a systematic approach to make vulnerability assessments regarding the future impacts of climate change on ecosystems, human health, and air and water quality.

The Cincinnati Division is responsible for developing the methods that drive the assessments used to determine the risks that certain pollutants pose to human health and the environment. This office also performs assessments of the toxicity found in chemicals for the Integrated Risk Information System (IRIS) program.

In the IRIS Division, which is run out of Arlington, Virginia, and Durham, North Carolina, staff members focus on developing peer-reviewed assessments of pollutants relating to EPA's regulatory mandates. These IRIS assessments are used throughout the EPA and other organizations around the world to inform regulatory action. The IRIS database is made up of over 550 assessments that can be accessed and searched by the public using chemical names, Chemical Abstract Services Registry Numbers, or keywords.

The Research Triangle Park Division, located in Durham, North Carolina, focuses on developing integrated science assessments (ISAs). Starting in 2008, these ISAs have been used for reviewing the National Ambient Air Quality Standards (NAAQS), which were established by the Clean Air Act Amendments of 1990. These standards were implemented to protect the public from six criteria pollutants—carbon monoxide, lead, nitrogen dioxide, ozone, particulate matter, and sulfur dioxide. The ISAs, representing evaluations of the most current scientific knowledge available, are essential to keeping the NAAQS up to date.

Another major initiative of the NCEA is the administration of HERO (Health and Environmental Research Online). HERO is a database of over 600,000 references to peer-reviewed scientific literature and data that are used by EPA researchers to inform regulatory and policymaking activity. The HERO database is part of the EPA's efforts to comply with the Obama administration's Memorandum on Transparency and Open Government. All citations from the HERO database are made publicly available for members of the public to actively participate in the rulemaking process. HERO staff members solicit members of the public to suggest additional studies to be included in the assessment process. Citations are generated from highly comprehensive and complex literature searches conducted by HERO personnel.

Anthony C. Holderied

See Also: Ambient Air Quality; Clean Air Act; Environmental Protection Agency; Integrated Risk Information System

Further Reading

President's Memorandum on Transparency and Open Government. The White House, Washington, DC, February 24, 2009. https://obamawhitehouse.archives.gov/the-press-office/transparency-and-open-government.

U.S. Environmental Protection Agency. *About the National Center for Environmental Assessment.* http://www.epa.gov/aboutepa/about-national-center-environmental-assessment-ncea (accessed December 21, 2015).

U.S. Environmental Protection Agency. *HERO: Health and Environmental Research Online.* http://hero.epa.gov/ (accessed November 30, 2015).

U.S. Environmental Protection Agency. *Integrated Risk Information System.* http://www.epa.gov/iris (accessed November 30, 2015).

NATIONAL ENVIRONMENTAL POLICY ACT

The National Environmental Policy Act (NEPA) requires federal agencies to assess the environmental and related social and economic effects of their proposed actions and to invite public review and comment on those assessments. Airports, federal buildings, military complexes, and highways are examples of projects ordinarily subject to NEPA review. NEPA was signed into law in 1970, and it applied to all federal agencies.

NEPA established the Council on Environmental Quality, which has three major duties: (1) ensuring federal agencies meet the requirements of NEPA, (2) providing oversight for the environmental impact assessment process, and (3) developing regulations and guidance for agencies complying with the provision of the act. (Many agencies supplement the CEQ regulations and guidance with their own internal NEPA procedures.) NEPA also requires federal agencies to take steps to ensure humans and nature exist in harmony and to include environmental considerations in their planning and decision-making processes. To consider the environmental consequences of a significant action, a federal agency may be required to prepare an environmental assessment (EA) and environmental impact statement (EIS).

A federal action can be categorically excluded from having to perform a detailed environmental analysis if the action is determined not to have a significant effect on the human environment. If not categorically excluded, the agency prepares an EA, which assesses whether the action has the potential to cause significant environmental effects. If no significant environmental effects are expected, the agency issues a finding of no significant impact, providing the rationale for this conclusion. On the other hand, if the EA determines that the action is expected to significantly affect the quality of the human environment, an EIS is prepared.

The steps to preparing an EIS include the following:

- Publishing a notice of intent in the *Federal Register* that notifies the public about plans to conduct an environmental analysis and how to get involved in the process
- Conducting a scoping process, where issues and potential alternatives are identified
- Publishing a draft EIS for public review and comment
- Considering all substantive public comments and conducting any additional analyses justified by the comments
- Publishing the final EIS
- Issuing a record of decision that explains the agency's final decision and alternatives considered and presents a plan for any mitigation and monitoring requirements

If a supplement to the EIS is required due to new circumstances or information justifying changes to the proposed action, the agency follows the same procedures required for approval of the initial EIS.

Federal agencies must consider environmental justice when complying with NEPA. The U.S. Environmental Protection Agency (EPA) defines "environmental justice" as "the fair treatment and meaningful involvement of all people regardless of race, color, national origin, or income with respect to the development, implementation, and enforcement of environmental laws, regulations, and policies." The EPA has a special role under NEPA, which is to review and comment on the EISs prepared by other agencies, including environmental justice concerns, and to maintain an EIS repository. Additionally, the EPA must prepare EISs for its own actions.

In the years following NEPA enactment, a variety of environmental advocacy groups, law firms, consulting engineers, research organizations, and university researchers have come to specialize in NEPA actions and analyses, representing a small but significant segment of the environmental health field in the United States.

Richard Crume

See Also: Environmental Impact Assessment; Environmental Justice; Environmental Protection Agency

Further Reading

Citizens Guide to the NEPA: Having Your Voice Heard. Washington, DC: Council on Environmental Quality, 2007.

National Environmental Policy Act of 1969. 42 U.S.C. §4321 et seq. (1969). https://www.gpo.gov/fdsys/pkg/USCODE-2010-title42/pdf/USCODE-2010-title42-chap55-sec4321.pdf.

Rom, William N. *Environmental Policy and Public Health Air Pollution, Global Climate Change, and Wilderness*. San Francisco, CA: Jossey-Bass, 2012.

U.S. Environmental Protection Agency. *National Environmental Policy Act*. https://www.epa.gov/NEPA (accessed March 23, 2017).

Wertz, Wendy R. *Lynton Keith Caldwell: An Environmental Visionary and the National Environmental Policy Act*. Bloomington: Indiana University Press, 2014.

NATIONAL ENVIRONMENTAL PUBLIC HEALTH TRACKING NETWORK

The National Environmental Public Health Tracking Network is a Web-based surveillance tool designed to track diseases related to environmental contaminant exposures. It is funded and managed by the U.S. Centers for Disease Control and Prevention's Tracking Network program. This online network of federal, state, and city surveillance systems enables users to query, chart, map, tabulate, and download standardized data on environmentally related diseases, environmental hazards, human exposures to those hazards, and population characteristics. Some individual surveillance systems include private portals where users can request access to confidential data for research purposes.

The Tracking Network was developed to fill an "environmental health gap" (i.e., the lack of standardized data to track and link environmental hazards with chronic diseases) identified by the Pew Environmental Health Commission in 2000. The list of Tracking Network indicators grows each year but currently includes measures to track (1) environmentally related chronic diseases (e.g., asthma, birth defects, cancer, childhood lead poisoning, developmental disabilities, and heart disease); (2) exposures to environmental hazards (e.g., exposure reports for pesticides and biomonitoring data for arsenic, benzene, cadmium, chloroform, cotinine, lead, mercury, naphthalene and pyrene metabolites, toluene, and uranium); (3) environmental hazards (e.g., air quality, water quality, toxic substances, and heat); and

(4) population vulnerability (e.g., vulnerability relative to climate change, community design, and housing and lifestyle risk factors). Funded programs may also track additional measures that are important to a state or city. For example, New York City's tracking system includes data on pedestrian and bicycle traffic-related injuries, and Maine's tracking system includes data on Lyme disease case rates.

Data from the Tracking Network have been used by researchers and government agencies to (1) facilitate data requests and analyses for epidemiologic studies that establish relationships between chronic diseases and environmental hazards; (2) support public health surveillance activities to identify at-risk populations and emerging threats and to respond to outbreaks; (3) inform and improve the public health basis for policy decisions, government planning, and prevention activities; (4) educate people about risks to their health and promote lifestyle changes; (5) support citizen rights to know about their environment and health; and (6) promote citizen involvement, oversight of polluters, and prompt industry compliance with environmental regulations.

As an example of the Tracking Network's public health relevance, Connecticut used the network to evaluate potential associations between excess cases of bladder cancer around a former manufacturing site and releases of asbestos, lead, and polychlorinated biphenyls. In South Carolina, Tracking Network staff worked with the state's occupational safety and health program to identify worksites with high rates of adult lead poisoning and to target them for inspection. Some Tracking Network programs have developed more advanced surveillance tools that are available for use with their tracking systems. For instance, California's Tracking Network staff developed a tool to identify high-traffic areas, and this tool is being used by San Francisco city planners to evaluate potential air contaminants near planned development projects.

The variety of surveillance tools and abundance of standardized data measures that are available in the Tracking Network make it a valuable information source and tool for researchers, communities, teachers, students, policymakers, and environmental and public health officials.

Adrienne L. Katner

See Also: Cancer Risk from Environmental Exposure; Environmental Epidemiology; Integrated Risk Information System; Socioeconomic Status and Health; Toxic Substances and Disease Registry, Agency for

Further Reading

America's Environmental Health Gap: Why the Country Needs a Nationwide Health Tracking Network. Baltimore, MD: The Pew Environmental Health Commission, 2000. http://healthyamericans.org/reports/files/healthgap.pdf.

Centers for Disease Control and Prevention. *Environmental Public Health Tracking Program*. http://ephtracking.cdc.gov/QueryPanel/EPHTNQuery/EPHTQuery.html?c=-1&i=-1&m=-1 (accessed April 18, 2016).

Centers for Disease Control and Prevention. *National Environmental Public Health Tracking Network*. http://ephtracking.cdc.gov/showHome.action (accessed April 18, 2016).

NATIONAL ESTUARY PROGRAM

The National Estuary Program (NEP) is a nonregulatory program administered by the U.S. Environmental Protection Agency (EPA). The NEP was authorized under the Clean Water Act to "protect and restore water quality and ecological integrity of estuaries of national significance." An estuary is a body of water partly surrounded by land where freshwater from rivers and streams meet and mix with saltwater from the oceans. Estuaries have characteristics of both freshwater and saltwater, and they represent one of the most fertile and productive ecosystems on the earth, providing habitat for a variety of wildlife.

The NEP is administered using a community-based approach. States identify nationally significant estuaries that are threatened by factors such as land use, development, and pollution, and then the EPA provides grants to develop management and restoration plans. Currently, there are 28 estuaries that have been identified as of national significance and participate in the NEP. These estuaries are listed in Table 10.

Table 10. Nationally significant estuary programs participating in the NEP.

Estuary Program Name
Albemarle-Pamlico National Estuary Program
Barataria-Terrebonne National Estuary Program
Barnegat Bay Partnership
Buzzards Bay National Estuary Program
Casco Bay Estuary Partnership
Charlotte Harbor National Estuary Program
Coastal Bend Bays and Estuaries Program
Delaware Center for the Inland Bays
Galveston Bay Estuary Program
Indian River Lagoon National Estuary Program
Long Island Sound Study
Lower Columbia Estuary Partnership
Maryland Coastal Bays Program
Massachusetts Bays National Estuary Program
Mobile Bay National Estuary Program
Morro Bay National Estuary Program
Narragansett Bay Estuary Program
New York-New Jersey Harbor Estuary Program
Partnership for the Delaware Estuary
Peconic Estuary Program
Piscataqua Region Estuaries Partnership
Puget Sound Partnership
San Francisco Estuary Partnership
San Juan Bay Estuary Partnership
Santa Monica Bay Restoration Foundation
Sarasota Bay Estuary Program
Tampa Bay Estuary Program
Tillamook Estuaries Partnership

Each estuary program develops and implements a Comprehensive Conservation and Management Plan that establishes long-term priorities and provides guidelines for environmental protection activities, funding, and research. These plans are developed and approved using a collaborative approach involving coalitions representing many stakeholders. Local priorities are established through consensus-building at management conferences, thus ensuring that unique plans are developed, tailor-made to address local conditions and needs.

The NEP is a critical program for protecting and restoring estuary ecosystems. It is also unique in terms of its coalition-building approach, which serves as a model for solutions to many other environmental challenges. This approach provides sustained cooperation among federal, local, and state governments and other stakeholders, ensuring that nation's critical estuaries are protected for future generations.

Ans Irfan

See Also: Clean Water Act; Ecosystems, Importance of; Environmental Protection Agency; Estuary Pollution; Stormwater Runoff; Wetlands and Healthy Waterways

Further Reading

Kennish, Michael J. *Estuary Restoration and Maintenance: The National Estuary Program.* Boca Raton, FL: CRC Press, 2000.

National Estuary Program Coastal Condition Report, EPA-842/B-06/001. Washington, DC: U.S. Environmental Protection Agency, 2006.

U.S. Environmental Protection Agency. *Overview of the National Estuary Program.* https://www.epa.gov/nep/overview-national-estuary-program (accessed January 3, 2017).

NATIONAL INCIDENT MANAGEMENT SYSTEM

The National Incident Management System (NIMS) is an approach used in the United States to manage emergencies, disasters, and other incidents that threaten life and property and require immediate response. The goal of NIMS is to provide a comprehensive national approach for managing incidents that improves the effectiveness of response for a wide range of possible threats and hazards. These include natural disasters like earthquakes and hurricanes, terrorist activities, and human-caused disasters such as accidental explosions and releases of toxic chemicals. NIMS is designed to address all U.S. threats and hazards, regardless of size, location, and complexity.

Incidents often involve multiple government jurisdictions and may require support from local agencies, nonprofit organizations, the private sector, and the federal government. When multiple agencies and organizations are involved, success depends on a common approach to sharing resources, integrating tactics, coordinating response activities, managing emergency personnel, and communicating with the public. NIMS provides this common approach by establishing a framework for coordination among all parties involved in a response so that the incident can be addressed in the most effective and efficient manner possible.

There are countless cases where the well-managed response to a serious incident has saved many lives.

The NIMS concept has evolved over the years, becoming more urgent in the aftermath of the September 11, 2001, terrorist attacks. Lessons learned by September 11 responders and public concerns about future attacks heightened awareness of the need for a system to standardize response structures, terminology, processes, and resources. Thus, NIMS was born several years later in 2004 by consolidating, expanding, and enhancing existing emergency response systems, policies, and guidelines.

To unify various emergency management and incident response programs across the United States, NIMS is designed around five focus areas:

- Command and Management: incident command, multiagency coordination, and public information systems
- Preparedness: planning, training, exercises, personnel qualification and certification standards, equipment acquisition and certification standards, and publication management processes and activities
- Resource Management: mechanisms and requirements to describe, inventory, mobilize, dispatch, track, and recover resources associated with an incident
- Communications and Information Management: standardized framework for communications, information management, and information-sharing
- Ongoing Management and Maintenance: strategic direction and oversight of NIMS, including routine review and continuous refinement

These components work together in an integrated manner to create a comprehensive incident response system that serves the entire country.

An important component of NIMS is the Incident Command System (ICS). The ICS is a management system that integrates the key response components—facilities, equipment, personnel, procedures, and communications—into a common organizational structure. The ICS concept is intended to help incident managers identify and manage critical response components, often during emergency conditions, without overlooking other important responsibilities. The ICS has been applied to many types of incidents, including hazardous material spills, natural disasters, serious fires, air and ground transportation system accidents, and search and rescue missions.

Although not part of NIMS, Congress passed related legislation in 1986 called the Emergency Planning and Community Right-to-Know Act (EPCRA), which requires state and local governments and private industry to plan and prepare for emergency releases of hazardous and toxic chemicals at industrial facilities and to make this information available to the community. The goal of the EPCRA is to improve the handling of chemicals and to protect public health and the environment. Among the EPCRA requirements are the preparation of emergency response and notification plans and safety data sheets. Additionally, the EPCRA establishes a toxics release inventory, to be compiled and maintained by the U.S. Environmental Protection Agency using data submitted by industries.

Richard Crume

See Also: Disaster Preparedness and Response; Emergency Planning and Community Right-to-Know Act; Environmental Protection Agency; Federal Emergency Management Agency; Natural Disasters; Safety Data Sheet; September 11 World Trade Center Attack; Toxics Release Inventory

Further Reading

Federal Emergency Management Agency. *National Incident Management System.* https://www.fema.gov/national-incident-management-system (accessed March 29, 2017).

Federal Emergency Management Agency. *National Preparedness System.* https://www.fema.gov/national-preparedness-system (accessed March 29, 2017).

Haraway, Mark. *Large Scale Incident Management.* Clifton Park, NY: Cengage Learning, 2009.

Walsh, Donald W. *National Incident Management System: Principles and Practice.* Sudbury, MA: Jones and Bartlett Learning, 2012.

NATIONAL INSTITUTE FOR OCCUPATIONAL SAFETY AND HEALTH

The National Institute for Occupational Safety and Health (NIOSH) is charged with researching and recommending measures to prevent injury and illness for more than 150 million Americans in the U.S. workforce. Along with the Occupational Safety and Health Administration, NIOSH has played a leading role in providing a safe and healthy workplace environment, which protects workers and strengthens families and communities. Additionally, by reducing lost workdays due to injury and illness, a healthy workforce helps companies be more competitive.

NIOSH Vision
Safer, healthier workers

NIOSH Mission
To develop new knowledge in the field of occupational safety and health and to transfer that knowledge into practice.

NIOSH was created by the 1970 Occupational Safety and Health Act, and it is part of the Centers for Disease Control and Prevention. Because of their multidisciplinary work, NIOSH hires experts from a wide range of professions, including chemistry, economics, engineering, epidemiology, industrial hygiene, medicine, nursing, psychology, safety, and statistics. NIOSH consults with private and public partners to identify the most important workplace safety and health issues, and then it pursues research aimed at finding solutions, including innovative technologies, protocols, and training materials.

NIOSH research covers the following areas:

- Agriculture, Forestry, and Fishing: Accomplishments include reducing child death rates from agricultural worksite risks, reducing fatalities from tractor rollovers, and helping the commercial fishing industry adopt lifesaving personal flotation devices.
- Construction: Projects include investigating the causes of falls and electrical hazards, studying musculoskeletal disorders in the construction industry, and examining health threats such as noise, asphalt fumes, silica dust, and welding fumes.
- Health Care and Social Assistance: In partnership with other organizations, NIOSH has helped to improve facility designs to minimize risks, and researchers have developed safe patient handling guidance to protect nurses from musculoskeletal disorders.
- Manufacturing: NIOSH's educational materials and programs have reduced injuries and fatalities from contact with equipment, falls, and other exposures, and NIOSH is actively pursuing worker safety and health issues in the new field of nanotechnology.
- Mining: Workers have benefited from NIOSH involvement with engineering controls to reduce mining noise levels, proximity detectors for mining equipment, LED lighting in miner caps, self-contained emergency oxygen devices, improved communication systems, training materials, and response protocols.
- Oil and Gas Extraction: NIOSH researchers have helped address the major causes of injury and illness among oil and gas extraction workers, including preparing training videos and safety checklists, and NIOSH is working with partner organizations to control silica exposure during hydraulic fracturing operations.
- Public Safety: NIOSH has prepared a large volume of literature and educational materials on safety and health in the law enforcement and wildland firefighting fields, and research has been conducted on integrating psychological, physiological, and subclinical measures of stress, disease, and mental dysfunction associated with policing.
- Services: For workers in the service industry, including hotels and fast-food restaurants, NIOSH has studied safety and health issues and prepared hazard evaluations, and other research has focused on health risks in the education sector.
- Transportation, Warehousing, and Utilities: Projects include developing guidance for commercial truck drivers, conducting research on safety ordinances for violence against taxi drivers, reducing the risk of musculoskeletal disorders among package drivers and airport baggage handlers, and establishing the Center for Motor Vehicle Safety.
- Wholesale and Retail Trade: Products developed include keyboards to improve work posture and a video to help identify risk factors for workplace violence, and research has resulted in nonskid mats being installed for warehouse workers handling liquids and in improved dust exhaust hoods at lumber stores.

America's population is aging, and it is estimated that by the year 2020, about one quarter of all workers will be over the age of 55. These changing demographics demand a new focus on the safety and health of an aging workforce. To address these concerns, NIOSH created the National Center for Productive Aging and Work (NCPAW), with the goal of promoting lifelong well-being for all workers and supporting productive aging throughout one's working life.

The NCPAW helps organizations identify interventions and strategies to promote safety and health for workers of all ages. Several strategies known to be effective as workers grow older are (1) encouraging workplace flexibility, particularly with regard to work schedule and location; (2) matching tasks to individual strengths and recognizing that some older workers thrive in self-paced work environments with fewer repetitive tasks; (3) avoiding or reducing sedentary work and providing, for example, sit/stand or walking workstations and breaks for physical activity; (4) providing optimal illumination and ergonomically designed workstations, chairs, and tools; (5) encouraging multigenerational teamwork, taking advantage of the insight and problem-solving experience of older employees; (6) providing training for all ages, including guidance for older employees in adapting to new technologies; and (7) encouraging return-to-work programs and reasonable accommodation following illness or injury.

Richard Crume

See Also: Centers for Disease Control and Prevention; Occupational Safety and Health; Occupational Safety and Health Administration

Further Reading

Centers for Disease Control and Prevention. *The National Institute for Occupational Safety and Health*. https://www.cdc.gov/niosh (accessed March 30, 2017).

Friis, Robert H. *Occupational Health and Safety: For the 21st Century*. Burlington, MA: Jones and Bartlett Learning, 2016.

National Institute for Occupational Safety and Health. *Productive Aging and Work: What Is NCPAW?* https://www.cdc.gov/niosh/topics/productiveaging/ncpaw.html (accessed March 30, 2017).

Reese, Charles D. *Occupational Health and Safety Management: A Practical Approach*. Boca Raton, FL: CRC Press, 2016.

NATIONAL INSTITUTE OF ENVIRONMENTAL HEALTH SCIENCES

The National Institute of Environmental Health Sciences (NIEHS) is one of 27 research institutes that make up the National Institutes of Health, part of the U.S. Department of Health and Human Services. The NIEHS is located in Research Triangle Park, North Carolina, and is focused on studying the impact that the environment has on human health.

One of the main research organizations at the NIEHS is the Intramural Research Division (IRD). This division consists of 11 branches and laboratories that conduct research on wide-ranging areas, including epidemiology, epigenetics, genomics, neurobiology, reproductive and developmental biology, and biostatistics. The IRD also houses the Clinical Research Branch, which is active in studying the interactions between genetic susceptibility and environmental factors in human disease. This branch is involved in identifying at-risk populations and developing strategies to prevent and treat disease. Additionally, it supports multiple research groups within the institute that are tasked with researching the impact of environmental conditions on a variety of common health problems, including asthma, cardiovascular diseases, and cancer.

The National Toxicology Program (NTP), headquartered at the NIEHS, is a federal interagency program responsible for testing and evaluating toxic substances found in the environment. The NTP division takes the lead in carrying out the overall goals of the NTP, and it consists of five branches and laboratories addressing biomolecular screening, cellular and molecular pathology, toxicology, program operations, and operation of the NTP laboratory.

The need for the NTP arose out of concern in Congress and the scientific community for the impact of chemical agents in the environment on human health. When the NTP was created, there was increasing evidence that many human diseases may be related to chemical exposures, and therefore, limiting or eliminating exposure to those chemicals could be a major factor in preventing disease and disability. To address these concerns, the NTP was designed to coordinate toxicology testing across the federal government, strengthen the science of toxicology, improve testing methods, and ultimately, provide information on potentially toxic substances to regulators, scientists, and the public.

The NIEHS funds a large portfolio of research each year across different disciplines within the environmental health sciences through its Extramural Research and Training Division. Grants from the division provide funding for investigators from a wide variety of organizations. Current research addresses a range of environmental health issues, including autism, bisphenol B exposure, breast cancer, oceans and human health, climate change, and nanotechnology. The NIEHS is currently leading a five-year, $25 million consortia research program with community and regional university partners to evaluate health effects stemming from the 2010 Deepwater Horizon oil spill in the Gulf of Mexico.

Anthony C. Holderied

See Also: Autism and Environmental Exposure; Bisphenol A (BPA); Breast Cancer and Environmental Exposure; Deepwater Horizon Incident; Environmental Epidemiology; Environmental Toxicology; Epigenetics; Nanomaterials; National Toxicology Program; Toxicogenomics

Further Reading

National Institutes of Health. *National Institute of Environmental Health Sciences.* https://www.niehs.nih.gov/ (accessed December 1, 2015).

National Institutes of Health. *Research at NIEHS.* https://www.niehs.nih.gov/research/atniehs/index.cfm (accessed December 1, 2015).

U.S. Department of Health and Human Services. *National Toxicology Program.* http://ntp.niehs.nih.gov/ (accessed December 1, 2015).

NATIONAL OCEANIC AND ATMOSPHERIC ADMINISTRATION

The National Oceanic and Atmospheric Administration (NOAA) is an agency under the U.S. Department of Commerce charged with marine and atmospheric affairs. NOAA's motto is "Science, Service, and Stewardship" and their mission is to (1) understand and predict changes in climate, weather, oceans, and coasts; (2) share that knowledge and information with others; and (3) conserve and manage coastal and marine ecosystems and resources.

Ocean Currents and Climate Change

We are only beginning to understand what changes in the Atlantic Ocean circulation may mean for future climate.

Interview with Dr. Julia Gottschalk

Paleoclimate Researcher, University of Bern

Dr. Julia Gottschalk conducts paleoclimate research at the Oeschger Center for Climate Change Research at the University of Bern, Switzerland. She completed her PhD in the Godwin Laboratory for Palaeoclimate Research at the University of Cambridge, where she was a Gates Cambridge Scholar. Dr. Gottschalk's latest research concerns how ocean processes, in particular in the Southern Ocean, are involved in shaping the observed variability of atmospheric carbon dioxide concentrations. Additionally, Dr. Gottschalk studies a variety of climate archives to understand the role of past abrupt climate events in the long-term evolution of glacial and interglacial climate states.

Recent studies have discovered that ocean currents in the Atlantic have slowed down during the past few decades. Is this a sign of climate change, and if the trend continues, what does this mean for the rate of climate change in the future?

The latest assessment report of the Intergovernmental Panel on Climate Change emphasizes that the lack of observations with sufficient spatial and temporal resolution is a challenge for identifying changes in the speed of ocean currents in the Atlantic Ocean. However, based on new data from the North Atlantic Ocean, it has been proposed that ocean currents over the last decades have weakened, causing cooling in the North Atlantic region, which is distinct from the global warming trend of mean annual land and sea surface temperatures. It has been suggested that the slowdown of the ocean circulation in the North Atlantic may be linked with freshwater input into the North Atlantic from the melting Greenland ice sheet, which may be associated with global warming. However, unequivocally determining the causes of these observations is still extremely difficult due to the lack of multi-annual and multi-decadal observational records, and we are only beginning to understand what changes in the Atlantic Ocean circulation may mean for future climate.

The last time the Gulf Stream was severely perturbed was at the end of the most recent ice age, about 12,000 year ago. Is there danger of this happening again this century, and if so, what would be the consequences for human health and the environment?

Model simulations and paleoclimate observations indicate that deep and surface ocean currents in the Atlantic Ocean (in fact, globally) are very sensitive to the freshwater injected into the North Atlantic stemming from the melting of ice sheets still in existence, such as on Greenland, and from those that no longer exist, such as the Fenno-Scandinavian ice sheet. A recent study has suggested a link between the freshening of the North Atlantic surface due to the decaying Greenland ice sheet and the slowdown of the currents. Further, freshening of the North Atlantic surface due to Greenland ice sheet melting or loss of Arctic sea ice may cause further changes in ocean currents—a process that is plausible but remains to be further investigated. Ocean circulation is very important for the distribution of heat and moisture, and therefore, for regional climate. Northward flowing western boundary currents, such as the Gulf Stream, provide heat to the northern hemisphere, resulting in year-round ice-free ports and mild winters along the U.S. East Coast and in Europe. Any changes in the strength or pathway of the Gulf Stream will ultimately have a substantial influence on regional climate, including changes in the water cycle and surface temperatures, which will affect, for instance, energy consumption and agriculture in these regions as well as global trade.

The oceans, which cover about 70 percent of the planet, are huge reservoirs of carbon dioxide, storing 60 times more carbon than the atmosphere. How much longer will the oceans be able to act as sinks for increasing atmospheric concentrations of carbon dioxide? Are we already approaching the saturation point?

The global ocean takes up excess carbon from the atmosphere (up to 40 percent over recent decades), and the carbon isotopic composition of atmospheric and oceanic carbon dioxide bears witness to this excess carbon being largely caused by the combustion of fossil fuels (e.g., for electric power generation). Although atmospheric carbon dioxide has already reached levels of more than 400 parts per million (by volume), present-day atmospheric carbon dioxide concentrations would be even higher, by about 55 parts per million (14 percent), in the absence of the oceanic buffer capacity of anthropogenic carbon dioxide. Global climate change alters the behavior of the ocean in taking up carbon from the atmosphere, and with increasing oceanic carbon dioxide uptake and rising atmospheric carbon dioxide levels, the buffer capacity of the ocean will decrease. As the ocean is a complex system, and its influence on atmospheric carbon dioxide levels is spatially and temporally variable, predicting the exact role of the ocean in shaping future atmospheric carbon dioxide concentrations remains a major challenge.

Looking back tens of thousands of years, changing ocean currents have been linked with abrupt climate events. Is there any evidence that this same phenomenon is happening now or could happen this century?

Ocean currents both in the surface and deep ocean, which are driven by winds and by temperature and salinity differences, distribute heat and the carbon stored in the ocean. This also determines which regions of the world are warm (e.g., Europe) and which are not (e.g., Antarctica). The paleoclimate record indicates that past global climate events were closely linked with perturbations of the ocean circulation in the Atlantic Ocean, causing changes in the redistribution of heat and carbon. However, it is still unclear whether this relationship is a cause or a consequence. Abrupt changes in the speed of ocean currents in the geological past predominantly occurred during glacial periods, when ice sheets were more extensive and the global ocean circulation was likely more sensitive to perturbations during glacial periods than at present-day due to larger ice sheets. Therefore, there is not a direct analog for the current period and events in the geological past. Nevertheless, there are few studies suggesting that the ocean currents are changing today, but whether this is a sign of global warming or natural climate variability, or a combination of both, is an open question.

What would be a good career path for a recent college or university graduate wanting to study ocean currents, climate change, and implications for human health?

Students wishing to understand the earth and climate system are advised to enroll in geosciences or the earth sciences programs at national or international universities that offer specializations in (Paleo-)Climatology or (Paleo-)Oceanography, or both. Interdisciplinary research connecting the earth and climate sciences with social sciences (including public health) may be appropriate for graduate and doctoral dissertation projects.

One of the most critical ways NOAA contributes to the field of environmental health is by collecting long-term measurements necessary to track and understand climate change. The National Center for Environmental Information is one repository of such data. Another resource widely used by the public, the National Weather Service, provides key insights into weather prediction, with a mission to provide (1) weather, water, and climate data and (2) forecasts and warnings for the protection of life and property and enhancement of the national economy.

NOAA also supports a number of programs at the cutting edge of coastal and marine environmental health research, including a few of the more prominent ones listed below:

- Center for Sponsored Coastal Ocean Research: supports a wide variety of extramural (e.g., university) research on coastal topics
- National Sea Grant College Program: provides direct support to selected universities that is then subawarded locally to support a broad national network of locally relevant environmental research and outreach
- Center for Coastal Environmental Health and Biomolecular Research: studies a variety of coastal environmental health topics, including harmful algal blooms and pollution impacts on marine ecosystems
- Northwest Fisheries Sciences Center: one of several regional hubs conducting research on issues relevant to coastal zone management, including characterizing blooms of harmful algal bloom toxins like domoic acid

In addition to its many contributions to science, NOAA also has key regulatory responsibilities. It is the chief agency tasked with implementing many federal laws, including the Marine Mammal Protection Act, the Coastal Zone Management Act, and the Magnusson-Stevens Fishery Conservation and Management Act. NOAA's Offices of Law Enforcement and General Counsel deal with a wide range of legal issues, including criminal prosecution.

Matthew O. Gribble

See Also: Air Pollution; Climate Change and Human Health; Estuary Pollution; Greenhouse Effect and Global Warming; Marine Pollution, International Treaties to Prevent; Marine Vessels, Pollution from; Naturally Occurring Toxins

Further Reading

National Oceanic and Atmospheric Administration. *Climate*. http://www.noaa.gov/climate (accessed January 5, 2017).

National Oceanic and Atmospheric Administration. *Coastal Zone Management Act*. https://coast.noaa.gov/czm/act (accessed January 5, 2017).

National Oceanic and Atmospheric Administration. *Home Page*. http://www.noaa.gov (accessed January 5, 2017).

National Oceanic and Atmospheric Administration. *Magnusson-Stevens Fishery Conservation and Management Act*. http://www.nmfs.noaa.gov/sfa/laws_policies/msa (accessed January 5, 2017).

National Oceanic and Atmospheric Administration. *National Centers for Coastal Ocean Science*. https://coastalscience.noaa.gov (accessed January 5, 2017).

National Oceanic and Atmospheric Administration. *National Weather Service*. http://www.weather.gov (accessed January 5, 2017).

National Oceanic and Atmospheric Administration. *Northwest Fisheries Sciences Center*. https://www.nwfsc.noaa.gov (accessed January 5, 2017).

National Oceanic and Atmospheric Administration. *Sea Grant*. http://seagrant.noaa.gov/Home.aspx (accessed January 5, 2017).

National Oceanic and Atmospheric Administration. *Text of the Marine Mammal Protection Act (MMPA)*. http://www.nmfs.noaa.gov/pr/laws/mmpa/text.htm (accessed January 5, 2017).

NATIONAL POLLUTION DISCHARGE ELIMINATION SYSTEM

The National Pollution Discharge Elimination System (NPDES) was added to the Federal Water Pollution Control Act (also known as the Clean Water Act, or CWA) in 1972 to limit and control pollution of waters in the United States. The NPDES is the primary permitting program that monitors and limits discharges of pollutants from industrial and municipal sources into surface waters, which are important for drinking water, recreation, and fishing. Thus, the NPDES plays a vital role in protecting public health and the environment.

When the CWA was first enacted in 1948, its purpose was to abate the pollution of waters to protect human health and welfare. However, the focus prior to 1972 was on the health of the water body itself. There were no uniform standards for controlling the discharge of pollutants to water and no regulatory mechanism to trace pollution found in water bodies back to its source. This made enforcement difficult. The 1972 CWA amendments strengthened existing water quality standards (which were based on human health), added new nationally uniform technology-based standards for wastewater discharges into water bodies, and established a robust permitting system aimed at controlling the quantities of pollutants allowed to reach the nation's surface waters. The NPDES made discharge requirements clearer to the dischargers (e.g., industrial facilities and municipal wastewater treatment plants) and easier for the U.S. Environmental Protection Agency (EPA) and other regulatory agencies to effectively enforce.

NPDES permits work by imposing "effluent limitations" on the discharger. "Effluent" is the term used to refer to the polluted wastewater that is discharged from a source into a water body, and "effluent limitations" are the permit terms that define the maximum quantity of pollutants allowed to be discharged from these "point sources" into certain water bodies. A point source is any identifiable structure that conveys the pollutants into surface waters, including a pipe, ditch, tunnel, well, and even a coal pile or heavy equipment.

The effluent limitations in NPDES permits are nationally uniform technology-based limits set by the federal government in industry-specific rulemakings or, in the absence of federal action for a particular industry, by individual federal or state permit writers directly applying the CWA's language. To establish technology-based effluent limitations, the EPA or individual permit writers review the pollution reduction that can be achieved by applying certain "best" technologies and then require the permitted discharger to meet that pollution reduction standard (i.e., the level of reduction achieved by the "best" technology). The discharger does not have to use the same technology the EPA used to develop the standard and only needs to achieve the same pollution reduction. Technology-based limits may differ depending on the type of discharger and pollutant. For example, new facilities are generally expected to invest more in the best pollution control technology available, whereas installing the same technology at an older facility may be cost-prohibitive for the industry, and consequently, a less stringent technology-driven standard may apply to these existing sources. Effluent limitations in NPDES permits also impose water quality-based effluent limitations to protect the specific water body to which a source discharges.

The NPDES program provides the foundation for enforcing effluent limitations and attaining water quality goals. The CWA makes it illegal to discharge pollutants into federal waters from a point source without an NPDES permit or in violation of the terms of a permit. The CWA also empowers the EPA, states, and even private citizens to enforce these requirements in the federal courts. Significant civil penalties can be levied for violations, and intentional violations may also be met with criminal sanctions.

States may apply for permission from the EPA to administer the NPDES program but must first establish that their state programs are at least as stringent as those required by the EPA under the CWA. The vast majority of the states currently administer their own NPDES permit programs.

The EPA and delegated states may issue both "general permits" and "individual permits" under the NPDES program. Individual permits authorize discharges from a single source, such as a specific city wastewater treatment plant or a manufacturing facility. General permits authorize discharges from an entire category of sources within a state or EPA region. Examples of the types of sources that are often authorized by general NPDES permits include concentrated animal feeding operations, seafood processing operations, and notably, the thousands of stormwater discharges that are regulated under the CWA.

NPDES permits are often very detailed in their requirements. In addition to imposing effluent limitations (defined in terms of maximum concentrations or mass of pollutants discharged), they also establish specific maintenance and inspection requirements, sampling and reporting procedures, and a variety of other notification and operational requirements designed to assure that compliance with the effluent limitations is maintained and that facility changes do not render the permit obsolete.

The NPDES permit program is generally recognized as a successful innovation in terms of improving surface water quality in the United States. It is the primary means of assuring attainment of human health-based water quality criteria, and it provides an effective mechanism for policing the extensive pollution reductions necessary to ensure the protection of human health and the environment. As science continues to identify water-borne risks to human health, the NPDES program stands ready to manage those risks to levels protective of the public, thereby ensuring that waters remain suitable for fishing and swimming and that drinking water sources are protected.

Leah A. Dundon and Richard S. Davis

See Also: Clean Water Act; Concentrated Animal Feeding Operations, Pollution from; Drinking Water Quality and Regulation; Environmental Protection Agency; Sewage Treatment and Disposal; Stormwater Runoff; Water Pollution

Further Reading

U.S. Environmental Protection Agency. *Federal Water Pollution Control Act, 33 U.S.C. §1251 et seq. (1972).* (Also known as the Clean Water Act.) http://www.epa.gov/laws-regulations/summary-clean-water-act (accessed January 1, 2016).

U.S. Environmental Protection Agency. *Learn about Effluent Guidelines*. http://www.epa.gov/eg/learn-about-effluent-guidelines (accessed January 1, 2016).

U.S. Environmental Protection Agency. *National Pollutant Discharge Elimination System (NPDES)*. http://www.epa.gov/npdes (accessed January 1, 2016).

NATIONAL RENEWABLE ENERGY LABORATORY

The National Renewable Energy Laboratory (NREL) was designated by President George H. W. Bush in 1991 to help study and research integration of renewable power into the utility grid so as to have a measurable impact in reducing fossil fuel emissions. Its predecessor, the Solar Energy Research Institute, was created several decades earlier as a result of the burgeoning environmental movement and the oil crises in the Middle East. The name was later changed to NREL to encompass energy efficiency and other renewable sources, including wind power. The NREL is funded through the U.S. Department of Energy.

The NREL's main campus and education center are located in Golden, Colorado, and the affiliated National Wind Technology Center is located nearby in Boulder. Examples of the research topics investigated by the NREL include (1) how to incorporate the expanding renewable energy infrastructure into the existing electric power grid, (2) how energy investors can access and understand data on resource potential and generation costs, (3) what the best practices are for governments to expand the renewable energy market, and (4) what research and development priorities are necessary to help the United States generate 80 percent of its electricity needs from renewable sources by 2050.

The health benefits that can be derived from the NREL's research include replacing fossil fuels for energy generation with cleaner renewable alternatives, with the result of reducing emissions of greenhouse gases and other air pollutants having adverse effects on human health. Carbon dioxide, the greenhouse gas contributing the most to climate change, is not directly harmful to humans, but the buildup of carbon dioxide and other greenhouse gases in the atmosphere will lead to adverse climate change effects, including more frequent and severe droughts and the spread of diseases. By replacing energy sources using fossil fuel with cleaner renewable energy alternatives, greenhouse gas emissions will be reduced, and air pollution like the smog that forms in urban areas will be less severe.

Recently, the NREL has been studying the use of microorganisms to convert methane into lactate, which can then be used to make bioplastics. By finding a use for methane, a potent greenhouse gas, less methane will be emitted into the atmosphere. The NREL is also developing less toxic, more efficient methods of producing biofuels like ethanol. Other research is aimed at making solar, wind, and fuel cell energy more efficient and less expensive. The ultimate goal is to make renewable energy sources cost competitive and ultimately preferable to traditional energy technologies, in particular those using fossil fuels.

The National Wind Technology Center has been working with wind power companies to make wind turbines safer for birds, a major concern among some environmentalists. For example, the center has been collecting flight pattern data that can be used in conjunction with radars to shut down turbines as flocks of birds approach. Work on issues surrounding offshore wind arrays is also in progress.

Aaron Dorman

See Also: Electric Power Generation, Health Implications of; Greenhouse Effect and Global Warming; Ozone and Smog in the Urban Environment; Renewable Energy, Health Implications of; Sustainable Development and Health

Further Reading

Brown, Lester R., et al. *The Great Transition: Shifting from Fossil Fuels to Wind and Solar Energy*. New York: Norton, 2015.

National Renewable Energy Laboratory. *Home Page.* https://www.nrel.gov (accessed March 10, 2017).

National Renewable Energy Laboratory. *National Wind Technology Center.* http://www.nrel.gov/nwtc (accessed March 10, 2017).

Peake, Stephen, ed. *Renewable Energy: Power for a Sustainable Future.* Oxford, UK: Oxford University Press, 2017.

NATIONAL TOXICOLOGY PROGRAM

The National Toxicology Program (NTP) comprises three federal agencies charged with coordinating toxicology research and testing on chemicals of public health concern in support of health regulatory and research agencies, scientific and medical communities, and the public. The three NTP agencies are the National Institute of Environmental Health Sciences (under the National Institutes of Health), the National Center for Toxicology Research (under the U.S. Food and Drug Administration), and the National Institute for Occupational Safety and Health (under the Centers for Disease Control and Prevention). The NTP places emphasis on the health and safety of industrial chemicals, pharmaceuticals, food additives, metals, and pesticides. The role of the NTP is to ensure the safety of these chemicals by determining safe exposure levels and identifying effects on human health during their use, manufacturing, distribution, and disposal and when present in air, water, and soil.

The NTP regulates the approximately 2,000 novel chemicals proposed for use in the United States annually, in addition to more than 80,000 currently registered chemicals. These new and existing chemicals are typically found in household products, prescription drugs, personal care items, foods, and lawn care products.

In the United States during the 1970s, increased attention was directed toward the effects of chemical agents prevalent in the environment. To learn more about how exposure to chemicals may contribute to human disease, regulatory agencies were tasked with studying human health issues, particularly related to cancer, reproductive and developmental disorders, genetic damage, and diseases of the cardiovascular, immune, and nervous systems. In 1978, Joseph A. Califano Jr., secretary of health, education, and welfare (later known as the Department of Health and Human Services), established the NTP, and in 1981, Secretary Richard S. Schwiker granted the program permanent status. The program's original goal, which remains today, was to establish an interagency effort to strengthen the scientific basis of toxicology, coordinate toxicology testing programs, improve current testing methods, and disseminate information about toxic chemicals.

The field of toxicology combines the disciplines of biology, chemistry, and pharmacology to study the potentially hazardous effects of chemicals in living organisms and biological systems by determining appropriate dose responses. The NTP strives to establish a scientific approach to addressing significant issues in toxicology by using best practices to design, conduct, and interpret scientific studies, thereby improving the ability to predict the toxicological impact of environmental agents. For example, NTP scientists study how exposure to common agricultural chemicals affects allergy and asthma symptoms and may contribute to the onset of Parkinson's disease.

The NTP is continually striving to use the most modern scientific research and methods to develop and apply new technologies, such as testing chemicals faster and more efficiently with robotics and computational models, while decreasing the use of animals in toxicity testing. Other objectives of the NTP are to increase the transparency of scientific inquiries, strengthen literature-based hazard assessments, and improve training for the next generation of toxicologists. Additionally, the NTP plays a role in creating database resources for scientists around the world for use in (1) standardizing toxicological terminology and (2) allowing toxicologists to formulate a comprehensive picture of toxicity with greater efficiency than with traditional methods. For example, the NTP supports the Chemical Effects in Biological Systems database, under the National Institute of Environmental Health Sciences, which presents data in the context of biology and study design and allows the integration of data across studies.

Simon Waldbaum

See Also: Allergens in the Environment; Asthma; Environmental Toxicology; National Institute for Occupational Safety and Health; National Institute of Environmental Health Sciences; Neurotoxicants; Parkinson's Disease and Environmental Exposure; Toxicogenomics

Further Reading

Centers for Disease Control and Prevention. *The National Institute for Occupational Safety and Health (NIOSH).* http://www.cdc.gov/niosh (accessed May 19, 2016).

Frank, Patricia, and M. Alice Ottoboni. *The Dose Makes the Poison: A Plain-Language Guide to Toxicology.* Hoboken, NJ: John Wiley and Sons, 2011.

Klaassen, Curtis, and John B. Watkins III. *Casarett and Doull's Essentials of Toxicology*. Columbus, OH: McGraw-Hill Education, 2015.

National Institutes of Health. *National Institute of Environmental Health Sciences.* https://www.niehs.nih.gov (accessed May 19, 2016).

U.S. Department of Health and Human Services. *National Toxicology Program.* http://ntp.niehs.nih.gov (accessed May 19, 2016).

U.S. Food and Drug Administration. *About the National Center for Toxicological Research.* http://www.fda.gov/AboutFDA/CentersOffices/OC/OfficeofScientificandMedicalPrograms/NCTR (accessed May 19, 2016).

NATURAL DISASTERS

Natural disasters increase suffering and cause great loss of life. Many natural disasters result from environmental conditions, such as hurricanes and floods, and they cause environmental health challenges, including the contamination of water sources following hurricanes or floods. A natural disaster is defined by three components: (1) it is a disruption of normal conditions; (2) it features significant human and property damage; and (3) it exceeds the capacity of the affected community or area to respond. Natural disasters often affect communities in many ways, such as by interrupting communication lines and community access, disrupting utilities, and causing long-term damage, such as medical casualties and reduced food sources.

Climate change, which will cause more heavy precipitation events and increased variability in temperature, is expected to result in more natural disasters. Therefore, there will be a greater need for disaster management and emergency preparedness programs. From the perspective of public health, disaster management must assess the needs of disaster-affected populations, match available resources, prevent further health effects, implement disease control strategies, evaluate effectiveness of disaster relief programs, and develop contingency plans for various disaster types. The medical and public health needs will vary for each disaster type. Better knowledge and prediction of causes of death and types of illness and injury during natural disasters will allow for better allocation of resources. Therefore, efficient planning and execution of disaster relief requires knowledge of which types of disaster may occur and the associated morbidity and mortality.

Floods are the most common natural disaster in the United States, causing more deaths than any other type of natural disaster. Flash floods cause most fatalities. Primary causes of death are drowning and impact by large debris in flood waters. Floods can also have longer-term public health impacts by disrupting water treatment and sewage disposal facilities and causing toxic waste site overflow. These events can increase the exposure to infectious pathogens, such as *E. coli* and *Cryptosporidium*.

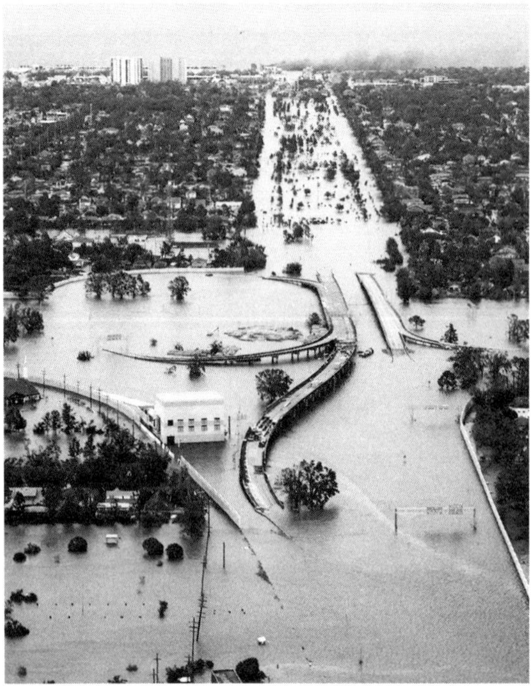

Aerial view of flooded New Orleans in the aftermath of Hurricane Katrina in 2005. Climate change is expected to cause heavier and more prolonged precipitation events, resulting in a greater need for disaster management and emergency preparedness programs. (U.S. Coast Guard)

Hurricanes and tornadoes are other natural disasters that can have significant public health impacts. Tornadoes are violent natural disasters that typically cause extensive property damage and can result in loss of life. North America is most prone to tornadoes, and it is estimated that over 700 tornadoes occur in the United States each year. Hurricanes, or tropical cyclones, can lead to tornadoes and flooding, which together with storm surge can cause high rates of morbidity and mortality. In the future, hurricanes are predicted to have greater impact as climate change leads to stronger hurricanes and coastal areas become more densely populated.

Volcanic eruptions and earthquakes are also natural disasters with considerable public health consequences. While most volcanoes are in thinly populated areas, the U.S. Geological Survey has identified 35 volcanoes that are likely to erupt in the future. Eruptions have immediate life-threatening health effects due to inhalation of airborne ash, burning steam from the eruption, and inability to escape mudflows. Indirect effects of volcanic eruptions include the toxic gases that are released during the eruption. Earthquakes can also result in significant loss of property and life. The greatest impacts from earthquakes are immediate due to injury and death from building collapse or falling debris. Public health preparedness efforts can rely on early warning systems for floods, hurricanes, and tornadoes. However, earthquakes are much more difficult to predict, and public health preparedness must focus on preventative efforts, such as strengthening buildings and instructing people in earthquake-prone areas to have emergency supplies on hand.

Jyotsna S. Jagai

See Also: Climate Change and Human Health; Disaster Preparedness and Response; Emergency Planning and Community Right-to-Know Act; Federal Emergency Management Agency; National Incident Management System; Sewage Treatment and Disposal

Further Reading

Haiti Earthquake 2010. Food and Agriculture Organization of the United Nations, Rome, Italy, 2017. http://www.fao.org/emergencies/crisis/haiti-earthquake-2010/en.

Harmon, Katherine. "Haiti Earthquake Disaster Little Surprise to Some Seismologists." *Scientific American* (January, 2010), https://www.scientificamerican.com/article/haiti-earthquake-prediction/.

Jenner, Lynn, and Brian Dunbar. *Hurricane Season 2005: Katrina*. National Aeronautics and Space Administration, Washington, DC, 2005. https://www.nasa.gov/vision/earth/lookingatearth/h2005_katrina.html.

Natural Disasters and Severe Weather. Centers for Disease Control and Prevention, Atlanta, GA, 2015. https://www.cdc.gov/disasters/alldisasters.html.

Robertson, Campbell, Richard Fausset, and Katy Reckdahl. "10 Years after Katrina." *New York Times*, August 26, 2015, https://www.nytimes.com/interactive/2015/08/26/us/ten-years-after-katrina.html.

World Health Organization. *Environmental Health in Emergencies: Natural Events*. http://www.who.int/environmental_health_emergencies/natural_events/en (accessed May 8, 2017).

NATURALLY OCCURRING TOXINS

The science of naturally occurring toxins, called toxinology, is a broad field that includes contributions by various professions, including microbiologists, mycologists, botanists, veterinarians, and marine biologists. Research on toxinology can be found in *Toxicon*, the official journal of the International Society on Toxinology, and in a wide variety of other professional publications. Naturally occurring toxins are important to the field of environmental health because they can cause serious health problems in humans and even death.

Perhaps the most lethal substance on the earth is botulinum toxin, produced by the bacterium *Clostridium botulinum*. It is also the active ingredient in a popular injection treatment to tighten muscles, which may be used cosmetically to offset the appearance of aging skin. This illustrates one common theme in toxinology: that there may be valuable uses (e.g., in pharmacy) for substances that are highly toxic in other contexts or at other doses. This is a major rationale for the interest pharmaceutical and bioengineering professionals have in discovering and characterizing naturally occurring toxic substances.

Toxins can have acute or chronic toxicity, as illustrated by some of the more infamous mycotoxins (toxins produced by fungi). For example, psilocybin, produced by "magic mushrooms" of the genus *Psilocybe*, and lysergic acid diethylamide (LSD), derived from the fungal genus *Claviceps*, are street drugs abused for their hallucinogenic effects, typically occurring 1.5 hours after consumption and lasting up to 12 hours. (These hallucinogenic mycotoxins activate the serotonin 5-HT_2 receptor.) A slower-acting, but far more deadly acute mycotoxin is α-amantin, produced by the mushroom *Amanita phalloides*, aptly nicknamed the "death cap" mushroom. This toxin disrupts the enzyme RNA polymerase II, leading to a cessation of new protein synthesis that results in liver damage and possible death. An example of a common mycotoxin contributing to chronic disease risk is aflatoxin, which may be responsible for 4.6 to 28.2 percent of hepatocellular carcinoma (HCC) cases worldwide and has synergistic toxicity with hepatitis B and C viruses for HCC risk. Aflatoxin is primarily produced by molds, such as *Aspergillus flavus*, which can grow on corn and peanuts.

Animals delivering toxins by injection (e.g., with fangs or stingers) are called venomous, while creatures delivering toxins more passively are called poisonous. Many poisonous creatures actually are carrying toxins produced by another organism. For example, the toxins from poison dart frogs are produced primarily by their insect prey.

Batesian mimicry is a defensive strategy whereby an organism imitates the appearance of another organism that is toxic (or sometimes just tastes bad). An example of this is how the nonvenomous scarlet kingsnake, *Lampropeltis elapsoides*, looks similar to the venomous American cobra, *Micrurus fulvius*, which shares a similar habitat.

Life began in the ocean, and over millennia, the evolutionary struggle to survive in the marine environment has given rise to particularly interesting and potent toxic species. One example is the cone snail, which produces offensive venoms to subdue prey and defensive venoms to deter predators. These "conotoxins" are secreted by different parts of the toxic gland and are released under different conditions. Another interesting example concerns algae, which under certain environmental conditions can proliferate, causing harmful algal blooms. A common consequence of algal blooms is depletion of oxygen from the water when the bloom of algae begins to die and decay, resulting in hypoxia and the subsequent deaths of large numbers of fishes. Additionally, sufficient doses of some algal toxins can produce very distinct toxidromes. For example, high doses of the domoic acid produced by the diatoms in genus *Pseudo-nitzschia* cause amnesiac shellfish poisoning, while high doses of the saxitoxins produced by *Alexandrium* cause paralytic shellfish poisoning. Even a low dose of ciguatoxins produced by *Gambierdiscus* can cause the disease ciguatera, which presents with a range of neurological, gastrointestinal, and sometimes even mental health symptoms in humans. The most distinctive symptom of ciguatera is reversed sensation of hot and cold. It is thought that ciguatera may be increasing in frequency due to climate change.

Matthew O. Gribble

See Also: Climate Change and Human Health; Environmental Toxicology; Neurotoxicants

Further Reading

Clark, V. C., et al. "Convergent Evolution of Chemical Defense in Poison Frogs and Arthropod Prey between Madagascar and the Neotropics." *Proceedings of the National Academy of Sciences*, vol. 102, no. 33 (August 2005): 11617–11622.
Dutertre, S., et al. "Evolution of Separate Predation- and Defense-Evoked Venoms in Carnivorous Cone Snails." *Nature Communications*, vol. 5, no. 3521 (March 2014).
Elsevier. *Toxicon*. https://www.journals.elsevier.com/toxicon (accessed January 7, 2017).
Gingold, D. B., M. J. Strickland, and J. J. Hess. "Ciguatera Fish Poisoning and Climate Change: Analysis of National Poison Center Data in the United States, 2001–2011." *Environmental Health Perspectives*, vol. 122, no. 6 (June 2014): 580–586.
International Society on Toxinology. *Home Page*. http://www.toxinology.org (accessed January 8, 2017).
Kikuchi, David W., and David W. Pfennig. "High Model Abundance May Permit the Gradual Evolution of Batesian Mimicry: An Experimental Test." *Proceedings of the Royal Society B: Biological Sciences*, vol. 277, no. 1684 (December 2009): 1041–1048.
Kloss, Brian T., and Travis Bruce. *Toxicology in a Box*. New York: McGraw-Hill Education, 2014.
Liu, Y., and F. Wu. "Global Burden of Aflatoxin-Induced Hepatocellular Carcinoma: A Risk Assessment." *Environmental Health Perspectives*, vol. 118, no. 6 (June 2010): 818–824.
Montecucco, C., and J. Molgó. "Botulinal Neurotoxins: Revival of an Old Killer." *Current Opinion in Pharmacology*, vol. 5, no. 3 (June 2005): 274–279.
Walsh, Patrick J., et al., eds. *Oceans and Human Health: Risks and Remedies from the Seas*. Amsterdam, the Netherlands: Academic Press, 2008.

NEUROTOXICANTS

Neurotoxicants are synthetic chemical compounds that cause damage to the central or peripheral nervous systems and to sense organs. Researchers have accumulated evidence that these compounds contribute to a wide range of neurological illnesses and conditions, including Parkinson's disease, Alzheimer's disease, and amyotrophic lateral sclerosis in adults as well as learning and developmental disorders in children. In addition to specific diseases and disorders, neurotoxicants also cause numerous general symptoms, such as nausea, dizziness, vertigo, irritability, physical incoordination, and impaired memory. Such general symptoms are typically reversible once exposure to the toxicant is stopped. However, many neurological, learning, and developmental disorders are permanent.

Neurotoxicants can cause neurological and developmental damage to the body in several ways, depending on the particular chemical. For example, they can (1) change enzyme activity and other biochemical balances; (2) lead to physiological changes through damage to the myelin sheaths of nerve fibers or changes to sensory organs; and (3) prompt morphological changes in nerve cells, including inflammation of cells, alterations within cells, and cell death.

Chemicals classified as developmental neurotoxicants are of special interest because they damage the fetal, infant, and child brain. Only a relatively small number of compounds have been conclusively demonstrated to cause neurodevelopmental disorders in immature humans, but many more compounds have suspected neurotoxicity characteristics based on animal studies and other research. Scientific research and clinical evidence have revealed links, both potential and proven, between prenatal and postnatal exposure to more than 100 chemicals and neurobehavioral and neurodevelopmental conditions, such as the following:

- Learning and memory disabilities
- Reduced intelligence quotient
- Autism spectrum disorders
- Attention-deficit/hyperactivity disorder
- Physical developmental delays (including delays in sexual development)

Such conditions have been diagnosed in as many as 20 percent of children in the United States, according to some estimates, with the number of diagnosed cases on the rise. Some research has even drawn associations between childhood exposure to certain developmental neurotoxicants, such as lead, and later antisocial and criminal behaviors. According to the National Research Council, 3 percent of neurodevelopmental disabilities can be attributed to direct environmental exposure to neurotoxicants, and 25 percent of neurodevelopmental disabilities can be linked to epigenetic interactions of environmental neurotoxicants with genetic factors.

Neurotoxicants are found in many common household products, including the cadmium metal in batteries and pigments (e.g., the colored designs on drinking glasses), the polybrominated diphenyl ether flame retardants in upholstered furniture and electronic circuitry, and various pesticides found in house and yard sprays and pet flea-and-tick killers. One of the best known neurotoxicants is lead, which was widely used in house paint until it was banned in the late 1970s, although it is still present in the paint of many older buildings. A number of suspected neurotoxicants have been found in cigarette smoke, urban air pollution, drinking water, foods, and drinks. Some neurotoxicant effects have been associated with certain pharmaceuticals and vaccines. Neurotoxicants are also among the hazardous chemicals encountered in many manufacturing facilities and other work environments.

Specific chemical compounds with evidence of neurotoxicant properties include the following:

- Acrylamide: used to make many plastic products and cosmetics. It is also produced during certain cooking processes, such as the roasting, baking, and frying of potatoes
- Aspartame: a common synthetic sweetener used as a substitute for sugar

- Benzene: incorporated into the plastics, resins, nylon, and synthetic fibers found in detergents, dyes (including food dyes), lubricants, rubber items, certain medicines, and other products
- Bisphenol A: found inside the resin lining and polycarbonate plastic of many beverage and food cans, baby bottles, and water bottles
- Fluoride: added to public drinking water supplies in most communities because it has been shown to reduce tooth decay, although some research identifies it as a developmental neurotoxicant
- Manganese: a metal used in the manufacture of aluminum drink cans, glass and rubber products, and fertilizers and fungicides
- Mercury: found in various products, including batteries, electronics, old thermometers, jewelry, light bulbs, and skin cream
- Monosodium Glutamate: one of the most widely used flavor enhancers (often listed under alternate names in food ingredients)
- Polychlorinated Biphenyls: production banned in the United States but may still be found in products manufactured before the ban, including electrical equipment, surface coatings, inks, paints, adhesives, and fire retardants
- Trichloroethylene: present in some cleaning and degreasing products

Some scientists suspect that there may be at least 200 neurotoxicants in many kinds of consumer products that have not yet been testing for evidence of neurotoxicity. Manufacturers create new products at a faster rate than researchers can evaluate them, and U.S. Environmental Protection Agency regulations allow companies to market certain kinds of products without first testing them for safety. Often tests of those items are conducted only after evidence develops of potential harm to humans following the marketing of the products. Toxicologists have called for greater testing of suspected neurotoxicants to provide more data relevant to public health and product safety.

A.J. Smuskiewicz

See Also: Bisphenol A (BPA); Environmental Protection Agency; Environmental Toxicology; Epigenetics; Heavy Metal Pollution; Lead Poisoning Prevention; Mercury Pollution; Pesticides and Herbicides; Polychlorinated Biphenyls

Further Reading

Costa, L. G., et al. "Neurotoxicants Are in the Air: Convergence of Human, Animal, and In Vitro Studies on the Effects of Air Pollution on the Brain." *BioMed Research International*, vol. 2014, no. 736385 (January 2014).

Kaplan, Sheila. *Investigative Reporting Workshop: EPA Develops Neurotoxicants List, New Testing*. American University School of Journalism, Washington, DC, 2010. http://investigativereportingworkshop.org/investigations/toxic-influence/story/epa-develops-neurotoxicants-list.

Miodovnik, A. "Environmental Neurotoxicants and Developing Brain." *Mount Sinai Journal of Medicine*, vol. 78, no. 1 (January–February 2011): 58–77.

Mundy, William R., et al. "Expanding the Test Set: Chemicals with Potential to Disrupt Mammalian Brain Development." *Neurotoxicology and Teratology*, vol. 52, part A (November–December 2015): 25–35.

NOISE POLLUTION

We ordinarily do not consider noise a form of pollution, but a noisy environment can lead to health issues, just like other forms of pollution. People exposed to excess noise often experience stress-related illnesses, high blood pressure, speech interference, sleep disruption, lost productivity, and hearing loss. A condition known as noise induced hearing loss (NIHL) is the most common effect of living and working in a noisy environment.

NIHL is a very common health condition in the United States, and unfortunately, hearing loss is ordinarily irreversible. Working in a loud factory can cause hearing loss, but so can going to a rock concert and even using a noisy leaf blower. Typically, the louder the sound and the longer the exposure, the greater the likelihood of permanent hearing loss. Among U.S. adults in the 20 to 69 age range, it is estimated that about 40 million suffer from NIHL. Half do not have noisy jobs, which means their hearing loss is associated with noise exposure at school or home or in the community. Of those adults who think their hearing is good to excellent, about 25 percent actually have some degree of hearing damage.

Instruments that measure noise levels use a unit of measure called the decibel (dB)—the higher the dB, the louder the noise. Hearing professionals generally consider noises louder that are about 85 dB in the range where extended exposure can cause hearing damage. Table 11 shows some common noises and associated dBs. As you can see, many noises we take for granted, such as running the washing machine or attending a sporting event, can result in high dB levels. According to the Centers for Disease Control and Prevention, exposure to a loud rock concert for as little as two minutes can cause hearing damage.

Over 45 million Americans suffer from tinnitus, a ringing or buzzing in the ears that is primarily associated with noise exposure and hearing loss. The likelihood of developing tinnitus increases with age, and it is estimated that roughly 30 percent of older adults experience tinnitus symptoms. Other groups at high risk for developing tinnitus are active military personnel and veterans, people working in loud workplace environments, musicians and music lovers, motor sports fans, hunters, and people with past behavioral health issues, such as depression, anxiety, and obsessive-compulsive disorder. Males tend to get tinnitus more than females,

Why So Little Concern over Noise Pollution?

Noise is around us almost all the time during our waking hours, and while it can be annoying at times, we usually do not consider it a danger to our health. But in fact, even a little unwanted noise can increase our stress level and lead to sleepless nights. We cannot see, taste, smell, or touch noise pollution, and perhaps, this is why it does not receive more attention. However, as with other forms of pollution, noise pollution can diminish our quality of life and even present a serious health hazard.

Table 11. Common noises and associated dB levels.

Activity	dB Level
Washing machine	70
Traffic noise while inside a car	80
Leaf blower	90
Sporting event	100
Rock concert	110
Emergency siren	120

perhaps because they have noisier jobs and participate in more hearing-risk behaviors like hunting. For unknown reasons, white, non-Hispanic people suffer more from tinnitus than other racial and ethnic groups.

There are several steps you can take to prevent hearing loss. Most important is simply limiting exposure to loud noises—walk away from the noise, lower the volume, or wear hearing protection, such as earplugs or earmuffs. And be careful wearing headphones and earbuds—there is increasing evidence they can cause hearing loss if the volume is too loud. Parents can help their children avoid hearing loss by turning the volume down on TVs and music players and requiring ear protection while working outside, for example, when using a noisy lawnmower or leaf blower.

Richard Crume

See Also: Centers for Disease Control and Prevention; Children's Environmental Health; Occupational Safety and Health; Quiet, Benefits of

Further Reading

American Tinnitus Association. *Home Page*. https://www.ata.org (accessed March 22, 2017).

Burkey, John M. *The Hearing-Loss Guide: Useful Information and Advice for Patients and Families*. New Haven, CT: Yale University Press, 2015.

Carroll, Yulia I., et al. "Vital Signs: Noise-Induced Hearing Loss among Adults—United States 2011–2012." *Morbidity and Mortality Weekly Report*, vol. 66, no. 5 (February 2017): 139–144.

Centers for Disease Control and Prevention. *Too Loud! For Too Long!* https://www.cdc.gov/vitalsigns/hearingloss/index.html (accessed March 22, 2017).

National Hearing Conservation Association. *Join the Experts*. http://www.hearingconservation.org (accessed March 22, 2017).

Noise and Its Effects on Children (EPA-410-F-09–003). Washington, DC: U.S. Environmental Protection Agency, 2009.

Prochnik, George. *In Pursuit of Silence: Listening for Meaning in a World of Noise*. New York: Anchor Books, 2011.

NOROVIRUS INFECTION

Norovirus is a highly contagious virus that causes inflammation of the stomach or intestines or both, a condition called acute gastroenteritis. Common symptoms are diarrhea, vomiting, nausea, stomach pain, and sometimes fever, headache, and body aches. Diarrhea and vomiting can lead to dehydration, particularly in children, older adults, and people having other illnesses. (Dehydration symptoms include decrease in urination, dry mouth and throat, and dizziness when standing up.) Following exposure, people develop symptoms within 12 to 48 hours, and most people begin to recover within one to three days. Of course, if you are concerned about exposure to norovirus or any other health condition, you should see your doctor.

The first known outbreak of norovirus occurred in 1968 at Norwalk-Bronson Elementary School in Norwalk, Ohio, where 150 students experienced nausea, vomiting, and diarrhea over a period of 12 to 24 hours. (The "noro" in norovirus is derived from Norwalk.) However, the viral agent was not actually identified until 1972, when the virus was first visualized using electron microscopy. This discovery was important because it was the first time a virus specifically associated with acute gastroenteritis had been identified. Following further investigation with sensitive molecular techniques, norovirus became the official genus name in 2002.

In the United States, norovirus infections are common and widespread. According to the Centers for Disease Control and Prevention, each year norovirus causes, on average, 19 to 21 million acute gastroenteritis cases, 1.7 to 1.9 million outpatient visits, 400,000 emergency room visits (mainly young children), 56,000 to 71,000 hospitalizations, and 570 to 800 deaths (mainly children and older adults). Only the common cold is more prevalent.

When a norovirus outbreak occurs, it often begins when an infected person spreads the virus to others. Additionally, norovirus can spread through contaminated food or by touching contaminated surfaces. (Because norovirus is resistant to many common disinfectants, it can persist on surfaces, even after they are

Staying Healthy on Your Cruise

While cruise ship viral infection outbreaks are uncommon, they do happen, and norovirus is usually to blame. To protect yourself, wash your hands frequently with soap and warm water, especially before and after meals and after using the restroom. Avoid touching your face after using the restroom and whenever your hands are dirty. Although an occasional handshake is acceptable, minimize contact with others as much as possible. Avoid eating uncooked food and touching unsanitized surfaces, drink bottled water, and do not share drinking glasses and eating utensils. Report any symptoms to the ship's medical clinic, and unless caring for a friend or loved one, stay away from other passengers who are sick. In other words, just use common sense to avoid situations where norovirus may be present—and wash your hands a lot!

cleaned and sanitized.) In the United States, about half of all food-related illnesses are caused by norovirus. Enclosed areas, such as daycare centers, nursing homes, schools, college dormitories, and cruise ships, are particularly conducive to the spread of norovirus. Around 50 percent of norovirus outbreaks in the United States are in long-term care facilities, and most outbreaks occur during the winter months.

Norovirus is particularly notorious for outbreaks on cruise ships, where it causes over 90 percent of diarrheal disease outbreaks. From 2008 to 2014, 133 cruise ship acute gastroenteritis outbreaks were reported for cruises sailing in U.S. jurisdiction (passenger vessels carrying 13 or more passengers and within 15 days of arriving in the United States), and almost all of the outbreaks were attributed to norovirus. While this may appear to be a large number of outbreaks, it actually represents only about 0.5 percent of voyages and 0.2 percent of passengers traveling during this period. Because cruise ships are required to submit detailed reports on norovirus outbreaks, we hear more about outbreaks occurring at sea than those occurring on land.

Currently, there are no medicines that are effective in treating norovirus infections. For example, antibiotics, which are used to treat bacterial infections, have no effect on viral infections. Furthermore, because there are many different types of noroviruses, being infected in the past and building up a resistance may not protect you from future infections from a different norovirus strain. Patients are often advised to drink plenty of fluids to help prevent dehydration, which can be a serious problem, even requiring hospitalization. If you believe you or someone you are caring for may be severely dehydrated, you should see a doctor.

There are several steps you can follow to avoid getting a norovirus infection and to prevent it from spreading to others. These include (1) washing hands frequently with soap and warm water, (2) washing fruits and vegetables and thoroughly cooking seafood, (3) throwing out any food that might be contaminated, (4) ensuring sick infants and children are kept away from food preparation areas, and (5) cleaning and disinfecting contaminated surfaces. If infected with norovirus, stop caring or preparing food for others for at least two days after symptoms disappear and stay home from school or work to avoid infecting others.

Richard Crume

See Also: Food Safety and Technology; Foodborne Diseases; Infectious Diseases

Further Reading

Brunette, Gary W., ed. *CDC Health Information for International Travel 2016*. Oxford, UK: Oxford University Press, 2015.

Centers for Disease Control and Prevention. *About Norovirus*. http://www.cdc.gov/norovirus/about/index.html (accessed June 30, 2016).

Centers for Disease Control and Prevention. *Morbidity and Mortality Weekly Report (MMWR): Acute Gastroenteritis on Cruise Ships—United States, 2008–2014*. https://www.cdc.gov/mmwr/volumes/65/wr/mm6501a1.htm?s_cid=mm6501a1_w (accessed June 30, 2016).

Centers for Disease Control and Prevention. *Outbreak Updates for International Cruise Ships.* http://www.cdc.gov/nceh/vsp/surv/gilist.htm (accessed June 30, 2016).

Chan, Paul K. S., Hoi S. Kwan, and Martin C. W. Chan, eds. *The Norovirus: Features, Detection, and Prevention of Foodborne Disease.* Cambridge, MA: Academic Press, 2016.

Hall, Aron J., et al. *Morbidity and Mortality Weekly Report (MMWR): Updated Norovirus Outbreak Management and Disease Prevention Guidelines.* Atlanta, GA: Centers for Disease Control and Prevention, 2011.

Prevention of Norovirus Infection in Schools and Childcare Facilities. Stockholm, Sweden: European Centre for Disease Prevention and Control, 2013.

NUCLEAR REGULATORY COMMISSION

The Nuclear Regulatory Commission (NRC) is an independent regulatory agency of the United States authorized by the Energy Reorganization Act of 1974. The NRC succeeded the Atomic Energy Commission (AEC) in 1975 due to calls by critics for the need to separate the AEC's conflicting roles of both promoting and regulating nuclear materials. Critics claimed that the AEC had been a victim of regulatory capture—a condition where regulators advance the interests of the industries and groups they regulate rather than the interests of the public they are mandated to protect. To remove any conflicts of interest, the AEC was disbanded, and the role of regulating nuclear materials was assigned to the NRC.

The NRC's ultimate responsibility is to protect public health and safety by ensuring the safe use and disposal of nuclear materials associated with civilian applications. The NRC's regulatory role is carried out through its powers to set and enforce rules and to license and inspect operations. While most often associated with the regulation of nuclear power plants, the NRC also oversees and regulates applications of nuclear materials in medicine, research, and other industries, and it regulates the storage and disposal of nuclear waste. Additionally, the NRC conducts research to inform regulatory decisions and develops public information and regulatory guidance.

One of the NRC's primary roles is to ensure the safe operation of nuclear power plants in generating nuclear energy. Operators of any facility proposing to use nuclear fuels and reactors to generate electricity must obtain permits from the NRC for both construction and operation. The NRC is also authorized to regularly inspect nuclear plants and enforce regulations when violations are found. The NRC's enforcement actions include issuing notices of violation, imposing monetary penalties, and modifying, suspending, or revoking licenses. Some issues confronting the NRC today are the renewal of licenses on aging plants, the decommissioning (dismantling) of older plants, and the storage and disposal of spent (used) nuclear fuel.

The NRC has several layers of controls to prevent outside influence from manipulating NRC activities and to ensure public trust in their decisions. The commission is headed by five members who must be appointed by the president of the United States and confirmed by the U.S. Senate. Neither the commission members nor the NRC staff may have any financial or personal interests in the entities they regulate. Regular reviews of NRC activities are conducted by an independent inspector general to ensure they are not only effective and efficient but also ethical. Prior to conducting any licensing activities, guidance must be considered from two advisory committees consisting of expert scientists. Finally, the public must be allowed to provide input prior to rulemaking, to access any materials used in decision making, and to attend any meetings in which decisions are made.

Adrienne L. Katner

See Also: Atomic Energy Commission; Electric Power Generation, Health Implications of; Nuclear Safety; Radiation, Ionizing and Nonionizing; Radiation Sickness

Further Reading

Fountain, Henry. "Amid a Graying Fleet of Nuclear Plants, a Hunt for Solutions." *New York Times*, March 21, 2016, https://www.nytimes.com/2016/03/22/science/nuclear-energy-power-plants-advanced-reactors.html.

Government Accountability Office. *Federal Oversight of Commercial Nuclear Power*. http://www.gao.gov/key_issues/federal_oversight_of_commercial_nuclear_power/issue_summary#t=0 (accessed December 12, 2016).

Nuclear Regulatory Commission. *Home Page*. http://www.nrc.gov/ (accessed December 12, 2016).

NUCLEAR SAFETY

Nuclear safety refers to the safety of nuclear power facilities and the waste generated by these facilities in terms of human health and the environment. Potential safety problems with nuclear power plants mainly involve the release of excessive amounts of radiation to workers or the public due to explosions or other mechanical failures. The most serious failures involve (1) partial meltdowns, where insufficient coverage by cooling water causes cracks and other damage to fuel rods, leading to the release of some radiation and (2) complete meltdowns, where the loss of all cooling water causes fuel pellets to fall to the bottom of the reactor and heat up to several thousand degrees, breaching the reactor vessel and leading to the release of massive amounts of radiation.

The Future Role of Nuclear Power

We need a meaningful price and trading regime on greenhouse gas emissions in all sectors, and then we'll see what a sensible role for nuclear power will be.

An Interview with Dr. Peter A. Bradford

Professor, Vermont Law School

Dr. Peter Bradford teaches Nuclear Power and Public Policy at Vermont Law School. He previously served on the U.S. Nuclear Regulatory Commission, and he chaired utility regulatory commissions in Maine and New York. Dr. Bradford also taught Energy Policy and

Environmental Protection at the Yale School of Forestry and Environmental Studies. He is currently vice chair of the Board of the Union of Concerned Scientists, and he is author of Fragile Structures: A Story of Oil Refineries, National Securities, and the Coast of Maine.

Because nuclear power plants do not emit greenhouse gases like carbon dioxide into the atmosphere, they do not contribute to climate change. As such, why are so many environmentalists opposed to further nuclear power development?

Having licensed about 20 plants and allowed funds to operate a dozen others during my regulatory career, I may not be the right person to answer. The problem faced by new reactors is the cost. Many low-carbon approaches appear to cost much less and to be available much more quickly, but a multibillion-dollar commitment to a new reactor ten or more years in the future crowds out these other solutions. As of this interview, a new nuclear power plant has not prevented a molecule of greenhouse gas emissions in the United States in this century, despite the proclamation of a nuclear revival by the Bush Administration in 2001 and the voting in by Congress and some states of every subsidy the industry requested a decade ago. This is not because of environmentalist opposition. Every one of the two-dozen or more plant cancellations and closings during that time has been for business reasons.

In the United States, the Clean Power Plan would have provided carbon-reduction credits for new nuclear power plants and allow existing nuclear plants to continue operating. Should nuclear power be viewed as an interim solution to reducing greenhouse gases, or will nuclear power inevitably be part of the final solution?

New reactors can't be an interim solution. They take too long to build in meaningful numbers. Wise energy policy is a matter of sound principles, not some gift of prophecy. We need a meaningful price and trading regime on greenhouse gas emissions in all sectors, and then we'll see what a sensible role for nuclear power will be. Neither the nuclear advocates nor their strongest opponents know nearly as much about the future as their claims suggest. That said, we also need to support research, development, and demonstration of new technologies that show promise of being able to reduce climate change cost-effectively.

Many nuclear power plants in Japan and several other countries shut down following the March 11, 2011, Great East Japan Earthquake and tsunami and subsequent meltdown of the Fukushima Daiichi reactors. As a result, Japan is now burning more coal for power production than ever before. Is this trade-off between nuclear power and coal power inevitable given the slow market penetration of renewable energy and challenges of infrastructure development?

Unplanned shutdowns of substantial nuclear capacity will inevitably cause other existing power plants to run longer hours and cause the construction of some capacity (as well as transmission and load control) on an emergency basis. However, given a little lead time and public policies that require low-carbon replacement, market-based approaches are usually fully capable of delivering such solutions. This should become even more feasible as storage technologies develop and their costs fall. Parts of the United States have closed nuclear plants without burning more coal, and recent marginal coal burning in Germany has been for export, not to replace the closed German nuclear units, which are increasingly being replaced by renewables.

What would be a good career path for a recent college or university graduate wanting to develop environmental law and policy and protect public health?

If such a student is inclined toward law or economics, the interplay between market performance and public policy is fascinating and crucial. If scientifically inclined, energy storage technologies and renewable resources seem likely to provide challenging, useful, and lucrative careers.

From 1952 to 2016, more than 30 serious accidents occurred at nuclear power plants around the world, ranging from relatively minor radiation releases that sickened a worker to partial meltdowns in which large amounts of radiation were released throughout the region surrounding the reactor, causing many illnesses and deaths. Six serious accidents have happened in the United States, the worst being the partial meltdown at the Three Mile Island facility in 1979.

Nuclear power plants in the United States, with some 60 years of experience and improvement in operations, are considered among the safest in the world. Their operations are regulated and overseen by the Nuclear Regulatory Commission (NRC), headed by five commissioners appointed by the president and confirmed by the Senate. Stringent government and industry regulations require these facilities to have multiple layers of security to protect workers, the public, and the environment. On-site inspectors with the NRC, who are independent from the facility's owners and operators, monitor a plant's performance regarding reactor safety, radiation safety, employee training and performance, and facility maintenance and security. The NRC establishes limits on the allowable annual amount of radiation to which nuclear plant workers can be exposed, which, on average, is lower than that airplane crews are exposed to due to background radiation.

Workers undergo extensive background checks, training, and federal licensing tests. All plants have detailed plans to respond to on-site and off-site emergencies, and these planned responses are practiced and tested every two years with the participation of local, state, and federal agencies. The NRC uses assessments made by the Federal Emergency Management Agency when evaluating a facility for operational approval.

Many of the technical systems in U.S. nuclear facilities are automated and redundant so that backup systems can quickly replace malfunctioning systems. Security procedures are tight to prevent terrorists or other intruders from entering facilities. Most reactors are surrounded by thick steel-reinforced concrete containment structures designed to withstand the impact of hurricanes, tornadoes, earthquakes, floods, and commercial airplane impacts. Cyberattacks are also taken into account in security strategies.

The most serious nuclear accident in the United States occurred at the Three Mile Island facility in Pennsylvania in March 1979. A malfunction in the cooling system and employee error led to a partial meltdown, in which about half of the reactor core melted, forming a puddle of radioactive material at the bottom of the reactor vessel. Although the vessel remained intact, a small amount of radiation escaped into the surrounding environment. This accident ranks 5 on the International Nuclear and Radiological Event Scale (commonly abbreviated INES), which ranges from 1 to 7, with 7 being the worst.

Internationally, the World Association of Nuclear Operators (WANO) collects, consolidates, and distributes the operational data of nuclear power plants in all countries. Annual evaluations are made by the WANO about the safety performance of these facilities. Data collected in 2015 revealed that 98.5 percent of facilities met targets for safety system performance, 87.7 percent met targets for radiation exposure, and 85.3 percent met targets for accident rate.

The April 1986 accident at the Chernobyl nuclear facility in Ukraine is considered the most serious nuclear accident in history, ranking 7 on the INES. A power surge caused an explosion in one of its reactors, resulting in the release of enough radiation throughout the region to lead to widespread and long-term health and environmental effects. Thirty workers at the facility died from radiation poisoning, and thousands of people in Ukraine, Belarus, and Russia are believed to have contracted thyroid cancer from the radioactive fallout.

An accident at Japan's Fukushima Daiichi nuclear power plant in March 2011, ranking 5 on the INES, involved the release of radioactivity into the surrounding environment. This was caused by a powerful earthquake and associated tsunami that led to explosions and the loss of electricity, requiring the subsequent decontamination and disassembly of all six reactors at the site, a process that could take four decades or longer.

The radioactive waste generated by nuclear power plants remains hazardous to humans and the environment for thousands of years. The management and disposal of this waste in the United States is regulated by the NRC's Office of Nuclear Material Safety and Safeguards. Most spent nuclear fuel is stored in specially designed steel-lined, concrete-walled pools of water at reactor sites throughout the country. Some fuel is stored in air-tight steel or concrete dry cask storage systems at current reactor sites, decommissioned reactor sites, or off-site interim storage facilities. A proposed permanent waste repository inside deep geological formations at Yucca Mountain in Nevada has yet to be approved by the NRC.

A.J. Smuskiewicz

See Also: Chernobyl Incident; Electric Power Generation, Health Implications of; Fukushima Daiichi Incident; Nuclear Regulatory Commission; Radiation, Ionizing and Nonionizing; Radiation Sickness; Radioactive Wastes; Three Mile Island Incident

Further Reading

Fountain, Henry. "A Look at the Mechanics of a Partial Meltdown." *New York Times*, March 31, 2011, http://www.nytimes.com/2011/03/14/science/earth/14meltdown.html.

International Atomic Energy Agency. *INES: The International Nuclear and Radiological Event Scale*. http://www-ns.iaea.org/tech-areas/emergency/ines.asp (accessed April 7, 2017).

Matson, John. "What Happens during a Nuclear Meltdown?" *Scientific American* (March 2011). https://www.scientificamerican.com/article/nuclear-energy-primer.

Nuclear Energy Institute. *Safety and Security*. https://www.nei.org/Issues-Policy/Safety-and-Security (accessed March 25, 2017).

Nuclear Power Plant Accidents: Listed and Ranked Since 1952. Guardian. https://www.theguardian.com/news/datablog/2011/mar/14/nuclear-power-plant-accidents-list-rank (accessed March 25, 2017).

Nuclear Regulatory Commission. *Home Page*. https://www.nrc.gov (accessed March 25, 2017).

World Association of Nuclear Operators. *Performance Indicators*. http://www.wano.info/en-gb/library/performanceindicators (accessed March 25, 2017).

O

OCCUPATIONAL SAFETY AND HEALTH

The field of occupational safety and health (OSH) involves protection of workers through identification and control of risks that arise from chemical, biological, physical, biomechanical, and psychosocial hazards in the workplace. As a multi-disciplinary field, exposure prevention calls upon industrial hygienists, occupational safety professionals, engineers, and ergonomists to monitor and mitigate adverse working conditions. (On the other hand, recognition, diagnosis, treatment, and management of occupational illnesses and injuries are the purview of health-care providers—physicians, nurses, psychologists, and other health professionals.) Engagement of managers, workers, and worker advocates is critical to ensuring safe operations that protect the health and safety of workers. Legislated oversight and support of the OSH system is provided by the governmental agencies listed in Table 12.

Table 12. Government agencies supporting occupational safety and health.

Agency	Occupational Oversight
Occupational Safety and Health Administration https://www.osha.gov	• Arm of the U.S. Department of Labor • Sets and enforces protective workplace standards • Provides information, training, and assistance to employers and workers
Mining Safety and Health Administration https://www.msha.gov	• Develops and enforces safety and health rules for all U.S. mines • Provides technical, educational, and other assistance to mine operators
Bureau of Labor Statistics https://www.bls.gov	• Collects, processes, analyzes, and disseminates statistical data (surveillance) related to employment, labor economics, and occupational illness and injury
National Institute for Occupational Safety and Health http://www.cdc.gov/niosh	• Responsible for conducting research and making recommendations for the prevention of work-related injury and illness
Environmental Protection Agency https://www.epa.gov https://www.epa.gov/pesticide-worker-safety/agricultural-worker-protection-standard-wps	• Protects human health and the environment by enforcing compliance with environmental laws • Oversees agricultural workplaces through the Worker Protection Standard, reducing risk of pesticide poisoning and injury

(Continued)

Table 12. Continued

Agency	Occupational Oversight
Workers' Compensation *State agencies:* https://www.dol.gov/owcp/dfec/regs/compliance/wc.htm *Federal agency:* https://www.dol.gov/owcp/dfec/ *Longshore and Harbor Workers' Compensation Act:* https://www.dol.gov/owcp/dlhwc/lhwca.htm	• A form of social insurance providing wage replacement and medical benefits to employees injured in the course of employment, in exchange for mandatory relinquishment of the employee's right to sue the employer for the tort of negligence
US. Department of Labor https://www.dol.gov	• Oversees employment laws regarding wages, hours, workers' compensation, and other workforce protections • Has specific programs for migrant and seasonal farm workers, temporary employment sector, immigrant workers, maritime workers, and federal employees

Workplaces include contained, indoor work environments (e.g., factories, hospitals, offices, warehouses, homes, and schools), outdoor settings (e.g., farms, construction sites, oil rigs, power line maintenance sites, and parks), and mobile containments (e.g., trucks, trains, airplanes, and automobiles). Health effects arising from hazards in these settings may be classified by hazard category, specific hazard, or health outcome, as illustrated in Table 13.

In the United States, workplace fatalities have gone from 6,217 in 1992 to a low of 4,551 in 2009, with a rise to 4,836 in 2015. Causes in 2015 were roadway and transportation incidents (42.5 percent); falls, slips, and trips (16.5 percent); contact with objects and equipment (14.9 percent); violence and other injuries by persons or animals (14.5 percent); exposure to harmful substances or environments (8.8 percent); and fires/explosions (2.5 percent). Construction remained the sector with the highest number of fatalities (935, representing 19.4 percent of the total), while agriculture had the highest rate per employed worker (22.8 per 100,000 full-time equivalent workers, compared with 3.4 per 100,000 full-time equivalent workers overall).

Why Is Worker Health Important?

Most of the population is employed, and "work" can contribute both positively and negatively to the health and well-being of the workers and their families and communities. Attention to worker health and safety through legislation has led to a greater awareness and a substantial decrease in occupational injuries and illnesses. In addition, the workplace is increasingly becoming recognized as a venue for *promoting* health. Nevertheless, on-the job illnesses and injuries cost workers, employers, insurance companies, and taxpayers billions of dollars each year in health care and work-time lost.

Table 13. Categories pertaining to adverse health outcomes from occupational hazard exposures.

Hazard Type	Examples
Chemical	• Solvents, metals, pesticides, simple irritants, fibers, particulates
Biological	• Infectious agents: bacteria, viruses, fungi, parasites
Physical	• Noise, radiation, heat, cold, vibration
Biomechanical	• Moving machinery, hand tools, vehicles
Psychosocial	• Shift work, low wages, part-time work, harassment, stress
Disorder by Organ System	
Musculoskeletal	• Acute traumatic injury: amputation, burn, head trauma, cumulative trauma (e.g., carpal tunnel syndrome)
Respiratory	• Acute inhalation injuries, asthma, chronic obstructive pulmonary disease, pneumoconiosis, hypersensitivity pneumonitis, metal fume fever, lung cancer
Neurologic/psychiatric	• Encephalopathy, cognitive defects, peripheral neuropathy, brain cancer
Dermatologic	• Irritant contact dermatitis, allergic contact dermatitis, chloracne, vitiligo, skin cancer
Reproductive	• Sexual dysfunction, fetal toxicity, poor reproductive outcomes
Cardiovascular	• Atherogenesis, cardiomyopathy, hypertension
Hematologic	• Methemoglobinemia, leukemia, aplastic anemia
GI/Hepatic	• Hepatitis due to infection, chemical toxicity, cirrhosis, cancer
Urinary tract	• Acute kidney disease, chronic kidney disease, cancer of bladder/kidney
Condition	
Cancer	• All organ systems, caused by chemical, biological, physical hazards
Infectious disease	• Systemic or organ system infection (e.g., healthcare workers)
Traumatic injury	• Machine operators, work at heights, vehicle drivers

The top five industries reporting the highest rates of nonfatal occupational injuries and illnesses with days away from work in 2015 were nursing and residential care facilities (6.8 per 100 full-time workers), hospitals (6.0 per 100 full-time workers), schools (4.8 per 100 full-time workers), and general merchandise stores (4.5 per 100 full-time workers). Public sector workers had a higher proportion of occupational injuries than their proportion in the workforce. Injuries represented 95 percent of reported cases, with the remaining 5 percent of cases made up of skin diseases (15.2 percent of the 2.9 million illness cases), hearing loss (12.7 percent of illness cases), respiratory conditions (8.4 percent of illness cases), and all other illnesses (i.e., systemic illnesses and cumulative trauma cases), representing 62.6 percent of illness cases.

There is increasing interest in health promotion among employers because of rising healthcare costs and recognition that a stable, highly skilled workforce is more profitable. Workplace health promotion activities include (1) worksite management of chronic conditions, such as diabetes and hypertension; (2) programs that promote physical activity, such as providing walking paths and longer lunch breaks, monetary incentives for going to the gym, fitness contests, and active transportation options; (3) lifestyle interventions to prevent smoking, such as smoke-free workplaces and smoking cessation programs; and (4) dietary support, including dietician counseling and healthy food choices.

Over the past several decades, the workforce has been downsized and outsourced, leading to many structural and practical changes. These include (1) increased size of single businesses (e.g., large agricultural producers with attendant hazardous operations, such as concentrated animal feeding operations that house hundreds to thousands of animals in a single facility); (2) decreased number of labor unions, resulting in fewer worker protections; (3) contracted labor, where the employee and the employer do not have a direct relationship and health insurance is not provided; (4) increased reliance on migrant labor, which is subject to lower wages and exploitive labor practices; and (5) more difficult work circumstances, including unstable employment, irregular work hours, and limited benefits. These conditions have led to increased safety and health risks for the American workforce, and they highlight the urgent need for professionals working in the field of OSH.

Linda Forst

See Also: Concentrated Animal Feeding Operations, Pollution from; Environmental Protection Agency; National Institute for Occupational Safety and Health; Occupational Safety and Health Administration; Safety Data Sheet

Further Reading

Bureau of Labor Statistics. *Census of Fatal Occupational Injuries (CFOI)—Current and Revised Data*. https://www.bls.gov/iif/oshcfoi1.htm#2015 (accessed January 3, 2017).

Bureau of Labor Statistics. *Nonfatal Occupational Injuries and Illnesses by Industry*. https://www.bls.gov/iif/oshsum1.htm (accessed January 3, 2017).

Friend, Mark A., and James P. Kohn. *Fundamentals of Occupational Safety and Health*. Lanham, MD: Bernan Press, 2014.

Friis, Robert H. *Occupational Health and Safety for the 21st Century*. Burlington, MA: Jones and Bartlett Learning, 2016.

LaDou, Joseph, and Robert Harrison. *Current Occupational and Environmental Medicine*. New York: McGraw-Hill, 2014.

Levy, Barry S., et al. *Occupational and Environmental Health: Recognizing and Preventing Disease and Injury*. Oxford, UK: Oxford University Press, 2011.

Plog, Barbara A., and Patricia Quinlan. *Fundamentals of Industrial Hygiene*. Itasca, IL: National Safety Council, 2012.

Quinlan, M., and P. Bohle. "Overstretched and Unreciprocated Commitment: Reviewing Research on the Occupational Health and Safety Effects of Downsizing and Job Insecurity." *International Journal of Health Services*, vol. 39, no. 1 (January 2009): 1–44.

World Health Organization. *Occupational Health: Workplace Health Promotion*. http://www.who.int/occupational_health/topics/workplace/en (accessed January 3, 2017).

OCCUPATIONAL SAFETY AND HEALTH ADMINISTRATION

The Occupational Safety and Health Administration (OSHA) is a federal agency of the U.S. Department of Labor charged with protecting the safety and health of workers in America. The OSHA was created by the Occupational Safety and Health Act (the act), signed into the law on December 29, 1970, by President Nixon.

The OSHA is headed by the assistant secretary for occupational safety and health, a presidential appointee, who is responsible for enforcing the act in the 50 states and certain territories and jurisdictions under federal authority. In the majority of states, territories, and jurisdictions, OSHA covers most private-sector workplaces but not those in the public sector operated by state and local governments. Exceptions to this arrangement are the six states and territories (Connecticut, Illinois, Maine, New Jersey, New York, and Virgin Islands) that have elected a hybrid option of mixing OSHA coverage of private-sector workplaces with state enforcement for governmental workplaces under an OSHA-approved state plan.

Twenty-two other states and territories chose to develop their own job safety and health programs through the OSHA state plan approval process, as strongly encouraged by Section 18 of the act. To be approved, a state program must be at least as effective as the federal OSHA program and cover both private- and public-sector employers and workers. Once approved by the OSHA, these states are responsible for enforcing the act in their own states. The states and territories with OSHA-approved state plans are Alaska, Arizona, California, Hawaii, Indiana, Iowa, Kentucky, Maryland, Michigan, Minnesota, Nevada, New Mexico, North Carolina, Oregon, Puerto Rico, South Carolina, Tennessee, Utah, Vermont, Virginia, Washington, and Wyoming. All federal employees fall under the jurisdiction of the federal OSHA and therefore are excluded from any state plan.

The OSHA is responsible for ensuring the safety and health of workers in American workplaces by setting and enforcing standards; monitoring the effectiveness of the OSHA-approved state plans; providing training, outreach, and education; and promoting workplace safety and health. OSHA health standards specify exposure limits for hazardous substances in the workplace, such as asbestos, cotton dust, benzene, lead, and blood-borne pathogens. OSHA safety standards establish requirements to prevent injuries, for example, standards for fall protection, trenching, and machine guarding. The OSHA issues fines to employers who violate the standards. The largest fine ever paid was $50.6 million by BP PLC in 2010 for failing to correct safety problems identified after a 2005 explosion at its Texas City refinery that killed 15 workers and injured 170.

The OSHA implements a complaint process whereby workers can file complaints with the OSHA about what they consider to be dangerous working conditions. Furthermore, the OSHA's whistle-blower protection program is designed to protect workers from retaliation for exercising their rights under the act. These rights include raising safety and health concerns with an employer, filing a complaint with the OSHA, requesting an OSHA inspection, or testifying related to an OSHA inspection. Critics point out that the OSHA has not been able to expand its capacity to respond to complaints in a timely manner.

To highlight its accomplishments, the OSHA points to statistics showing that work-related fatalities and injuries declined more than 65 percent since 1971, while the size of the workforce population nearly doubled during the same period. However, critics contend that this downward trend began well before the OSHA was created, and therefore, the OSHA's accomplishments may not be as impressive as they claim. Nevertheless, it is undisputable that the OSHA plays a key role in making the American workplace safer and healthier.

Yoko S. Crume

See Also: Asbestos; Black Lung Disease; Indoor Environment; Lead Poisoning Prevention; National Institute for Occupational Safety and Health; Occupational Safety and Health

Further Reading

Moran, Mark M. *The OSHA Answer Book for General Industry*. Fleming Island, FL: Moran Associates, 2014.

U.S. Department of Labor. *All about OSHA*. https://www.osha.gov/Publications/about-osha/3302-06N-2006-English.html#TheStandardsSettingProcess (accessed May 1, 2016).

U.S. Department of Labor. *Occupational Safety and Health Administration*. https://www.osha.gov (accessed May 1, 2016).

U.S. Department of Labor. *The Occupational Safety and Health Administration: A History of Its First Thirteen Years, 1971–1984*. http://www.dol.gov/dol/aboutdol/history/mono-osha13introtoc.htm (accessed May 1, 2016).

OCEAN ACIDIFICATION

Carbon dioxide (CO_2) is a gas that has both natural and human sources. The issue with CO_2 today is that it is a widespread greenhouse gas, contributing more than all other atmospheric gases to climate change. There is near-unanimous agreement in the scientific community that CO_2 concentrations in the atmosphere are on the rise and that these elevated levels are causing long-term climate change, a trend that at this point may be difficult if not impossible to reverse.

In addition to climate change, the increasing concentrations of CO_2 in the atmosphere are having another impact, perhaps less recognized, but every bit as troubling: the acidification of the oceans. Ocean water is a CO_2 sink, which means it absorbs CO_2 from the atmosphere, including up to one-third of the CO_2 emitted into the atmosphere from human activities like the combustion of fossil fuels for electric power generation. If it were not for the carbon uptake capacity of the oceans, scientists have calculated atmospheric CO_2 concentrations would be about 20 percent greater than they presently are, and as a consequence, the earth would be a much warmer place.

The continued absorption of greater and greater quantities of CO_2 into the ocean is concerning. Once dissolved in seawater, CO_2 gas reacts with water to form carbonic acid (H_2CO_3), which then dissociates by losing hydrogen ions to form bicarbonate (HCO_3^-) and carbonate ($CO_{3\_}^{2}$) ions:

$$CO_{2(atmos)} \leftrightarrow CO_{2(aq)} + H_2O \leftrightarrow H_2CO_3 \leftrightarrow H^+ + HCO_3^- \leftrightarrow 2H^+ + CO_3^{2-})$$

The more CO_2 that is added to ocean water, the more hydrogen ions increase and the more acidic the water becomes. Since preindustrial times, the average ocean surface pH has fallen by approximately 0.1 units, from about 8.21 to 8.10. Projections show that a further decrease of 0.3 to 0.4 pH units can be expected by the end of the century at the current trajectory.

What impacts will manifest from such changes in ocean chemistry? The potential consequences to marine life and also to economic activities that depend on a healthy marine ecosystem are difficult to assess and predict but potentially devastating. Reduced carbonate ion concentrations would provide less body building material for marine calcifiers, and experiments show stunted growth in marine organisms, subjecting them to potentially greater predation. The shells of some organisms dissolve more quickly in the low pH environment, potentially disrupting vital food webs in the oceans. Entire marine species in these food webs could become extinct if ocean acidification continues, further altering the ocean ecosystem. Acidosis from increasing carbonic acid concentrations in the body fluids of larger animals may cause problems with respiration, growth, and reproduction.

Of more immediate concern, declining oyster beds along the West Coast of the United States and declining coral reefs around the world are suspected to be related to the ocean acidification phenomenon. Coral reefs provide habitat to many species and are often regarded by ecologists as centers of biodiversity in the oceans. Mathematical modeling suggests that ocean acidification will generally reduce fish biomass and catch, and fisheries, tourism, and coastal protection will all be impacted.

While the chemistry of ocean acidification is well understood and verified by field measurements, the long-term impacts and potential adaptation of the marine environment is not. Models and other research suggest that the impact of rising CO_2 levels on marine biota will be varied, with both ecological winners and losers. However, the acidification of oceans impacts processes so fundamental in the marine ecosystem that the consequences, like those of climate change, could have far-reaching consequences. Geo-engineering solutions that attempt to slow global warming based on, for example, solar radiation management will not abate acidification. Reduction of atmospheric CO_2 is the most effective method to mitigate ocean acidification, but unfortunately, CO_2 concentrations continue rising at an accelerating pace.

John K. Borén

See Also: Carbon Dioxide and the Carbon Cycle; Climate Change and Human Health; Greenhouse Effect and Global Warming; Mauna Loa Observatory, Carbon Measurements at

Further Reading

Climate Change 2014: Impacts, Adaptation, and Vulnerability. Geneva, Switzerland: Intergovernmental Panel on Climate Change, 2014.

Doney, Scott C., et al. "Ocean Acidification: The Other CO_2 Problem." *Annual Review of Marine Science*, vol. 1 (December 2009): 169–192.

Eisler, Ronald. *Oceanic Acidification: A Comprehensive Overview*. Boca Raton, FL: CRC Press, 2012.

Gattuso, Jean-Piere, and Lina Hansson. *Ocean Acidification*. Oxford, UK: Oxford University Press, 2012.

National Oceanic and Atmospheric Administration. *NOAA Ocean Acidification Program*. http://oceanacidification.noaa.gov (accessed May 1, 2017).

Raisman, Scott, and Daniel T. Murphy. *Ocean Acidification: Elements and Considerations*. Hauppauge, NY: Nova Science Publishers, 2013.

U.S. Environmental Protection Agency. *Climate Change Indicators: Ocean Acidity*. https://www.epa.gov/climate-indicators/climate-change-indicators-ocean-acidity (accessed May 1, 2017).

OCEAN DUMPING AND THE PACIFIC GARBAGE PATCH

Ocean dumping and other human activities cause ocean pollution, including the Pacific garbage patch. As a result, the ocean is contaminated with a wide variety of toxic chemicals and plastic trash that harm wildlife and accumulate in fish and shellfish. This creates a health risk for people who eat seafood.

Garbage Patches—Not Just the Pacific

The North Pacific garbage patch has the largest and densest amount of plastic debris, but plastic trash is also found in the Atlantic and Indian Oceans. The Atlantic Ocean garbage patch, first documented in 1972, has an estimated 11,700 tons (10,600 metric tons) of plastics, and the Indian Ocean garbage patch, discovered in 2010, contains an estimated 2,200 tons (2,000 metric tons) of plastics. To raise awareness about ocean pollution, Italian artist Maria Cristina Finucci proclaimed the State of Garbage Patch at UN Educational, Scientific, and Cultural Organization (UNESCO) headquarters in 2013. The UNESCO subsequently granted Garbage Patch symbolic statehood status.

Throughout the industrial period, ships could dump treated and untreated sewage, industrial and radioactive wastes, and military munitions into the ocean without restriction. The United States banned ocean dumping in 1972, and in later international treaties, other countries agreed to stop dumping industrial products. As of 2015, practically every country with shipping had banned dumping. However, illegal dumping still occurs, and waste also enters the ocean through rivers. In particular, nitrogen fertilizer from agricultural runoff causes "dead zones" resulting from eutrophication (a process whereby algae and cyanobacteria grow rapidly and eventually deplete the oxygen supply). In these areas, excess algae or bacteria deplete the oxygen in the water. Other ocean pollution comes from offshore mining and oil/gas exploration.

Are Plastics in Your Diet?

Did you know that if you eat ocean fish, you may also be ingesting tiny particles of plastic? This is because the 8.8 million tons (8 million metric tons) of plastics that end up in our oceans every year (equivalent to one garbage truck each minute) eventually break down into minute pieces that are ingested by fish. According to a study by the Scripps Institution of Oceanography, about 9 percent of fish sampled near the North Pacific Subtropical Gyre contained plastics, and the researchers believe this to be a low estimate. And another study by researchers at the University of California–Davis found plastics and textile fibers in about 25 of the fish sampled at one California fish market. Plastics in the oceans may absorb toxic chemicals that are released into a fish's bloodstream or tissues while being digested, and one common plastic ingredient, styrene, is considered a possible human carcinogen by the International Agency for Research on Cancer. Furthermore, the volume of amount of plastics in the oceans is dramatically increasing, such that by 2050, there may actually be more plastics in the ocean (on a weight basis) than fish! Despite these concerns, the consensus of most public health professionals, at least for now, is that the health benefits of eating these ocean fish generally outweigh the potential risks. (On the other hand, be cautious about eating certain species of fish known to have high mercury concentrations, including swordfish, shark, mackerel, and tuna.)

Healthy Oceans and Human Health

I just worry that in a hundred years, people will look back at our generation and say, "They knew, they had a choice, but they did nothing."

An Interview with Dr. Iain Kerr

Chief Executive Officer, Ocean Alliance

Dr. Kerr, chief executive officer of the Ocean Alliance, is an international leader in whale research and ocean conservation. He has led oceanographic expeditions all over the globe, including the Voyage of the Odyssey, *which provided the first complete set of data on the concentration and distribution of synthetic contaminants and effects on top predator species in the world's oceans. The Ocean Alliance collects information on whales and other ocean life, with the goal of educating policymakers and the public on wise stewardship of the oceans to prevent the collapse of marine mammal populations and promote ocean and human health.*

You have said humans are "utterly dependent" on preserving the marine environment. Why is a healthy marine environment important to human health?

It is popular to talk about preserving "planet earth," but we should really be discussing "planet ocean." Over 70 percent of the world is covered with water, and almost all of this is in the oceans. And about 70 percent of the oxygen in our atmosphere comes from marine plants, mainly phytoplankton (Prochlorococcus).

Over half the world's population lives within about 125 miles (200 kilometers) of a coastline, and about three billion people rely on wild-caught and farmed seafood for their primary source of meat protein. As land resources continue to be depleted, humans will increasingly turn to the oceans for essential resources, especially food. Thus, the critical importance of the oceans to human health and survival is undeniable.

You also believe that environmental conservation should be a "state of mind." What exactly does this mean, and how can humanity's general apathy about the oceans be reversed?

I met an astronaut once who told me I would never meet another astronaut who is not a rabid environmentalist after seeing our fragile planet from space. We spend a lot of time protecting ourselves with safer cars, home security systems, and healthy diets, but few people appreciate the connection between healthy oceans and their own health. This is probably because environmental degradation in the oceans is hard to see for the average person. There are dead zones all over the oceans, but we just don't see them. There are fish die-offs in the oceans all the time, but we usually are not aware. Environmental issues are complex, and none of us are perfect citizens when it comes to protecting the environment, but if 90 percent of everyone would do just one thing for the environment every day (like picking up trash or recycling a bottle), we would live in a very different world.

Much of your current research focuses on whales, specifically studies of toxicology, behavior, bioacoustics, and genetics. Are there any lessons from your research that can be applied to protecting the human species?

Humanity is a cosmopolitan species at the top of the food chain, and research shows that it is the most complex species that are most at risk from environmental pollution. We have learned that whales and other mammals bioaccumulate toxins and pass them on to their offspring. I believe whales serve as excellent bioindicators for the health of the planet, and when whales suffer from toxins, plastics, and other ocean pollutants, we are all at risk.

The Ocean Alliance promotes wise stewardship of the oceans. Is there any hope for the future of the oceans given the problems that are already occurring, such as coral reef bleaching, ocean acidification, dead zones, invasive species, mercury pollution, and giant gyres of trash?

I believe in humanity, and I try to see every crisis as an opportunity. Many organizations are working very hard to solve our environmental issues, and a number of large corporations are showing leadership in protecting the environment. Working together, we can solve this problem. I just worry that in a hundred years, people will look back at our generation and say, "They knew, they had a choice, but they did nothing." Let's not let that happen!

What would be a good career path for a recent college or university graduate wanting to make a real difference in preserving the oceans and protecting public health?

Whatever career one pursues, do pro bono work for the environment, pick up trash when you see it, and most importantly, believe you can make a difference!

Dumping materials into the ocean can endanger marine ecosystems and human health. For instance, mercury from industrial dumping accumulates in the bodies of marine animals, resulting in contaminated seafood. The highest mercury concentrations are found in swordfish, shark, mackerel, and tuna. Women of childbearing age are encouraged to limit their consumption of these fish because mercury can cause neurological problems in developing infants. The World Health Organization lists mercury as one of 10 chemicals of "major public health concern."

The Pacific garbage patch is a vast area in the northern Pacific Ocean with a high density of plastic trash. This area contains items such as bottles, plastic bags, fishing nets, and cigarette lighters, but most of the patch is a "soup" consisting of tiny pieces of plastic. The patch was first discovered in 1997 by Captain Charles Moore, who has since established the Algalita Foundation to investigate the scope and significance of this floating debris. Recent estimates of the size of this debris field range between 270,000 and 5.8 million square miles (700,000 and 15 million square kilometers). This represents an area covering up to 8 percent of the entire Pacific Ocean. The density of plastic in the northern Pacific Ocean is estimated to be 64,700 pieces per square mile (25,000 pieces per square kilometer).

Worldwide, the ocean receives an estimated 8.8 million tons (8 million metric tons) of plastic trash every year. In the Pacific Ocean, a large circular system of currents known as a gyre transports and concentrates the plastics into one large area, the Pacific garbage patch. Plastics are generally not biodegradable, so sunlight and other weathering processes break down plastic trash into increasingly smaller pieces. Most of the plastics retrieved from the ocean are less than the size of a person's smallest fingernail. Some of the smallest pieces, called microplastics, come from strands of rope, nets, textiles, and microbeads found in exfoliating soaps and some toothpastes.

This trash is harmful to many species of birds and fish as well as humans. A well-documented case concerns albatross chicks on Midway Atoll, a national marine sanctuary that receives up to 20 tons (18 metric tons) of plastic debris every year. These chicks die when their parents feed them bottle caps and other trash. Additionally, other animals get stuck in large pieces of trash and cannot free themselves. The plastics also present risks to human health. For example, plastics absorb from the seawater toxic chemical pollutants like polychlorinated biphenyls and the pesticide dichlorodiphenyltrichloroethane (better known as DDT), and when these plastics are ingested by jellyfish and small fish, the absorbed toxins are passed up the food chain to larger fish and finally humans. Additionally, bacteria, algae, and other microbes grow on the plastic trash, creating what has been termed the "plastisphere." The impact of the plastisphere is relatively unknown, but one study of the microbial life on plastic trash in the ocean has identified bacteria in the genus *vibrio*, which includes the bacteria that cause cholera.

Efforts to clean up ocean pollution, including plastic debris, are expected to be costly. The National Oceanic and Atmospheric Administration sponsors the Marine

Debris Program to support locally driven marine debris prevention and removal projects, benefiting coastal habitats, waterways, and wildlife. The Ocean Cleanup is a foundation established in 2013 to remove plastics from the oceans and prevent future contamination. They have designed a passive removal system of barriers that funnels debris to extraction platforms, and they plan to begin large-scale trash removal in 2020. However, reducing consumption of plastic in the form of throwaway utensils, water bottles, and synthetic textiles is key in preventing future trash from entering the garbage patches of the world.

Alisha K. Newton

See Also: Estuary Pollution; Fish Consumption Advisories; Marine Pollution, International Treaties to Prevent; Mercury Pollution; National Estuary Program; National Oceanic and Atmospheric Administration

Further Reading

How Plastic in the Ocean Is Contaminating Your Seafood. National Public Radio, Washington, DC, 2013. http://www.npr.org/sections/thesalt/2013/12/12/250438904/how-plastic-in-the-ocean-is-contaminating-your-seafood.

Jambeck, Jenna R., et al. "Plastic Waste Inputs from Land into the Ocean." *Science*, vol. 347, no. 6223 (February 2015): 768–771.

Kostigen, Thomas M. "The World's Largest Dump: The Great Pacific Garbage Patch." *Discover Magazine* (July 2008), http://discovermagazine.com/2008/jul/10-the-worlds-largest-dump.

Rochman, Chelsea M., et al. "Anthropogenic Debris in Seafood: Plastic Debris and Fibers from Textiles in Fish and Bivalves Sold for Human Consumption." *Scientific Reports*, vol. 5, no. 14340 (September 2015).

Scripps Institution of Oceanography. *Scripps Study Finds Plastic in Nine Percent of "Garbage Patch" Fishes.* https://scripps.ucsd.edu/news/1928 (accessed December 12, 2016).

Smithsonian Museum of Natural History. "Pollution." *Smithsonian Ocean Portal.* http://ocean.si.edu/conservation/pollution (accessed December 12, 2015).

Teuten, Emma L., et al. "Transport and Release of Chemicals from Plastics to the Environment and to Wildlife." *Philosophical Transactions of the Royal Society B: Biological Sciences*, vol. 364, no. 1526 (July 2009): 2027–2045.

Worm, Boris. "Silent Spring in the Ocean." *Proceedings of the National Academy of Sciences*, vol. 112, no. 38 (September 2015): 11752–11753.

ODOR POLLUTION

If it smells bad, it must be bad for you. This is what many people believe about odors, but this is not always the case. Countless substances having a pungent smell are harmless, while other odorless substances may cause serious health problems. Regardless, no one likes being around something that smells bad. Historically, odor complaints represent a large fraction of the citizen complaints made to local environmental health agencies.

Keeping a Personal Odor Diary

Are you bothered by an odor in your community? If so, try keeping an odor diary. Odor diaries provide information that help local environmental health officials identify the source of the odor and take action to reduce or eliminate the offensive smell. The information typically found in an odor diary includes the date the odor was detected, start and end times, location, odor type and severity, effects on normal activities, weather conditions, and any comments that may be helpful in locating the source. With this information, combined with other data about air pollution emissions and air quality, local officials can assess the problem and formulate a solution, for example, ordering the source of the odor to modify or cease operations or requiring technology to capture, disperse, or destroy the odor.

Many odors are associated with human activities, for example, making compost, treating sewage, collecting garbage, or operating diesel-fueled vehicles. Other odors emanate from industrial operations, including oil refineries, landfills, paper mills, and wastewater treatment plants. Concentrated animal feeding operations (agricultural operations where animals are kept and raised in confined situations) can also be sources of offensive odors.

Among the five senses, our ability to smell is the most complex. Humans can distinguish over 10,000 different odors, some of which are perceived as pleasant and others the opposite. Pleasant odors help us enjoy a delicious meal at our favorite restaurant or a walk through the woods on a cool spring morning, while unpleasant odors can sometimes indicate a hazard, for example, a gas leak. Having to live with unpleasant odors in a community can diminish the quality of life and sense of well-being. While humans are excellent in distinguishing odors, it is an interesting fact that we almost always have great difficulty describing them in words.

There are four characteristics that determine our perception of odors, for example, how strong the odor is and whether it is pleasant or unpleasant. The first characteristic is *detectability*, which refers to the minimum concentration of the substance in the air that we can smell. (In other words, our noses cannot detect concentrations lower than this minimum level.) Because detectability varies from person to person, someone may be able to detect a faint odor that someone else misses. Nevertheless, the ability to detect odors is similar for most people.

The second characteristic of odor is *intensity*, which refers to whether the odor is perceived as strong or weak. Intensity increases with concentration of the substance in the air. The third characteristic is *character*, which is what the odor smells like or reminds us of. Odors often have a smell described as fishy, hay, nutty, creosote, turpentine, rancid, sewer, and ammonia. Sometimes we can recognize specific chemicals or sources from their smell.

The fourth characteristic of odor is *hedonic tone*, which represents subjective judgment about whether an odor is pleasant or unpleasant. (The word "hedonic" is derived from the Greek word *hedone*, which means "pleasure.") A variety of factors influence hedonic tone, including the odor intensity, character, duration, and frequency of occurrence. Location and time of day can also be factors. For example, freshly baked bread may smell wonderful in a bakery but may be annoying if we are trying to fall asleep.

Odors can cause various adverse health experiences, depending on the substance causing the odor, the concentration in the air, how long and often exposure occurs, and a person's age, general health condition, and sensitivity to the substance. Some examples of odor symptoms are headaches, nasal congestion, sore throat, coughing and wheezing, chest tightness, shortness of breath, heart palpitations, nausea, and irritation of the eye, nose, and throat. Strong odors can interfere outdoor activities and sleep, and if the odor is associated with a toxic chemical, serious health episodes may occur. In some cases, the substance causing an odor can worsen asthma, chronic obstructive pulmonary disease, and emphysema. In general, children, older adults, and pregnant women tend to be more sensitive to odors than the general population.

Some hazardous substances have no odor, making detection difficult. For example, natural gas (methane), which is widely used in the United States for heating and cooking, is odorless, colorless, and tasteless, making leak detection difficult. This is a problem because if a natural gas leak occurs, for example, in the furnace that heats your home, and if gas concentrations build up, a fire and explosion can occur. To make natural gas leaks more easily detectable, a harmless but smelly substance called mercaptan (also known as methyl mercaptan and methanethiol) is routinely added, giving the mixture an odor similar to rotten eggs.

Carbon monoxide (CO) is another example of a substance that has no detectible odor. CO occurs when fuels are combusted in engines, stoves, lanterns, grills, fireplaces, gas ranges, and furnaces. If the fuels are used in an enclosed area with poor ventilation, the CO can build up to dangerous levels, resulting in CO poisoning that can kill you. Common symptoms of CO poisoning include headache, dizziness, vomiting, chest pain, and confusion, and sometimes CO symptoms are described as flu-like. People who are asleep or drunk can die from CO poisoning before knowing they have symptoms. According to the Centers for Disease Control and Prevention, over 400 Americans die each year from accidental CO poisoning (excluding fires), and more than 20,000 visit emergency rooms.

The U.S. government does not regulate odors per se, but some air quality regulations reduce concentrations of pollutants that happen to be odorous. For example, sulfur dioxide gas, which has a strong, pungent odor, is regulated by a National Ambient Air Quality Standard. Additionally, many cities and local governments have nuisance codes for odors that residents find objectionable.

Richard Crume

See Also: Air Pollution; Ambient Air Quality; Concentrated Animal Feeding Operations, Pollution from; Respiratory Disease and Air Pollution

Further Reading

Agency for Toxic Substances and Disease Registry. *Environmental Odors*. http://www.atsdr.cdc.gov/odors/index.html (accessed June 24, 2016).

Centers for Disease Control and Prevention. *Carbon Monoxide Poisoning*. http://www.cdc.gov/co (accessed June 24, 2016).

McGinley, Charles M., Michael A. McGinley, and Donna L. McGinley. "'Odor Basics,' Understanding and Using Odor Testing." *Twenty-Second Annual Hawaii Water Environment Association Conference* (June 2000), http://www.fivesenses.com/Documents/Library/33%20%20Odor%20Basics.pdf.

Public Broadcasting Service. *NovaNext: Why We're Good at Identifying Smells, But Horrible at Describing Them*. http://www.pbs.org/wgbh/nova/next/body/good-identifying-smells-horrible-describing.

Reference Guide to Odor Thresholds for Hazard Air Pollutants Listed in the Clean Air Act Amendments of 1990 (EPA/600/R-92/047). Research Triangle Park, NC: U.S. Environmental Protection Agency, 1992.

OIL SPILLS, HEALTH CONSEQUENCES OF

Oil spills have provided some of the worst man-made disasters in history, resulting in devastating impacts on human health and the environment. While many of the oil spills making headlines are offshore, a number of oil spills have also occurred on land. But regardless of where the oil spill occurs, the potential exists for harmful human health effects. While workers and volunteers who respond to spills and assist in the cleanup are at greatest risk, the surrounding population may also be threatened with adverse health consequences, depending on the extent of the spill and the nature of the exposure.

Oil spills can generally be grouped into two different categories: accidental and deliberate. Accidental spills often occur during the storage, handling, and transportation of oil. Many of the well-known oil spill disasters, such as the *Exxon Valdez* oil spill, happened during transportation over ocean waters, but oil spills also occur on land from pipelines and storage tanks. A common example of a storage-related spill is a gasoline leak from an underground storage tank at an automobile

World's Worst Oil Spill

The world's worst oil spill occurred during the 1991 Gulf War as Iraqi forces retreating from Kuwait set fire to oil wells and opened oil rig and pipeline valves to try to slow advancing American troops, releasing 252 to 336 million gallons (0.95 to 1.27 million cubic meters) of oil into the Persian Gulf. The resulting oil slick covered an area about the size of the island of Hawaii. In contrast to other oil spills, this incident was a *deliberate* wartime act. On the other hand, the 2010 Deepwater Horizon explosion and subsequent oil leak, releasing 134 million gallons (0.51 million cubic meters) into the Gulf of Mexico, is world's largest *accidental* oil spill.

fueling station. Depending on how old the gasoline storage tanks are and how long they have been underground, these tanks can leak gasoline into the surrounding soil and even contaminate groundwater. Accidental oil spills can also happen from routine maintenance activities, such as cleaning ships and trucks, and from offshore drilling operations. These types of spills are often caused by carelessness, negligence, or recklessness by those responsible for the oil at various stages of its production and sale.

In contrast to accidental oil spills, deliberate spills are purposeful releases of oil into the environment by a polluter. Two examples of deliberate oil spills are discharges of oil from ships in international waters, where the enforcement of international oil pollution laws is difficult, and from automobile service stations, where oil may be discharged directly into drains and sewers. While accidental oil spills, particularly large releases by offshore oil tankers, typically receive the most attention in the press, deliberate oil spills by industries and even individuals (e.g., disposing of automobile or lawnmower oil down the sewer drain) account for much more of the oil discharged into the environment globally.

Oil is also released into the environment from natural sources. For example, crude oil and natural gas, which occur naturally underground, often seep into both marine and terrestrial environments from cracks and fissures in the ground. However, such releases generally pale in comparison to the accidental and deliberate releases described previously.

The severity of an oil spill, the resulting cleanup effort, and the impact on human health all depend, in part, on the type of oil that spilled. Oil is characterized by its viscosity (a measure of a substance's resistance to flow) and volatility (a measure of how quickly a substance evaporates). Heavy crude oils typically have a high viscosity and low volatility, meaning that they move and evaporate very slowly. Conversely, light oils, such as gasoline or jet fuel, have a very low viscosity and high volatility, meaning that they move and evaporate quickly. Very heavy crude oils, such as Fuel Oil No. 6, which is used in industrial processes and power plants, are difficult to clean up and can cause widespread contamination along a shoreline, often coating animals and birds with a thick oily film. Because heavy oils biodegrade and weather slowly, they have a high risk of causing severe health effects. The medium and light oils also pose significant risks, but their cleanup can be more effective if done efficiently and quickly. Very light oils, like gasoline, are toxic to the environment and difficult to cleanup, but due to their high viscosity, they will evaporate in just a few days.

Once an oil spill has occurred, a number of methods can be used to respond to, clean up, and remediate the spill. If an oil spill was caused by an accident at an oil tanker at sea, booms are often deployed to contain the oil slick. (Booms are floating barriers that prevent the oil from spreading.) Skimmers (boats that skim or collect oil from the surface) can be used to remove oil from the water, or the oil can be set on fire and burned away. Burning is a safe and efficient way for removing oil from the water, although the technique results in air pollution. Dispersants can also be used on oil spills to help decompose the oil into smaller particles so that microorganisms such as bacteria can more efficiently break down the oil. This process also causes the oil particles to sink, which prevents the oil from washing up on coasts and inflicting more damage to coastal ecosystems. Dispersants were widely used in the Deepwater Horizon oil spill in 2010.

For oil spills that reach a coastline, sorbents are often used in coastal areas that skimmers cannot reach. Sorbents are insoluble (will not dissolve in water), oleophilic (oil-attracting), and hydrophobic (water-repellent) materials that both *absorb* and *adsorb* the oil. Sorbents absorb by drawing the oil into the material itself, much like a sponge absorbing water. Sorbents adsorb oil by attracting it to the sorbent surface, like a magnet. Other cleanup methods include vacuuming the oil, washing the oil with high-pressure or low-pressure hoses, and removing contaminated soil from the site. Deciding which method to use depends on numerous variables, such as the weather, type of oil, area of contamination, soil type, and local ecology.

The severity of the health effects associated with an oil spill is related to the amount of exposure to the oil and the specific type of oil. The contaminants found in oil that pose the most severe health risks to humans are polycyclic aromatic hydrocarbons, volatile organic compounds, and heavy metals. Many of these contaminants are carcinogenic and have the potential to disrupt important physiological systems, such as the endocrine and immune systems. Many oil spill health studies target cleanup workers and volunteers who may come into direct contact with the oil. Additionally, the general population may also be at risk during an oil spill by breathing contaminated air, contacting skin with oil, and consuming contaminated food and water. Acute effects can include dermal irritation, respiratory discomfort, nausea, vomiting, light-headedness, and headaches. The vast majority of acute effects are experienced by workers and volunteers who are directly involved with the cleanup. Some studies of workers and volunteers have documented altered blood profiles and liver function.

Other studies have documented psychological effects in the years following an oil spill. For example, one study involving the *Exxon Valdez* oil spill found that those who had high exposure to the contamination were 3.6 times more likely to suffer from general anxiety disorder and 2.9 times more likely to suffer from posttraumatic stress disorder. A similar trend was also observed following the Deepwater Horizon oil spill.

Adverse health effects can be caused not only by the oil spill itself but also by how the cleanup is conducted. For example, in situ burning releases harmful toxins and particulate matter into the air that can cause respiratory discomfort. While the consequences of dispersant exposure are not fully understood, questions have been raised about the safety of these chemicals. While more research is needed, most scientists believe that the health risks posed by an oil spill can be severe and have the potential to cause significant harm, particularly to those who participate in the response and cleanup efforts.

Anthony G. Papetti

See Also: Deepwater Horizon Incident; Disaster Preparedness and Response; Fish Consumption Advisories; Ocean Dumping and the Pacific Garbage Patch; Water Pollution

Further Reading

Grattan, Lynn M., et al. "The Early Psychological Impacts of the Deepwater Horizon Oil Spill on Florida and Alabama Communities." *Environmental Health Perspectives*, vol. 119, no. 6 (June 2011) 838–843.

National Oceanic and Atmospheric Administration. *How Do Spills Happen?* http://response.restoration.noaa.gov/training-and-education/education-students-and-teachers/how-do-spills-happen.html (accessed March 13, 2016).

National Oceanic and Atmospheric Administration. *Oil Types*. http://response.restoration.noaa.gov/oil-and-chemical-spills/oil-spills/oil-types.html (accessed March 13, 2016).

Oil Spills, What Is Oil Used For, and How Much Do We Use? (Fact Sheet). Saskatoon, Canada: Safe Drinking Water Foundation, n.d.

Solomon, Gina M., and Sarah Janssen. "Commentary: Health Effects of the Gulf Oil Spill." *Journal of the American Medical Association*, vol. 304, no. 10 (September 2010): 1118–1119.

UN Environmental Programme (Global Marine Oil Pollution Information Gateway). *Facts on Marine Oil Pollution*. http://oils.gpa.unep.org/facts/facts.htm (accessed March 13, 2016).

U.S. Environmental Protection Agency. *Sorbents*. http://www.epa.gov/emergency-response/sorbents (accessed March 13, 2016).

ONE HEALTH

Environmental and human health are inextricably connected, and a comprehensive understanding of emerging health issues in human populations requires analysis of both the human and environmental aspects. For example, urbanization of formerly unpopulated areas has increased contact between humans and wild animals, offering more opportunities for diseases to hop from animals to humans. About 75 percent of emerging infectious diseases are now zoonotic (transferred between animals and people), resulting in the beginnings of a public health crisis. To understand these diseases and their impact, we cannot solely focus on human health. One Health is a collaborative effort that hinges on the idea that human, animal, plant, and ecosystem health are all interdependent—that when considering the health challenges of a population, we must also consider how that population interacts with its ecosystem. This approach requires systems thinking and coordinated actions to solve and to prevent health problems at the local, national, and global scale.

The One Health approach integrates multiple disciplines, sectors, and scales. While this may be challenging, the increasing pressures of pollution, disease, food and water security, poverty, conflict, and extreme weather have motivated agencies and organizations to launch One Health initiatives. This can be observed at various levels of training and research. For example, human and veterinary medical colleges are enhancing curricula with One Health training, and researchers are working at landscape scales to benefit the people and animals who live there.

This integration helps us understand, prevent, and treat conditions common to both people and animals, including cancer, heart disease, and diabetes.

While the label is new, the idea of One Health has been around since the 19th century. Rudolph Virchow (1821–1902), Louis Pasteur (1822–1895), William Osler (1849–1919), Rachel Carson (1907–1964), and Calvin Schwabe (1927–2006) all wrote about connections between health and environmental conditions. However, the concept has gained significant momentum in recent years. Veterinary and human medical colleges are increasingly engaged in One Health research and conservation medicine. Public health agencies at the federal level are also leading One Health efforts. Agencies with active One Health programs include the Centers for Disease Control and Prevention, National Institute for Environmental Health Sciences, Department of Agriculture, and Geological Survey.

One Health is also gaining traction globally. The One Health Commission, formed in 2009, serves as a world health network, linking multiple disciplines and sectors and promoting a shared One Health agenda. Since 2010, the International One Health Congress has been held biannually at various locations, with topical discussions on the intersection of health with peace, shelter, education, food, income, and social well-being. This conversation is particularly relevant for underserved, subsistence cultures, where people live off the land in close proximity to domestic animals and wildlife. The One Health approach hopes to advance research and projects that help people in subsistence cultures to improve health, overcome poverty, reduce wildlife conflicts, and preserve ecosystems.

Progress will require breaking down barriers to implementation, including academic traditions of tenure and specialization, isolation within government agencies, international language barriers, and lack of specific funding allocations. Despite these hurdles, the One Health approach presents a potential strategy for collaboratively addressing the growing pressures on human, animal, and environmental health.

Gwen Griffith

See Also: Carson, Rachel; Centers for Disease Control and Prevention; Infectious Diseases; National Institute of Environmental Health Sciences; Zoonotic Diseases

Further Reading

Aguirre, Alonso A., et al. "One Health-Transdisciplinary Opportunities for SETAC Leadership in Integrating and Improving Health of People, Animals, and the Environment." *Environmental Toxicology and Chemistry*, vol. 35, no. 10 (October 2016): 2383–2391.

American Association of Veterinary Medical Colleges. *One Health: Promoting a One Health Approach to Global Wellbeing*. http://www.aavmc.org/Strategic-Plan/One-Health.aspx (accessed April 29, 2017).

Centers for Disease Control and Prevention. *One Health*. http://www.cdc.gov/onehealth (accessed April 29, 2017).

Mackenzie, John S., et al. *One Health: The Human-Animal-Environment Interfaces in Emerging Infectious Diseases*. Berlin, Germany: Springer, 2016.

One Health Commission. *Home Page.* https://www.onehealthcommission.org (accessed April 29, 2017).

Wendee, Nicole. "Seeing the Forest for the Trees: How 'One Health' Connects Humans, Animals, and Ecosystems." *Environmental Health Perspectives*, vol. 122, no. 5 (May 2014): A122–A129.

OPEN BURNING OF WASTE

Open burning of waste is the combustion of discarded material in various environments that are not enclosed. Typically, the material being combusted is household or commercial waste, including yard waste and items such as paper, cardboard, plastic, and construction debris. Open waste combustion often occurs in barrels, open pits, outdoor stoves and fireplaces, and fields. Burning waste is common in rural areas and can be an effective waste management tool when completed in an appropriate enclosed burn unit, such as an incinerator. Improper burning can result in wildfires and increased pollution. Open burning is typically not recommended because it is harder to contain and control.

Under ideal burning conditions, adequate mixing of fuel (i.e., waste) and air occurs over a sufficient time period to ensure the waste fully burns. This situation minimizes the quantity and toxicity of combustion by-products. Lack of adequate mixing results in incomplete combustion, which can produce toxic chemicals that pose health risks to those exposed to the fumes. The release of these toxic chemicals can have an especially adverse impact on people with sensitive respiratory systems as well as on children and the elderly. Many of these toxic chemicals can also end up in the ash that is left behind from open burning. These constituents can leach into the soil, where they are adsorbed by plants or deposited into streams, lakes, and ponds.

Some of the pollutants contained in the smoke and fumes from open burning of waste can include:

- Carbon Monoxide: a product of the incomplete combustion of trash. Carbon monoxide is a colorless, odorless gas that prevents oxygen from being absorbed by the blood and lungs. It is especially dangerous when breathed by young children with immature lungs, the elderly, and people with chronic heart conditions or lung disease.
- Dioxin: one of the most harmful pollutants released during the burning of trash. Dioxin is a known carcinogen and associated with birth defects. It can be inhaled directly or deposited on soil, water, and crops, where it becomes part of the food chain.
- Hexachlorobenzene: a highly persistent toxin that degrades slowly in the air and can travel long distances in the atmosphere. It bioaccumulates in fish, marine animals, birds, lichens, and animals that feed on fish and lichens. Hexachlorobenzene is a probable human carcinogen and may damage a developing fetus, lead to kidney and liver damage, and cause fatigue and skin irritation.
- Formaldehyde: a product of combusting pressed wood products, paints, coatings, siding, urea-formaldehyde foam, and fiberglass insulation. Exposure to formaldehyde can result in watery eyes, a burning sensation in the eyes and throat, nausea, difficulty in breathing (e.g., coughing, chest tightness, and wheezing), and skin rashes. Prolonged exposure to formaldehyde may cause cancer.

- Hydrogen Chloride Gas: or hydrochloric acid, a by-product of burning polyvinyl chloride plastic. Hydrogen chloride can cause fluid buildup in the lungs and ulceration of the respiratory tract.
- Visible Smoke: tiny particles (particulates) that occur due to incomplete combustion. Smoke often contains toxic pollutants, and if inhaled, these microscopic particles can reach deep into the lungs and remain there for months to years. Breathing particulates increases the chances of respiratory infection, can trigger asthma attacks, and causes problems like coughing, wheezing, chest pain, and shortness of breath.

Virtually all state and many local agencies have developed rules prohibiting open burning or restricting the types of materials that can be burned under unenclosed environmental conditions. To complement these rules, some agencies require that individuals and organizations obtain permits prior to burning solid waste. Some agencies also conduct awareness training and outreach on the deployment of less impactful alternatives. For example, when it comes to managing fallen leaves, state and local agencies encourage residents to mulch leaves into the lawn with a mower, or alternatively, to compost them in their backyards or through an organics collection program.

The quantity of open waste burning can be reduced when both household and commercial entities implement waste minimization and pollution prevention practices. Some basic principles include:

- Reduce: Avoid disposable items. Buy products in bulk instead of individually wrapped or single-serving sizes. Buy durable products and products that can be recharged, repaired, or refilled.
- Reuse: Donate items you no longer need, such as clothing, furniture, books, magazines, and toys. Mend and repair items rather than discarding or replacing them.
- Recycle: Separate the recyclable items from your garbage for collection or drop-off at a local recycling depot.
- Compost: Install a backyard compost bin for composting your kitchen and yard waste, and if available, participate in your community's organics collection program.
- Dispose: Put your garbage out for collection or take it to your local landfill.

Richard F. Pandullo

See Also: Dioxin Pollution; Formaldehyde; Hazardous Air Pollutants; Persistent, Bioaccumulating, and Toxic Chemicals; Pollution Prevention; Respiratory Disease and Air Pollution; Three Rs of Waste Management

Further Reading

U.S. Environmental Protection Agency. *Requirements and Regulations for Open Burning and Fire Training*. https://www.epa.gov/large-scale-residential-demolition/requirements-and-regulations-open-burning-and-fire-training (accessed May 7 2017).

Wiedinmyer, C., R. J. Yokelson, and B. K. Gullett. "Global Emissions of Trace Gases, Particulate Matter, and Hazardous Air Pollutants from Open Burning of Domestic Waste." *Environmental Science and Technology*, vol. 48, no. 16 (August 2014): 9523–9530.

Wisconsin Department of Natural Resources. *Open Burning*. http://dnr.wi.gov/topic/Open Burning (accessed May 7 2017).

ORGANIC AGRICULTURE

Organic agriculture is a food production method that helps protect the health of humans, animals, and the farmed land by using practices that conserve the diversity of life and promote ecological well-being. It focuses on the long-term view of promoting human health and the environment through sustainable farming methods.

The demand for organic agriculture has been increasing as public awareness grows of the possible risks of traditional farming methods to human health, biodiversity, and ecological systems. Since the dawn of the organic agriculture industry nearly three decades ago, the demand for organic food has grown faster than supply, with sales increasing 20 percent annually.

There are many common organic agricultural practices, including crop rotation, the use of natural pest control methods in place of chemical pesticides, and avoidance of growth hormones and antibiotics when caring for farm animals. Many studies indicate that organic agriculture produces food with fewer pesticide residues and higher nutritional value—more essential amino acids, vitamins, and minerals.

Organic agricultural practices are more sustainable over time. Because the practices take a long-term view of overall soil health, organic farming alters the environment much more slowly than conventional farming practices, and it does so in a way that minimized damage to the local ecology. Organic practices help to prevent disease while producing hardier plants without the need for genetic modification to resist certain pesticides.

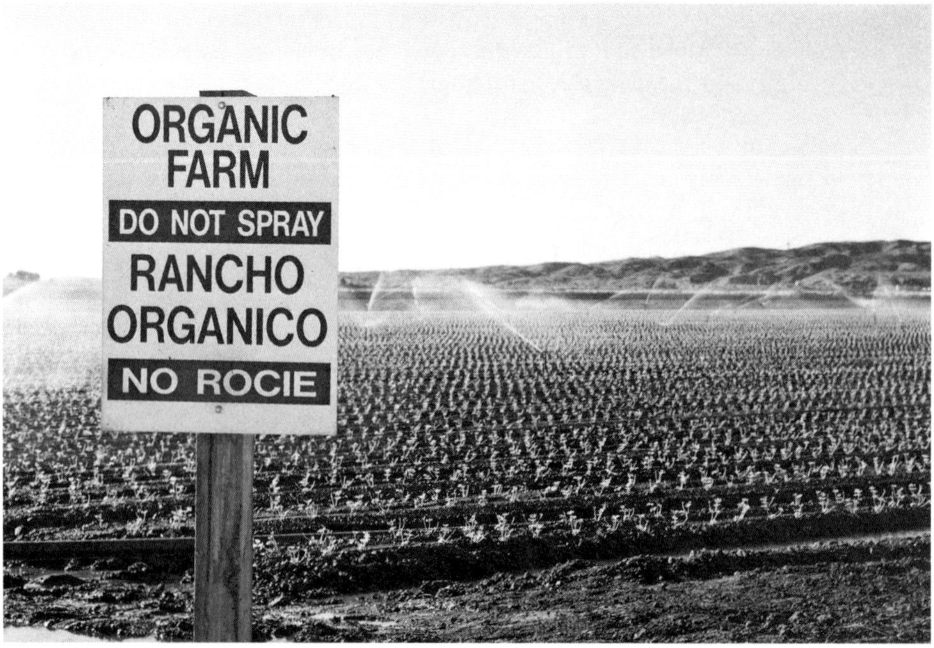

A sign identifying an organic farm and warning against spraying of pesticides. Organic farming uses sustainable farming methods that conserve the diversity of life and promote ecological well-being. (Elswarro/Dreamstime.com)

In addition to direct benefits to plants, organic methods for farming positively impact the environment surrounding the organic farm. For example, stormwater runoff has fewer pesticides and other chemicals, and pollination methods, crop rotation, soil conditioning, and other practices work to minimize harm to the ecosystem.

Organic animal agricultural practices focus on the welfare of the animal by avoiding antibiotics and growth hormones, providing a more humane living environment, and ensuring animals are fed healthy diets. These practices protect animals from cruelty, avoid contamination of meat products with antibiotics and drug-resistant bacteria, and keep the environment free of chemicals.

Studies have demonstrated that biodiversity within a farm and the surrounding area increases when organic agricultural practices are used. This increase in biodiversity includes more types of foliage and animals, as habitat and species diversity improve compared with similar conventional agricultural sites.

In 2015, there were 2.4 million organic farmers globally, an increase of over 7 percent from the previous year, and the United States continues leading the world in organic product production. While there is debate over the ability of sustainable and organic agricultural practices to produce adequate food supplies for the nation (particularly for grain production), increasing funding for research is helping organic farmers improve practices and increase yields.

Ronda Bowen

See Also: Food Supply, Environmental Threats to; Genetic Engineering and GMOs; Intensive Farming Practices and Health; Pesticides and Herbicides; Stormwater Runoff

Further Reading

Gabriel, Doreen, et al. "Food Production vs. Biodiversity: Comparing Organic and Conventional Agriculture." *Journal of Applied Ecology*, vol. 50, no. 2 (April 2013): 355–364.

Obach, Brian K. *Organic Struggle: The Movement for Sustainable Agriculture in the United States*. Cambridge: Massachusetts Institute of Technology Press, 2015.

Reganold, John P., and Jonathan M. Wachter. "Organic Agriculture in the Twenty-First Century." *Nature Plants*, vol. 2, no. 15221 (February 2016).

Sustainable Agriculture Research and Education. *What Is Organic Farming?* http://www.sare.org/Learning-Center/Bulletins/Transitioning-to-Organic-Production/Text-Version/What-is-Organic-Farming (accessed May 2, 2017).

U.S. Department of Agriculture. *Introduction to Organic Practices.* https://www.ams.usda.gov/publications/content/introduction-organic-practices (accessed May 2, 2017).

OZONE AND SMOG IN THE URBAN ENVIRONMENT

Smog is a type of air pollution that is found in many metropolitan areas and sometimes in rural areas. It consists primarily of a pollutant called ozone, which can adversely affect human health. Smog is also composed of several other air pollutants, including nitrogen oxides (NOx), sulfur dioxide, carbon monoxide, volatile organic compounds (VOCs), and small particles. These pollutants are caused by industrial operations and by electric power plants that burn coal, oil, or natural gas. Additionally, they are found in the exhausts of motor vehicles, such as automobiles, trucks, and buses, that are powered with gasoline or diesel fuel.

Good Ozone, and Bad

The ground-level ozone in polluted metropolitan areas is often referred to as the *bad* ozone because breathing it can cause adverse health effects, like coughing, shortness of breath, chest pain, and irritation of the lungs, and it can also aggravate asthma. However, ozone also occurs in the stratosphere, which is a layer of the atmosphere about 32 miles (50 kilometers) above the earth's surface. Stratospheric ozone is often referred to as the *good* ozone because it helps block harmful ultraviolet radiation from the sun.

Ozone, the main ingredient in smog, is not emitted directly into the air. Instead, it is formed at ground level when NOx and VOCs react in the presence of sunlight, particularly on warm summer days. The major sources of NOx and VOCs include nonnuclear power plants, motor vehicles, manufacturing facilities, chemical plants, and oil refineries. The ground-level ozone discussed here should not be confused with the ozone that occurs naturally in the stratosphere and helps shield the earth from harmful ultraviolet radiation from the sun.

Breathing ozone and the other components of smog can cause a variety of adverse health effects. In particular, ozone can irritate the respiratory system, cause chest pain, aggravate asthma, and reduce lung function. ("Lung function" is a term the medical profession uses to characterize the volume of air inhaled when taking a full breath and the speed at which the air is exhaled.) Ozone can also inflame and even damage the linings of the lungs, similar to sunburn on exposed skin. Shortness of breath and coughing on a warm day could be a sign of elevated ozone concentrations in the surrounding air.

About one of every three Americans is at a higher risk of experiencing adverse health effects due to ozone. These Americans include children, adults who are active outdoors, people with respiratory diseases, and other adults who for unknown reasons show unusual sensitivity to ozone. Children are especially at risk from ozone exposure because their lungs are still developing, they are likely to be active outdoors when ozone levels are high, and many children suffer from asthma. Ozone inhalation by older adults is also a serious concern if they already suffer from respiratory disease or spend significant time outside.

Ozone can also harm sensitive vegetation, especially during the growing season. Black cherry, quaking aspen, ponderosa pine, and cottonwood trees are notable for their sensitivity, as are certain crops. Ozone damages vegetation by entering the leaves and interfering with food production and storage. Exposure to ozone over long periods can increase the susceptibility of plants to diseases and insect damage.

According to the U.S. Environmental Protection Agency (EPA), over 50 million Americans live in areas where ozone levels exceed government standards intended to protect public health. To help the public know when levels of ozone and other pollutants are elevated, the EPA has set up a website called AirNow, which provides daily reports on air quality. Another EPA service, EnviroFlash, delivers daily e-mail alerts about air quality, with suggested safety measures when local air pollution levels are high.

Richard Crume

See Also: Air Pollution; AirNow and the Air Quality Index; Ambient Air Quality; Asthma; Children's Environmental Health; Crops and Vegetation, Air Pollution Damage to; Environmental Protection Agency; Respiratory Disease and Air Pollution; Stratospheric Ozone Depletion; Volatile Organic Compound Pollution

Further Reading

Godish, Thad, Wayne T. Davis, and Joshua S. Fu. *Air Quality*. 5th ed. Boca Raton, FL: CRC Press, 2014.

Seinfeld, John H., and Spyros N. Pandis. *Atmospheric Chemistry and Physics: From Air Pollution to Climate Change*. 3rd ed. Hoboken, NJ: John Wiley and Sons, 2016.

U.S. Environmental Protection Agency. *AirNow: Ozone Facts*. https://www.airnow.gov/index.cfm?action=ozone_facts.index (accessed May 19, 2016).

U.S. Environmental Protection Agency. *Ozone Pollution*. www.epa.gov/ozone-pollution (accessed May 19, 2016).

Vallero, Daniel. *Fundamentals of Air Pollution*. 5th ed. Cambridge, MA: Academic Press, 2014.

P

PARKINSON'S DISEASE AND ENVIRONMENTAL EXPOSURE

Parkinson's disease is a neurodegenerative disease believed to be caused by the interaction of genes and the environment. People with Parkinson's disease experience a loss of neurons in the midbrain, resulting in a reduction of dopamine, a neurotransmitter responsible for coordinating muscle movement with other parts of the brain. The disease progresses more rapidly in some patients than in others, and while some patients may become severely disabled, the disease may cause only minor motor interferences in others. People with Parkinson's disease generally have a shorter life expectancy compared with the general population.

Because there are no blood or laboratory tests to confirm the presence of Parkinson's disease, the rate of misdiagnosis may be relatively high. Nevertheless, it is estimated that at least one-half to one million Americans have Parkinson's disease, and the prevalence of the disease is increasing as the population ages. The disease can be found among all races, ethnic groups, nationalities, and income levels.

The symptoms of Parkinson's disease include tremors (trembling in the hands, arms, legs, jaw, and face), rigidity (stiffness of limbs and trunk), bradykinesia (slowness of movement), and instability (problems with balance and coordination). As these symptoms worsen, patients may have difficulty walking, talking, and completing simple tasks. Patients may also experience a poor sense of smell, constipation, depression, cognitive impairment, and fatigue, and these symptoms may occur years before motor problems become evident.

Michael J. Fox Battles Parkinson's

Michael J. Fox, a popular professional actor appearing in award-winning theater and television shows, was diagnosed with young-onset Parkinson's disease in 1991. As his symptoms became more severe, he stopped acting in 2000 and launched The Michael J. Fox Foundation for Parkinson's Research. The foundation is the largest nonprofit funder of drug development for Parkinson's disease and "the most credible voice on Parkinson's research in the world," according to the *New York Times*. Finding he could control his symptoms with drug treatments, Fox returned to acting in 2012, playing various roles, including a character with Parkinson's disease. Fox has received several lifetime achievement awards for acting as well as numerous honorary degrees and humanitarian awards, and he is the best-selling author of three books.

The causes of Parkinson's disease are unknown despite many years of study and research. It is possible that the disease is primarily caused by genetic factors in some people and by illness or environmental toxins in others. It is known that age is a factor, with people over 60 years old at greater risk of developing the disease. It is also believed that most Parkinson's cases are not directly inherited. At present, there is no cure for the disease, although medications can lessen the severity of symptoms. In cases where the patient does not respond well to medications, surgery may be appropriate (e.g., implanting electrodes, connected to a pulse generator, into the brain). By understanding what causes the loss of dopamine-producing cells, many researchers are optimistic about finding treatments to slow down or even reverse the disease.

While most scientists believe that Parkinson's is caused by interaction between a person's genetic makeup and the environment, this interaction is quite complex and poorly understood. Some environmental factors may increase the risk of Parkinson's disease, while others decrease the risk, and the same may be said for genetic makeup. The research challenge has been to identify the combinations of environmental factors and genetic makeup that cause the disease.

Some evidence of an association with Parkinson's disease has been found for the following potential risk factors: age (about 1 percent of people over age 60 have Parkinson's disease), gender (it is more common in men than women), history of traumatic brain injury, the geographical area where one lives, occupation, and genetic predisposition. There may also be an association with exposure to solvents, polychlorinated biphenyls (PCBs), and certain pesticides, herbicides, fungicides, and metals, which is of particular interest to the environmental health field because these are all common environmental pollutants. However, presently there is no conclusive evidence that environmental factors acting alone can actually cause Parkinson's disease.

In addition to the factors associated with an increased risk of Parkinson's disease, there are also factors associated with a reduced risk of the disease. These potential protective factors include drinking coffee and tea, certain fats in a person's diet, higher levels of uric acid in blood, use of anti-inflammatory drugs, cigarette smoking (nicotine may be a factor), higher vitamin D levels, and regular exercise. However, as with the potential risk factors, more research is needed to assess these potential protective factors, and you should always consult a medical professional before taking any steps to prevent Parkinson's disease or slow its progression.

Richard Crume

See Also: Heavy Metal Pollution; Neurotoxicants; Pesticides and Herbicides; Polychlorinated Biphenyls

Further Reading

Aschner, Michael, and Lucio G. Costa. *Environmental Factors in Neurodevelopmental and Neurodegenerative Disorders*. Amsterdam, the Netherlands: Elsevier/Academic Press, 2015.

Mayo Clinic. *Diseases and Conditions: Parkinson's Disease*. http://www.mayoclinic.org/diseases-conditions/parkinsons-disease/basics/definition/con-20028488 (accessed October 26, 2016).

The Michael J. Fox Foundation for Parkinson's Research. *Purpose. Partnership. Progress.* https://www.michaeljfox.org (accessed October 26, 2016).

National Institute of Neurological Disorders and Stroke. *NINDS Parkinson's Disease Information Page*. http://www.ninds.nih.gov/disorders/parkinsons_disease/parkinsons_disease.htm (accessed October 28, 2016).

Noceranov, Joe. "Taking Science Personally." *New York Times*, November 10, 2008, http://www.nytimes.com/2008/11/11/giving/11SICK.html.

Pahwa, Rajesh, and Kelly E. Lyons. *Handbook of Parkinson's Disease*. London: CRC Press, 2013.

Stetka, Bret. "Parkinson's Disease and Pesticides: What's the Connection?" *Scientific American* (April 2014). https://www.scientificamerican.com/article/parkinsons-disease-and-pesticides-whats-the-connection.

Weiner, William J., Lisa M. Shulman, and Anthony E. Lang. *Parkinson's Disease: A Complete Guide for Patients and Families*. Baltimore, MD: Johns Hopkins University Press, 2013.

PARTICULATE MATTER AND BIOAEROSOLS POLLUTION

Particulate matter is defined as solid and liquid particles suspended in the air. These particles can be generated directly through emissions from cars and factories or indirectly through chemical reactions of pollutants in the atmosphere. Once particulate matter has entered the body through inhalation, it can cause disease in a variety of ways. Additionally, fine particulate matter (particles with a diameter of less than 2.5 microns) is the primary cause of reduced visibility (i.e., haze) in many areas of the United States. Particulate matter pollution is regulated by the Environmental Protection Agency, which sets standards to reduce particulate matter emissions and improve the air quality.

Particulate matter is classified into three categories: PM_{10}, $PM_{2.5}$, and $PM_{0.1}$. The subscripts refer to the maximum diameter of particles in each class in microns. PM_{10}, $PM_{2.5}$, and $PM_{0.1}$ are often referred to as coarse, fine, and ultrafine particulate matter, respectively. Each size class necessarily includes those smaller than it—that is, $PM_{2.5}$ includes $PM_{0.1}$, and PM_{10} includes $PM_{2.5}$ and $PM_{0.1}$. Damage from inhalation of particulate matter depends on the size of the particles. Larger particles can lodge in the respiratory tract and cause inflammatory reactions. Fine and ultrafine particulate matter can lodge deep in the lungs and cause respiratory disease and other serious medical problems.

Bioaerosols are organic molecules that have been aerosolized in the environment and contribute to both indoor and outdoor pollution. Types of bioaerosols include bacteria, fungi, viruses, pollen, and endotoxins. Viable (active) bioaerosols can cause illnesses, such as the flu, tuberculosis, and smallpox. Occupational settings, like farms, slaughterhouses, and furniture factories, can subject workers to illness-causing bioaerosols, where health outcomes often depend on an individual's immune response to the bioaerosol. Nosocomial infections (hospital-acquired infections) are a huge cause of morbidity and mortality, and these are often caused by bioaerosols. Hospitals typically try to combat bioaerosols by using isolation techniques (e.g., wearing masks, gowns, and gloves). Pet dander, dust, germs, and viruses are some bioaerosols found in the home that can also cause severe reactions and illnesses.

Andrew P. Barefield

See Also: Air Pollution; AirNow and the Air Quality Index; Ambient Air Quality; Asthma; Bioterrorism; Healthcare-Associated Infections; Legionnaires' Disease; Respiratory Disease and Air Pollution

Further Reading

Bakand, Shahnaz, and Amanda Hayes. "Toxicological Considerations, Toxicity Assessment, and Risk Management of Inhaled Nanoparticles." *International Journal of Molecular Sciences*, vol. 17, no. 6 (June 2016): 1–17.

Environmental Protection Agency. *Particulate Matter (PM) Basics*. https://www.epa.gov/pm-pollution/particulate-matter-pm-basics (accessed May 7, 2017).

Gilbert, Yan, and Caroline Duchaine. "Bioaerosols in Industrial Environments: A Review." *Canadian Journal of Civil Engineering*, vol. 36, no. 12 (December 2009): 1873–1886.

Lu, Senlin, et al. "Comparison of Cellular Toxicity Caused by Ambient Ultrafine Particles and Engineered Metal Oxide Nanoparticles." *Particle and Fibre Toxicology*, vol. 12, no. 1 (March 2015).

Thurston, George D., et al. "Ambient Particulate Matter Air Pollution Exposure and Mortality in the NIH-AARP Diet and Health Cohort." *Environmental Health Perspectives*, vol. 124, no. 4 (April 2016): 484–490.

PERCHLORATE

Perchlorate is both a naturally occurring and a manufactured chemical typically found as perchloric acid, ammonium perchlorate, potassium perchlorate, or sodium perchlorate. Perchlorate can form naturally in the atmosphere, leading to low levels of perchlorate in precipitation, and high levels of perchlorate occur naturally in some areas such as west Texas and northern Chile. However, most exposure to perchlorate is not from natural sources but from manufactured sources. It is a concern to health professionals because it is ubiquitous in the environment and known to adversely affect human health.

The most common use for perchlorate today is as an oxidizer in rocket fuel, munitions, fireworks, vehicle airbag initiators, matches, and signal flares. Additionally, it is used in some disinfectants and herbicides and in some electroplating operations. Perchlorate was once used by the medical profession to treat hyperthyroidism, but that use was discontinued in the United States due to adverse health effects.

The most common route of exposure for perchlorate compounds is through the ingestion of contaminated food and water. Common foods contaminated with perchlorate are eggs, milk, fruits, and leafy green vegetables. Additionally, small amounts of perchlorate can be inhaled through contaminated soils and dust.

Because perchlorate is very soluble in water, the potential for perchlorate to contaminate groundwater and surface water is a growing concern. It is often found in drinking water and food, and it is known to interfere with thyroid gland's ability to make hormones. Perchlorate can also irritate the eyes, nose, throat, skin, and gastrointestinal tract, and inhaling ammonium perchlorate has been associated with respiratory irritation and pulmonary edema. In 2011, the U.S. Environmental Protection Agency designated perchlorate as a contaminant, thereby permitting regulation under the Safe Drinking Water Act.

Given its widespread distribution in the environment, many sites contaminated with perchlorate require remediation. Some of the common techniques for perchlorate remediation rely on ion exchange technology, bioremediation, and soil remediation. While ion exchange is most cost-effective, it is not suitable for all situations.

Elizabeth Ann Glass Geltman and Nichole LeClair

See Also: Bioremediation for Waste Treatment; Children's Environmental Health; Drinking Water Quality and Regulation; Environmental Protection Agency; Food Safety and Technology; Safe Drinking Water Act

Further Reading

California Department of Toxic Substances Control. *Perchlorate*. http://www.dtsc.ca.gov/hazardouswaste/perchlorate (accessed March 4, 2017).

Leung, Angela M., Elizabeth N. Pearce, and Lewis E. Braverman. "Environmental Perchlorate Exposure: Potential Adverse Thyroid Effects." *Current Opinion in Endocrinology, Diabetes, and Obesity*, vol. 21, no. 5 (October 2014): 372–376.

Lewandowski, Thomas A., Michael K. Peterson, and Gail Charnley. "Iodine Supplementation and Drinking-Water Perchlorate Mitigation." *Food and Chemical Toxicology*, vol. 80 (June 2015): 261–270.

National Institutes of Health. *Tox Town: Perchlorate*. https://toxtown.nlm.nih.gov/text_version/chemicals.php?id=75 (accessed March 4, 2017).

Trumpolt, Clayton W., et al. "Perchlorate: Sources, Uses, and Occurrences in the Environment." *Remediation*, vol. 16, no. 1 (December 2005): 65–89.

U.S. Environmental Protection Agency. *Perchlorate in Drinking Water*. https://www.epa.gov/dwstandardsregulations/perchlorate-drinking-water (accessed March 4, 2017).

U.S. Environmental Protection Agency. *Technical Fact Sheet—Perchlorate*. https://www.epa.gov/fedfac/technical-fact-sheet-perchlorate (accessed March 4, 2017).

PERSISTENT, BIOACCUMULATING, AND TOXIC CHEMICALS

Persistent organic pollutants (POPs) are hazardous organic (carbon-based) compounds that resist degradation. Many industrial products fall into this category. For example, incomplete combustion generates polycyclic aromatic hydrocarbons, which can enter the food chain through precipitation (rain, snow, sleet, or hail) depositing the particulate matter in soil and water. Exposure to polycyclic aromatic hydrocarbons has been strongly linked with cancer. Another common POP is polychlorinated biphenyl, which is primarily deposited in the food chain as a by-product of industrialization and can cause skin rashes, fatigue, and liver damage. Resistance to degradation means that these chemicals can accumulate in the environment, magnifying their potential effects on human health.

Health hazards posed by POPs are amplified by the phenomena of bioaccumulation and biomagnification. Bioaccumulation occurs when a POP enters the food chain more quickly than it can be removed, resulting in an accumulation of the pollutant that can lead to disease. This effect can be compounded by biomagnification, the concentration of a substance in an organism as a result of it eating other organisms that have ingested the substance. For example, mercury is a heavy metal introduced to the food chain through industrialization. This metal accumulates in water and is subsequently consumed by sea life. Bioaccumulation of this metal is concentrated in adipose (fat) tissue, and consequently, pregnant women are advised to avoid consuming fatty fish (tuna, swordfish, and shark) so that they will not ingest the mercury accumulated in the fish.

Lead is another product of industrialization that bioaccumulates. A recent epidemic of lead poisoning cases occurred in Flint, Michigan, where the city began sourcing the city's drinking water from the Flint River without using appropriate corrosion inhibitors. The pipes carrying the water from the river to the city were lined with lead, which leached into the public water supply. This resulted in lead levels of up to 13,000 parts per billion (ppb) in home water sources. (The federal limit is 15 ppb.) While the lead concentration has since returned to acceptable levels, the long-term effects, especially upon the children who were exposed to extremely high concentrations of lead, are still unknown.

Many persistent organic pollutants are endocrine disruptors (EDCs). The endocrine system is a series of glands and organs that serve as a long-range signaling system for the body by secreting hormones into the circulatory system. These hormones convey biochemical "messages" to various organs, thereby regulating processes like metabolism, development, and reproduction. An EDC is any chemical or substance that can affect the endocrine system by acting as an agonist (increasing hormonal effects), an antagonist (reducing hormonal effects), or both. EDCs often mimic the sex hormones (estrogen and testosterone). However, EDCs can also affect the thyroid, pancreas, and other organs. Furthermore, EDCs can alter the development of the reproductive tract and cause cancer later in life, and the effects of EDCs can be passed from one generation to another, depending on when they are introduced into the developmental life cycle (prenatally or before the child reaches puberty). Some schools of thought propose that obesity is the result of a perpetual cycle in which the EDCs are a causative factor of obesity, and accumulation in adipose tissue increases the effects of the EDC, resulting in further adipose tissue buildup (and, therefore, further bioaccumulation).

Andrew P. Barefield

See Also: DDT Exposure; Endocrine Disruptors; Fish Consumption Advisories; Heavy Metal Pollution; Lead Poisoning Prevention; Mercury Pollution; Polychlorinated Biphenyls; Polycyclic Aromatic Hydrocarbons

Further Reading

Proffitt, Fiona. "U.N. Convention Targets Dirty Dozen Chemicals." *Science*, vol. 304, no. 5674 (May 2004): 1093c.

U.S. Environmental Protection Agency. *Persistent Bioaccumulative Toxic (PBT) Chemicals Covered by the TRI Program*. https://www.epa.gov/toxics-release-inventory-tri-program/persistent-bioaccumulative-toxic-pbt-chemicals-covered-tri (accessed April 29, 2017).

U.S. Environmental Protection Agency Region 9. *Persistent, Bioaccumulative and Toxic Chemicals (PBTs)*. https://www3.epa.gov/region9/waste/p2/projects/pbts.html (accessed April 29, 2017).

Young, Alvin L., and Paul F. Cecil. "Agent Orange Exposure and Attributed Health Effects in Vietnam Veterans." *Military Medicine*, vol. 176, no. 7S (July 2011): 29–34.

PERSONAL CARE PRODUCTS, HEALTH ISSUES WITH

Personal care products are used to cleanse and beautify the human body. These products include shampoo and conditioner, toothpaste, soap, deodorant, lip balm, sunscreen, body lotion, hair dye, and makeup. Many of the chemicals found in personal care products have been linked to possible adverse health effects, ranging from mild allergic reactions to disruption of the endocrine system and even cancer. However, most of these concerns are not strongly supported by scientific evidence.

The Food and Drug Administration (FDA) classifies most personal care products as cosmetics, which are distinct from drugs (products that are intended to treat or prevent disease). Some personal care products are both cosmetics and drugs, such as fluoridated toothpaste, antiperspirant, dandruff shampoo, and sunscreen. These products must be labeled with their active ingredients, which must be approved by the FDA.

According to a survey by the Environmental Working Group (EWG), a consumer-safety advocacy group, the average woman uses 12 personal care products every day, the average man uses 6, and the average teenager uses 17. The EWG survey found that consumers are exposed to hundreds of unique chemicals on a daily basis from the application of these products. These chemicals can be absorbed by the skin, inhaled from sprays or powders, or ingested.

Almost any product applied to the skin can cause an allergic reaction, from mild redness and irritation to burning and itching. Manufacturers cannot guarantee that a product will or will not cause an allergic reaction, so many products carry warning labels that instruct users to first test the product on a small patch of skin. Additionally, products with fragrances can cause respiratory allergies or aggravate asthma. The label "hypoallergenic," often taken to mean the product does not cause an allergic reaction, is not regulated by the FDA.

Three chemical groups in particular are currently under scrutiny: parabens, phthalates, and triclosan. These chemicals have been widely used in personal care products for the past 40 to 50 years. Parabens in personal care products act as preservatives by preventing bacterial growth. They have been found in tissue samples of breast cancer tumors, but no study has found a direct connection between exposure to parabens and increased risk of breast cancer. Phthalates are found in some nail polishes, perfumes, lotions, and hair sprays. Various studies have linked phthalate exposure to low testosterone levels, low-quality sperm, and even obesity and insulin resistance in adult men. In 2008, Congress banned phthalates in children's toys, but they are still legal in personal care products. More than three-quarters of the U.S. population have detectable phthalates in their urine. Finally, triclosan, an antimicrobial chemical in soap and toothpaste, is thought to disrupt hormones and has been linked to weakened cardiac function. It may also promote bacterial resistance to medicine. Additionally, triclosan is a persistent environmental pollutant that is toxic to aquatic life, especially algae.

Other chemicals of concern include formaldehyde, coal tar, and hydroxy acids. Formaldehyde may be found in nail polish, and it is also formed as a by-product of chemical interactions. The National Toxicology Program considers formaldehyde as a known carcinogen. Coal tar, linked to cancer, may be found in darker hair dyes. Alpha and beta hydroxy acids are applied to the skin to reduce the appearance of wrinkles, but they can increase skin sensitivity to ultraviolet rays from sunlight.

Some people believe that aluminum in antiperspirants mimics estrogen and thus increases risk for breast cancer. However, the link between antiperspirants and cancer is not supported by scientific research, according to the National Cancer Institute. In general, studies exploring the risks of chemicals in personal care products are currently limited in scope. Animal studies often show endocrine disruption after high levels of exposure to certain chemicals, but there are few conclusive studies in humans.

Not every chemical in personal care products is listed on the ingredients label. For instance, the ingredient "fragrance" may contain phthalates, which may not be listed separately. Additionally, many terms found on product labels do not have a specific definition, and terms such as "natural," "alcohol-free," and "fragrance-free" are not regulated by the FDA. If consumers wish to avoid certain chemicals, they should look for product labels that say "no phthalates" or "no parabens." Consumer-safety advocate groups like the EWG believe that regardless of whether these chemicals cause cancer, all products should be clearly labeled with their actual ingredients.

Despite the limited nature of studies on the toxic effects of chemicals in personal care products, the European Union (EU) has taken a precautionary stance. The 2013 EU Cosmetics Directive banned 1,328 ingredients that are either known or suspected to disrupt hormones or cause cancer. Hundreds of products sold in the United States contain these same chemicals (see Table 14). The EU also requires products to be approved and registered before they are sold.

In the United States, 11 chemicals are banned from cosmetics, including chlorofluorocarbons (CFCs), chloroform, mercury, and zirconium, and no chemicals have been banned since 1989. (In cosmetics, the FDA only has authority to regulate color additives in hair dyes.) The FDA does not approve products before they go to market, although manufacturers may voluntarily register their products with the Agency. Therefore, products cannot be labeled or marketed as "FDA-approved." The FDA can only recall a product if it proves harmful under the label's

Table 14. Chemicals banned in the EU by use and health concern.

Chemical	Use	Health Concern
Selenium sulfide	Dandruff shampoo	Probable carcinogen
Hydroquinone	Skin/hair bleach	Probable carcinogen
p-Phenylenediamine	Dark hair dyes	Asthma, allergic reactions
Salicylic acid	Acne treatment, preservative	Possible salicylate poisoning
Talc	Loose powder	Asbestos, possible carcinogen
Titanium dioxide	Sunscreen	Possible carcinogen when inhaled
Zinc stearate	Anticaking agent	Respiratory problems when inhaled
Lead acetate	Hair dye	Lead poisoning when ingested
Quaternium-15	Preservative	Releases formaldehyde
Triclosan	Toothpaste, antibacterial soaps	Possible endocrine disruption
Butylparaben	Preservative	Possible endocrine disruption

directions or if it is improperly labeled. In 1976, the FDA supported the creation of the Cosmetic Ingredient Review (CIR), an independent panel that evaluates personal care products. The CIR, funded by the Personal Care Products Council (an industry trade group), researches the health effects of chemicals in personal care products and recommends whether their use should continue.

Several large retail stores and manufacturers have recently decided to phase out certain chemicals from their personal care products, including triclosan, diethyl phthalate, and compounds that release formaldehyde. For example, the major retailers Target and Walmart are working in conjunction with the global manufacturing companies Procter and Gamble and Johnson and Johnson to modify certain product ingredients. This market-based regulation preempts possible future federal rulings, as industries themselves ban potentially harmful chemicals in personal care products.

Alisha K. Newton

See Also: Cancer Risk from Environmental Exposure; Chlorofluorocarbons; Consumer Product Safety Commission; Environmental Toxicology; Formaldehyde; Mercury Pollution; Nanomaterials; National Toxicology Program; Phthalates

Further Reading

Antiperspirants/Deodorants and Breast Cancer. National Cancer Institute, Bethesda, MD, 2008. http://www.cancer.gov/about-cancer/causes-prevention/risk/myths/antiperspirants-fact-sheet.

Barrett, Julia R. "Chemical Exposures: The Ugly Side of Beauty Products." *Environmental Health Perspectives*, vol. 113, no. 1 (January 2005): A24.

Chemical Widely Used in Antibacterial Hand Soaps May Impair Muscle Function. University of California-Davis Health News Service, Davis, CA, 2012. http://news.ucdavis.edu/search/news_detail.lasso?id=10301.

Clancy, Heather. "How Target and Walmart Led a Push to Make Over Makeup." *GreenBiz*, December 2015, http://www.greenbiz.com/article/how-target-and-walmart-lead-push-make-over-makeup.

Dodson, Robin E., et al. "Endocrine Disruptors and Asthma-Associated Chemicals in Consumer Products." *Environmental Health Perspectives*, vol. 120, no. 7 (July 2012): 935–943.

Food and Drug Administration. *Cosmetics*. http://www.fda.gov/Cosmetics/default.htm (accessed December 14, 2015).

Phthalates Now Linked to Fat, Related Health Risks. University of Rochester Medical Center, Rochester, NY, 2007. https://www.urmc.rochester.edu/news/story/1405/phthalates-now-linked-to-fat-related-health-risks.aspx.

PESTICIDES AND HERBICIDES

Pesticides are anthropogenic chemicals used to control or eliminate pests. Pesticides include insecticides, fungicides, herbicides, and rodenticides, and they target plant diseases, weeds, insects, rodents, and animal vectors of disease. By preventing pest-related crop loss, pesticides can improve crop yield and farm productivity. Pesticides can also prevent the spread of infectious diseases by killing, for example, disease-carrying mosquitoes. However, some pesticide ingredients are dangerous to human health and must be used carefully. The health effects of pesticides vary according to the type of pesticide and the level and duration of exposure. Pesticides can irritate eyes and skin and adversely affect the nervous and endocrine systems of the human body. Other pesticides may be carcinogens.

Dichlorodiphenyltrichloroethane (DDT) is a well-known insecticide and a persistent organic pollutant. While still used in some parts of the world, DDT was banned in the United States in 1972 when its registration was canceled by the newly formed Environmental Protection Agency. As a persistent organic pollutant, DDT has a long half-life, which means that it can survive in the environment a long time without degrading. DDT also bioaccumulates in the food chain, and storage in adipose (fatty) tissue can result in biomagnification. This causes humans and large predators to inadvertently accumulate high concentrations of DDT, with possible adverse effects on health. The degradation products of DDT, dichlorodiphenyldichloroethane (DDD) and dichlorodiphenyldichloroethylene (DDE), are also toxic. While DDT use has been banned in the United States, traces of DDT, DDD, and DDE can still be found in the environment and in human adipose tissue. DDT, DDD, and DDE are believed to cause adverse developmental, endocrine, hepatic, neurological, and reproductive effect, and they are reasonably anticipated to be human carcinogens.

One of the better known herbicide incidents involved Agent Orange, which was sprayed during the Vietnam War as a tactical defoliant (a chemical that removes the leaves from trees). Agent Orange has been associated with numerous health complaints from veterans present in the areas that were sprayed. Health effects attributed to Agent Orange include acute and subacute peripheral neuropathy, AL amyloidosis, chloracne, chronic lymphocytic leukemia, B cell leukemia, type 2 diabetes, Hodgkin's lymphoma, prostate cancer, respiratory cancers, soft tissue sarcomas, Parkinson's disease, and spina bifida in offspring. The Veterans Administration alerts veterans to possible long-term health effects related to Agent Orange exposure during military service, and it offers eligible veterans a free health assessment for health issues related to their exposure.

Andrew P. Barefield

See Also: Children's Environmental Health; DDT Exposure; Endocrine Disruptors; Environmental Protection Agency; Environmental Toxicology; Zika Virus

Further Reading

Agency for Toxic Substances and Disease Registry. *DDT, DDE, DDD.* https://www.atsdr.cdc.gov/substances/toxsubstance.asp?toxid=20 (accessed May 7, 2017).

Ahmed, G., et al. "Environmental Assessment of Fate, Transport, and Persistent Behavior of Dichlorodiphenyltrichloroethanes and Hexachlorocyclohexanes in Land and Water Ecosystems." *International Journal of Environmental Science and Technology*, vol. 12, no. 8 (April 2015): 2741–2756.

Blair, Aaron, et al. "Pesticides and Human Health." *Occupational and Environmental Medicine*, vol. 72, no. 2 (February 2015): 81–82.

Conis, Elena. "Debating the Health Effects of DDT: Thomas Jukes, Charles Wurster, and the Fate of an Environmental Pollutant." *Public Health Reports,* vol. 125, no. 2 (March 2010): 337–342.

"Eat the Peach, Not the Pesticide: A Shopper's Guide." *Consumer Reports*, vol. 80, no. 5 (March 2015): 29–32.

U.S. Department of Veterans Affairs. *Agency Orange*. https://www.publichealth.va.gov/exposures/agentorange (accessed May 7, 2017).

U.S. Environmental Protection Agency. *Pesticides*. https://www.epa.gov/pesticides (accessed May 7, 2017).

PHARMACEUTICALS IN THE ENVIRONMENT

Human and animal health greatly benefited from the development of pharmaceutical and personal care products, collectively known as PPCPs. Pharmaceuticals are natural or synthetic compounds used to treat illness and promote wellness. The most common examples include antibiotics, antidepressants, analgesics (pain killers), hormone therapies, and lipid regulators. Their production is regulated for safety and effectiveness in people and animals but not for their presence in the environment. With growing populations and increasing use of human and veterinary medications, the release of pharmaceutical compounds into the environment has become a significant concern.

Pharmaceutical chemicals and their metabolic by-products are now being found in the waters of cities around the world, including surface water, groundwater, and treated drinking water, as well as some soils and food products. In addition to medications, there is a growing list of personal care products entering the environment with natural or synthetic active ingredients that induce biologic effects. The expanding array of these products includes soaps, shampoos, moisturizers, cosmetics, nutritional supplements, fragrances, bug repellant, and sunscreens.

What Is Triclosan?

Triclosan is one example of a ubiquitous bioactive compound found in many personal care products. It is recognized as one of many emerging contaminants that is detectable but not regulated in the environment. Triclosan is best known as the antibacterial ingredient in many hand soaps. Originally created for surgical scrubs in the 1940s, it has since been incorporated into a long list of products, including hand sanitizers, toothpastes, body washes, cosmetics, deodorants, and even countertops, textiles, and kitchenware. At one point, triclosan was present in 76 percent of liquid and 29 percent of bar soaps in the United States. Laboratory studies showed triclosan to be an endocrine disrupter with adverse effects on frogs and rats. In September 2016, the U.S. Food and Drug Administration (FDA) recognized triclosan and 18 other antibacterial compounds in soaps as being unnecessary and potentially dangerous, and the FDA issued a ban of those 19 substances, giving companies one year to remove the chemicals or take their products off the market. The ban applies only to hand soaps, so other products may continue to include this and other antibacterial compounds under the current rules.

As with medications, these active ingredients in personal care products are emerging contaminants of concern. Yet, they too are not commonly monitored or regulated in the environment. The release of this plethora of chemical compounds into the environment poses potential health risks to people, wildlife, and ecosystems. Allergic reactions, increases in antibiotic-resistant bacteria, and disruptions to hormonal systems are all possible. Adverse effects to ecological systems are also a major concern, with effects on fish and aquatic organisms already being detected in many cities around the world.

Pharmaceuticals are designed to have an effect on the body at the lowest possible dose and to persist so that their medical benefits last as long as possible. These are good qualities in the body, but they become a problem when these chemicals enter the environment, where they can have a persistent effect on animals and ecosystems even at very low concentrations.

The most commonly detected pharmaceuticals in waters are human and veterinary medications, including antibiotics, estrogenic steroids (e.g., oral contraceptives and hormone therapies), antidepressants, and chemotherapy agents. However, there are many other unregulated compounds that are being released into the environment, and we do not yet know their effects. The study of emerging contaminants is a burgeoning new field of research working to determine what and where these chemicals are, their potential for harmful effects on people and nature, and how to reduce those negative consequences.

The same is true for the compounds in hundreds of personal care products, which end up in the wastewater stream after they are washed down the drain from sinks, tubs, washing machines, and many other sources. The highest concentrations of these compounds in nature are found downstream of the discharge pipes of municipal wastewater treatment plants. These waters continue downstream and become the source for human drinking water for the next city. Drinking water treatment plants usually reduce the concentrations of these chemicals, but they rarely remove 100 percent. Trace levels have been found to persist in up to 30 percent of public drinking water sources.

Another important source of environmental release is the improper disposal of unused or expired medications or supplements, either by flushing or as leachate that leaks into the groundwater from municipal landfills. Manufacturing facilities for drugs or personal care products are also significant sources of PPCPs in the environment. This is especially true in countries without strict regulatory limits on pollution discharges. Other significant sources for direct environmental releases are farm fields where treated sewage sludge has been used as fertilizer or for sewage disposal. The compounds may run off into streams or be absorbed into crops and return to people or animals through food products grown on those fields.

Sources of contamination from personal care products vary widely depending on the intended use. The primary source tends to be wastewater from homes and buildings. Significant sources beyond homes include healthcare facilities, nursing homes, pharmacies, veterinary operations, meat processors, landfill leachate, and septic sewage tank haulers. The chemicals from PPCPs may come from cleaning supplies, deodorants, cosmetics, disinfectants, and pesticides, along with soaps, shampoos, and hair conditioners. In fact, almost any xenobiotic substance (chemical foreign to living organisms) that enters the environment has the potential to persist and create adverse biological effects.

In people, there are more questions than answers about the effects of these emerging contaminants on health. As researchers get better at detecting very small amounts of contamination, their presence is being found widely throughout the environment. These trace levels are usually in the nanogram or microgram per liter range, which is well below amounts thought to have an effect on people. Most research to date focuses on antibiotics and hormone products for their effect on people and the environment. Antibiotic resistance is already a concern in human health due to prevalent use of prescriptions for people and their use in livestock as growth enhancers. There is concern that chronic, low-level environmental exposure to antibiotics will exacerbate an already existing problem of antibiotic resistance and encourage "superbugs" that are even harder to fight.

Perhaps an even greater concern is the various compounds found in oral contraceptives, hormonal therapies, and certain industrial products, such as Bisphenol A. Unlike most medications, these chemicals are shown to have significant effects on hormonal systems even at the extremely low concentrations found in the environment. They are referred to as endocrine disrupters because of their hormonal effects on people and animals. The risks are increased when exposure occurs during the early developmental stages of children and animals. These medications are designed specifically to persist, bioaccumulate (increase) in the food chain, and resist degradation. Studies have shown effects on aquatic organisms, even at extremely low concentrations in water. This raises concerns about the effects of even trace amounts in human drinking water, especially on children. In addition to the concerns about single ingredient exposures, humans and the environment are being exposed to mixtures of multiple chemicals over a long period of time. The complexity of this system poses tremendous challenges for researchers trying to understand and predict potential harm to people or nature.

There are also measurable effects in land animals from environmental pharmaceuticals. The most dramatic example is the near extinction of three species of Asian vultures caused by feeding on carcasses of livestock treated with the anti-inflammatory drug, diclofenac. Unexpectedly, the vultures were exquisitely sensitive to ingesting small amounts of this drug. A major population collapse and near extinction occurred before the cause was determined and steps taken to stop this exposure of the birds to diclofenac. Another passage of chemicals up the terrestrial (land-based) food chain has been observed when birds eat insects from a field treated with contaminated sewage sludge fertilizer and are affected by those chemicals. These health effects on animals suggest that these chemicals may affect people too, especially as people are potentially exposed to multichemical mixtures in water and food at low levels over a period of many years.

Addressing these emerging contaminants calls for efforts on several fronts. First, at the source of the problem, pharmaceutical products themselves can be redesigned through the use of green chemistry techniques to have less environmental impact. Green chemistry is the design of chemical products and processes that reduce or eliminate the use and generation of hazardous substances. For pharmaceuticals, that would mean products that do not persist in the environment or bioaccumulate in the food chain and that break down into inert compounds when released into the environment. Improvements in water treatment techniques that can remove 100 percent of PPCPs from wastewater discharge and from drinking water would also greatly reduce exposure to people and nature. Finally, preventing improper disposal of medications that results in environmental release can be helped through awareness, behavior changes, and organized drug take-back programs.

Gwen Griffith

See Also: Antibiotic Resistance; Bisphenol A (BPA); Drinking Water Quality and Regulation; Endocrine Disruptors; Medical and Infectious Waste Management; Personal Care Products, Health Issues with; Sewage Treatment and Disposal; Water Pollution

Further Reading

Boxall, A. B., et al. "Pharmaceuticals and Personal Care Products in the Environment: What Are the Big Questions?" *Environmental Health Perspectives*, vol. 120, no. 9 (September 2012): 1221–1229.

Disposal of Unused Medicines: What You Should Know. Federal Drug Administration, Washington, DC, 2017. https://www.fda.gov/drugs/resourcesforyou/consumers/buyingusingmedicinesafely/ensuringsafeuseofmedicine/safedisposalofmedicines/ucm186187.htm.

Khetan, Sushil K., and Terrence J. Collins. "Human Pharmaceuticals in the Aquatic Environment: A Challenge to Green Chemistry." *Chemical Reviews*, vol. 107, no. 6 (May 2007): 2319–2364.

Pharmaceutical and Personal Care Products in Drinking Water and Aquatic Environments: Answers to Frequently Asked Questions. Concord, NH: New Hampshire Department of Environmental Services, 2010.

PHTHALATES

Phthalates are chemicals used to create plastic products, and they help make plastics flexible and durable. Polyvinyl chloride (better known as PVC) pipe is a common example of a plastic product made from a phthalate. Health professionals are concerned about phthalates because of adverse effects associated with their use.

Phthalates are ubiquitous in modern life. Most Americans use plastic products containing phthalates repeatedly during the day. Common plastics that contain phthalates include building materials, clothing, cosmetics, perfumes, food packaging, toys, and vinyl products (e.g., flooring, shower curtains, and raincoats). Phthalates are also used extensively in plastic medical devices, such as bags and tubing for blood transfusions and intravenous therapy drips. Additionally, phthalates are added to lubricating oils, solvents, and detergents.

Numerous adverse health effects are associated with phthalates. Studies suggest that phthalates can act as endocrine disruptors or hormonally active agents, and exposure can result in increased incidence of developmental abnormalities in humans, including cleft palate and skeletal malformation. Extensive studies document phthalate exposure having adverse effects on the male reproductive tract, including increased incidence of undescended testes, decreased testes weight, and decreased anogenital distance. Phthalate exposure has been shown to cause increased fetal death in experimental animal studies, and new scientific evidence suggests phthalate exposure in humans may lead to allergies and asthma, neurological and metabolic health effects, and adverse outcomes on pregnancy and female reproduction.

Growing public concern centers on what happens to children exposed to phthalates. Of particular concern is exposure to phthalates in medical supplies, food wrapped in plastic packaging, and plastic toys, cups, bowls, and bottles. Because everyday exposure to phthalates is extensive, phthalate metabolites can be found in the blood and urine of most Americans, and these metabolites have also been found in human breast milk and commercial milk from cows. Thus, infants and small children can be exposed to phthalates regardless of whether the caretaker nurses or feeds the child infant formulas.

The U.S. Congress acted to reduce phthalate exposure by passing the Consumer Product Safety Improvement Act (CPSIA) of 2008, which banned six specific types of phthalates (DEHP, DnBP, BBzP, DINP, DIDP, and DnOP) from use in toys and items sold to children in concentrations of greater than 0.1 percent. In addition, when enacting the CPSIA, Congress tasked the Consumer Product Safety Commission with appointing a Chronic Hazard Advisory Panel to examine the cumulative health risks of both phthalates and phthalate substitutes and to recommend whether any other phthalates or phthalate substitutes should be banned.

The U.S. Food and Drug Administration (FDA) issued guidance restricting the use of two phthalates (DBP and DEHP) in protective coatings for pills for both prescription and over-the-counter medicines. Although the FDA determined DBP and DEHP are not safe or suitable as inactive ingredients in prescription and over-the-counter medicines, the agency did not restrict use or impose labeling requirements for DBP and DEHP in cosmetics.

The U.S. Environmental Protection Agency (EPA) has developed an action plan for phthalates due to concern over their toxicity, widespread use, and human exposure. The EPA regulates the levels of DEHP in drinking water under the Safe Drinking Water Act, lists DEHP and DEP as hazardous pollutants under the Clean Air Act, and regulates phthalates as hazardous wastes under the Resource Conservation and Recovery Act.

California, Vermont, and Washington each have standards exceeding those set by the federal government for the allowable content of certain phthalates in children's items. Additionally, the American Public Health Association and other public health professional groups have urged government regulators to replace PVC in medical care settings, schools, public housing, and building materials.

Elizabeth Ann Glass Geltman and Henry Babatunde Akinleye

See Also: Children's Environmental Health; Clean Air Act; Consumer Product Safety Commission; Drinking Water Quality and Regulation; Endocrine Disruptors; Environmental Protection Agency; Hazardous Air Pollutants; Reproductive Health and Environmental Exposure; Resource Conservation and Recovery Act; Safe Drinking Water Act

Further Reading

Limiting the Use of Certain Phthalates as Excipients in CDER-Regulated Products. Washington, DC: U.S. Food and Drug Administration, 2012.

Meeker, J. D., S. Sathyanarayana, and S. H. Swan. "Phthalates and Other Additives in Plastics: Human Exposure and Associated Health Outcomes." *Philosophical Transactions of the Royal Society B: Biological Sciences*, vol. 364, no. 1526 (July 2009): 2097–2113.

Phthalates Action Plan (Revised). Washington, DC: U.S. Environmental Protection Agency, 2012.

Phthalates and Cumulative Risk Assessment: The Tasks Ahead. Washington, DC: National Academy of Sciences, 2008.

Policy Number 20119: Reducing PVC in Facilities with Vulnerable Populations. Washington, DC: American Public Health Association, 2011.

U.S. Food and Drug Administration. *Phthalates.* https://www.fda.gov/Cosmetics/ProductsIngredients/Ingredients/ucm128250.htm (accessed March 6, 2017).

POLLUTION PREVENTION

Environmental solutions are often prescriptive, dealing with problems after they happen. Even recycling and effective disposal methods deal with products or materials at the end of their life cycle. A better approach is to prevent the pollution from occurring in the first place. This is what the field of pollution prevention is all about—preventing pollution so that costly pollution controls and cleanups are not required.

Pollution prevention, also known as source reduction, is defined by the U.S. Environmental Protection Agency (EPA) as any practice that reduces, eliminates, or prevents pollution at its source. The EPA considers source reduction at the top of its environmental protection hierarchy, which means that we should try to prevent pollution before taking other measures, such as recycling, treatment, disposal, or release.

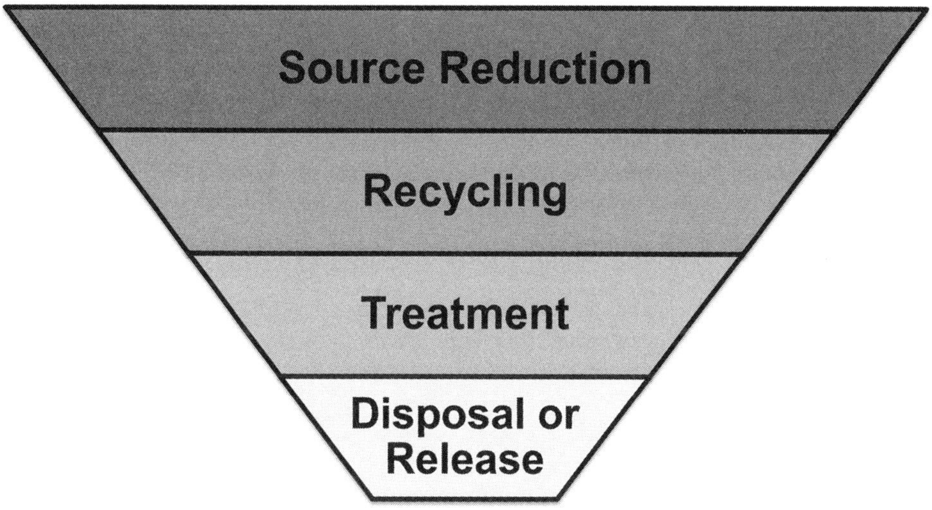

Source reduction is at the top of the environmental protection hierarchy. (U.S. Environmental Protection Agency, Pollution Prevention)

Some specific ways pollutants can be prevented from entering the environment are (1) using improved equipment or technology that pollute less or not at all; (2) redesigning products so that their compositions are less toxic or nontoxic; (3) using recycled materials instead of extracting raw materials; (4) relying on less water and chemicals in agricultural applications; and (5) switching to renewable energy sources like solar, wind, and geothermal power. Individuals can also take actions in their own homes to help prevent pollution, for example, turning off lights when not in use, drinking out of reusable water bottles, and purchasing Energy Star (energy-efficient) appliances.

The need for specific laws and measures to control and prevent pollution became clear after the United States experienced a number of environmental crises in the 1960s and 1970s, resulting in formation of the EPA and passage of several landmark environmental legislations, including the Clean Air and Water Acts. It later became apparent that preventing pollution deserved more attention, and in 1990, the Pollution Prevention Act was enacted. More recently, the EPA has developed a pollution prevention strategic plan, and there have been several executive orders reinforcing the importance of sustainable practices within government.

One of the most successful pollution prevention programs is the grant-funded Pollution Prevention Resources Exchange, created in 1997 by the EPA. Under this program, eight regional centers share information among experts and the public, increase awareness about pollution prevention, and evaluate the impact of various pollution prevention tools. There are nearly 100 participating organizations that help collect data, including state and local environmental agencies, academic institutions, and other nonprofit organizations. Among the findings for the years 2010 through 2012, the economic benefits associated with pollution prevention amounted to $5.4 billion nationwide, and 4.5 million tons (4.1 million metric tons) of pollution were minimized or eliminated.

Aaron Dorman

See Also: Energy Star; Environmental Protection Agency; Pollution Prevention Act; Recycling; Three Rs of Waste Management

Further Reading

Dupont, R. Ryan, Kumar Ganesan, and Louis Theodore. *Pollution Prevention: Sustainability, Industrial Ecology, and Green Engineering*. Boca Raton, FL: CRC Press, 2017.

National P2 Results Data System, 2010 to 2012. Washington, DC: National Pollution Prevention Roundtable, 2015.

25 Years Preventing Pollution: A Retrospective Report. Seattle, WA: The Pacific Northwest Pollution Prevention Resource Center, 2015.

U.S. Environmental Protection Agency. *Pollution Prevention (P2)*. https://www.epa.gov/p2 (accessed March 11, 2017).

U.S. Environmental Protection Agency. *Summary of the Pollution Prevention Act, 42 U.S.C. §13101 et seq. (1990)*. https://www.epa.gov/laws-regulations/summary-pollution-prevention-act (accessed March 11, 2017).

POLLUTION PREVENTION ACT

The Pollution Prevention Act (PPA) is a federal law, promulgated in 1990 by the U.S. government, that established a new national policy based on the belief that "pollution should be prevented or reduced at the source whenever feasible." Thus, the prevention or reduction of waste was placed at the top of the waste management hierarchy. Furthermore, the act declared that if pollution could not be prevented, it should be recycled. And if recycling is not feasible, the pollution should be treated and, if necessary, disposed of "in an environmentally safe manner" as a last resort.

This policy reflected a shift in the national attitude toward environmental protection in that the focus moved to waste reduction and prevention. Prior to enactment of the PPA, environmental statutes generally focused on "end of pipe" cleanups (i.e., the control, treatment, and disposal of pollution). However, over time it was found that the costs associated with control, treatment, disposal, and responsibility for risks to human health and the environment were not sustainable. Thus, the primary impetus behind this law was the need to reduce costs related to pollution control and liability and to minimize risks to public health and safety. This idea is similar to the central theme of the field of public health—prevention of disease is a preferable strategy to treatment of the disease after it has been acquired.

The PPA authorized the U.S. Environmental Protection Agency (EPA) to establish an independent office to develop and promote strategies to prevent pollution and reduce contaminant sources. The EPA's Office of Pollution Prevention and Toxics (now the Office of Chemical Safety and Pollution Prevention) was formed to carry out the provisions of the PPA, which include funding state pollution prevention activities and developing and disseminating information about source reduction strategies. The PPA defines source reduction as any activity that reduces the release of contaminants into the environment before they are treated, recycled, or disposed of. Source reduction methods can include improved technologies, equipment, industrial processes, materials, and housekeeping. Training on these methods is also important.

The PPA also required certain facilities to report their source reduction and recycling activities each year to the EPA. This report includes information about how much of each reported chemical is recycled or released into the environment as well as source reduction practices employed. These data are used by the EPA to measure source reduction activities and evaluate the success of the program. All such data reported to the EPA are publicly accessible on EPA's pollution prevention website.

Implementing the PPA has been fraught with difficulty due to the small budget authorized for implementation and a lack of mechanisms to force compliance upon the business community. Because business participation in PPA activities is voluntary, the EPA can only offer incentives to ensure its success. Other barriers to success of the PPA include (1) the lack of technical expertise among businesses in how to shift from pollution treatment to pollution prevention and (2) possible economic impacts of imposing pollution prevention strategies on influential industry stakeholders.

Adrienne L. Katner

See Also: Environmental Protection Agency; Marine Pollution, International Treaties to Prevent; Municipal Solid Waste Management; Pollution Prevention; Recycling; Three Rs of Waste Management; Waste Incineration; Water Reuse and Recycling

Further Reading

Johnson, Barry L. *Environmental Policy and Public Health*. Boca Raton, FL: CRC Press, 2006.

Pollution Prevention Act of 1990. 42 U.S.C. 13101, as amended through December 31, 2002. https://www.gpo.gov/fdsys/pkg/USCODE-2010-title42/pdf/USCODE-2010-title42-chap133.pdf.

U.S. Environmental Protection Agency. *Pollution Prevention (P2) and TRI*. https://www.epa.gov/toxics-release-inventory-tri-program/pollution-prevention-p2-and-tri (accessed April 18, 2016).

U.S. Environmental Protection Agency. *Summary of the Pollution Prevention Act, 42 U.S.C. §13101 et seq. (1990)*. https://www.epa.gov/laws-regulations/summary-pollution-prevention-act (accessed April 18, 2016).

POLYCHLORINATED BIPHENYLS

Polychlorinated biphenyls (PCBs) are man-made organic chemicals that are pervasive throughout the environment despite manufacturing being banned in the United States in 1979 due to health concerns. Because PCBs are chemically stable and have excellent electrical insulating properties, they were used in a wide range of products, materials, and industrial processes before 1979, including:

- Electrical equipment, such as transformers and capacitors
- Oils for motors and hydraulic equipment
- Plasticizers in paints, plastics, and rubber products
- Insulating materials, such as fiberglass and foam
- Adhesives, tapes, caulking, floor finish, and carbonless copy paper

In addition to banning the manufacturing of PCBs, imports of PCB-containing products were also banned in 1979, and PCBs were banned internationally in 2001 through the Stockholm Convention on Persistent Organic Pollutants. PCB chemicals were often known by their commercial names (e.g., Arochlor).

PCBs are considered probable carcinogens. Exposure is also associated with heart disease, suppression of the immune system, endocrine disruption, asthma, and birth defects, including impaired cognitive ability in children exposed to PCBs *in utero*.

Although banned for many years, PCBs are still prevalent in buildings and machinery used today that were built or manufactured prior to 1977. Additionally, PCBs are commonly found in abandoned, illegal, or poorly maintained hazardous waste sites, where leaks from PCB-containing electrical transformers are a common source contamination. Improper disposal of PCB-containing consumer products has resulted in contamination of some municipal and public landfills not designed for hazardous waste.

PCBs continue to enter the environment due to the improper disposal practices of the past. The persistence of the chemical, coupled with bioaccumulation in wildlife, has often resulted in the contamination of food, especially predatory fish and wild game. Also, studies have detected low levels of PCBs in the breast milk of women who consume large amounts of predatory fish.

Elizabeth Ann Glass Geltman

See Also: Cancer Risk from Environmental Exposure; Hazardous Waste Disposal; Land Disposal of Waste Materials; Persistent, Bioaccumulating, and Toxic Chemicals

Further Reading

Polychlorinated Biphenyls: Human Health Aspects. Geneva, Switzerland: World Health Organization, 2003.

Polychlorinated Biphenyls and Polybrominated Biphenyls: IARC Monographs on the Evaluation of Carcinogenic Risks to Humans. Lyon, France: International Agency for Research on Cancer, 2016.

Toxicological Profile for Polychlorinated Biphenyls (PCBs). Atlanta, GA: Agency for Toxic Substances and Disease Registry, 2000.

U.S. Environmental Protection Agency. *Integrated Risk Information System: Polychlorinated biphenyls (PCBs)*. https://cfpub.epa.gov/ncea/iris2/chemicalLanding.cfm?substance_nmbr=294 (accessed March 7, 2017).

U.S. Environmental Protection Agency. *Polychlorinated Biphenyls (PCBs)*. https://www.epa.gov/pcbs (accessed March 7, 2017).

POLYCYCLIC AROMATIC HYDROCARBONS

Polycyclic aromatic hydrocarbons (PAHs) result from the incomplete combustion of garbage, petroleum products, coal, and other organic substances, and they are also found in tobacco smoke. PAHs can be generated through both natural and man-made processes. Volcanic eruptions and wildfires are examples of natural processes, and car exhaust, coal burning, asphalt production, and various industrial operations are examples of man-made processes.

PAHs can be found in soil and water, and in the air, they contribute to smog. People can also be exposed to PAHs through products like shampoos, cigarettes, and skin creams as well as by eating the char on burnt meat. The health effects from low-level exposure to PAHs are unknown, but higher concentrations can irritate eyes and breathing passages, and some workers have developed blood and liver abnormalities. Skin contact with PAHs can cause reddening and peeling of the skin and sometimes even blistering. Several PAHs and PAH mixtures are considered carcinogenic.

There is a wide diversity of PAHs, with some more toxic than others. They are known to remain in the environment for a long time. Additionally, because many are insoluble, they will biomagnify, allowing concentrations to build up to higher levels. The most studied PAH is perhaps benzo[a]pyrene (BaP), which is associated with a host of potential acute and chronic health effects, including cancer. BaP results from the combustion of plants, wood, and coal, and it is emitted from gasoline and diesel motor vehicles. Indoor sources of BaP include fireplaces, stoves, and tobacco smoking.

Andrew P. Barefield

See Also: Air Pollution; Cancer Risk from Environmental Exposure; Hazardous Air Pollutants; Ozone and Smog in the Urban Environment; Personal Care Products, Health Issues with

Further Reading

Boone, Clifford. *Polycyclic Aromatic Hydrocarbons*. New York: Nova Science, 2015.

Centers for Disease Control and Prevention. *Fact Sheet: Polycyclic Aromatic Hydrocarbons (PAHs)*. https://www.cdc.gov/biomonitoring/PAHs_FactSheet.html (accessed April 9, 2017).

Haines, Pierre A., and Milton D. Hendrickson. *Polycyclic Aromatic Hydrocarbons: Pollution, Health Effects and Chemistry*. New York: Nova Science, 2009.

U.S. Environmental Protection Agency. *Integrated Risk Information System: Polycyclic Aromatic Hydrocarbon (PAH) Mixtures*. https://cfpub.epa.gov/ncea/iris2/chemicalLanding.cfm?substance_nmbr=1033 (accessed April 9, 2017).

Zelinkova, Z., and T. Wenzl. "The Occurrence of 16 EPA PAHs in Food—A Review." *Polycyclic Aromatic Compounds*, vol. 35, no. 2–4 (March 2015): 248–284.

POPULATION TRENDS, HEALTH IMPLICATIONS OF

The year 2015 saw the greatest forced displacement of people since World War II and the highest death rate for migrants on record. Globally, 65.3 million people were displaced by conflict and violence, and 21.3 million of those displaced crossed international borders. Women were the largest group of migrants, accounting for 48 percent of the migrant population, and individuals under 20 made up 15 percent. Approximately one in three of the 21.3 million refugees crossing borders were minors, a quarter without parents.

In addition to conflict and violence, an estimated 19.2 million people were displaced by natural disasters. This displacement, mostly weather-related, is 60 percent more likely now than it was in the previous four decades, partly due to the earth's changing climate.

Human trafficking is a huge risk to the health and safety of more than 21 million people who are forced into labor or sexual exploitation. Over one-third of the victims of trafficking are children, and in the case of sex trafficking, most victims are women and children. Men are more likely to be victims of labor trafficking. Undocumented migrants crossing the U.S. southern boarder are most vulnerable to becoming human trafficking victims.

Mental health is a key issue for people subject to forced migration. Many migrants are moving in response to real or potential trauma in their home country, and mental health resources are key to helping them resettle. Moreover, when individuals can break free from human trafficking bonds, they need trauma counseling.

Poverty is another concern when discussing population trends. Densely populated areas tend to suffer more from the effects of poverty, including hunger and limited shelter. Such areas draw migrants due to their perceived promise of opportunity, but access to health care and education is often a problem, and crime threatens their health and safety. Until individuals become naturalized citizens of the country they have migrated to, it may be very difficult for them to obtain quality health care, and the healthcare system itself may become increasingly taxed as the migrant population grows. Communicable diseases can also spread faster through migrant populations when health care is limited.

The causes of migration are complex, often involving geopolitical conflicts that result from or are exacerbated by limited resources. In particular, drinking water and food shortages are brought about by population growth combined with land use practices and climate change that increase the frequency of floods and droughts and expand desertification. Many governments and international aid agencies are providing assistance to those most in need, but as the world's population grows from today's 7.5 billion to perhaps 9.7 billion by 2050, the fate of tens of millions of future migrants remains uncertain.

Ronda Bowen

See Also: Climate Change and Human Health; Communicable Diseases; Deforestation; Drought and Desertification, Health Consequences of; Natural Disasters

Further Reading

Global Migration Trends Factsheet 2015. Geneva, Switzerland: International Organization for Migration, 2016.

Newbold, K. Bruce. *Six Billion Plus: World Population in the Twenty-First Century*. Lanham, MD: Rowman and Littlefield Publishers, 2007.
Rechel, Bernd, et al. "Migration and Health in an Increasingly Diverse Europe." *The Lancet*, vol. 381, no. 9873 (April 2013): 1235–1245.
Schenker, Marc B., and Heather E. Riden. "FACTS Special Issue on Migration and Health." *The Journal of Field Actions: Field Actions Science Reports*, Special Issue 10 (March 2014).

PRENATAL EXPOSURE TO POLLUTANTS

We need to begin with the reasons for the sensitivity and susceptibly differences of prenatal (before birth) and postnatal (after birth) exposures to pollutants. The greater likelihood of detrimental outcomes from prenatal exposures requires an understanding of early development.

After fertilization of the egg (ovum), the single cell develops into the blastocyst (about 200 cells). The cell proliferation and differentiation takes 6 to 10 days before the blastocyst implants into the highly vascularized endometrium of the uterine wall, which begins the maternal supply of oxygen and nutrients. Prior to implantation, the embryo relies on a low supply of nutrients, maternal hormones, and factors in seminal fluid. Any additional stress from pollutants would be highly detrimental because cell division is occurring in a relatively unprotected environment, the embryo is already undergoing hypoxic stress, and any additional stress could lead to modified intracellular organelles, mutations, and epigenetic modifications that can affect the offspring for a lifetime.

There has been minimal research on toxicant effects during the early transitions within the first trimester. By approximately the 10th gestational week of human development, all organs have begun to develop, although they may not be in their final locations. If exposure to pollutants occurs, the pollutants could disseminate more readily and diversely throughout the fetus than they could in a neonate or adolescent because innate protective barriers (e.g., skin, blood brain barrier, and gut blood barrier) have not fully formed and are leaky. Thus, cell expansions and differentiation within multiple organs are susceptible during prenatal development.

Throughout gestation, the fetus is reliant on nutrients and oxygen passed from the maternal system through the placenta to the fetus. Therefore, placental development is critical for fetal growth, and it is dependent on how well the embryo implanted into the uterine wall, which is dependent on maternal hormones and immune activities. Pollutants such as endocrine-disrupting chemicals (e.g., bisphenol A, phthalates, dichlorodiphenyltrichloroethane, and perfluorooctanoic acid) and chemicals inducing inflammation and immune alterations (e.g., metals such as arsenic, cadmium, and lead and alcohols) interfere with placental growth, and thus, the health of the fetus. Sensitivity to pollutants can differ due to sex because 15 percent of genes on the Xi (inactivated X) chromosome of female trophoblasts are not inactivated, giving females (XX) a double dose of enzymes over those of males (XY) to positively or negatively deal with stress. Pollutants are often thought of as chemicals that contaminate the air, water, or soil. However, pollutants affecting maternal-placental-fetal interactions that can modify prenatal or postnatal health can also be biological (toxins and pathogens) and even physical (e.g., noise and light).

The development of the fetus is dependent on prior and current maternal exposures to pollutants, diet, and physical/psychological stresses that affect the placenta's delivery of nutrients. The maternal supply of nutrients versus toxicants and the placental organization affecting this supply will determine how well the fetus develops and reaches full-term development. Pollutants are known to shorten the gestational period and lower the birth weight of the fetus due to intrauterine growth restriction. Prenatal exposure to single pollutants has been suggested to reduce fetal growth, and multiple combinations of pollutants or pollutants combined with physical or psychological stressors have been noted to worsen offspring health outcomes. Additionally, depending on genetic and environmental influences, some neonates born at lower size and weight due to environmental stressors have become overweight with high inflammatory conditions later in life, leading to cardiovascular disorders and type 2 diabetes.

Prenatal pollutant exposures affect long-term health because of early alteration of cells dispersing into organs undergoing development. For example, prenatal exposure to diesel exhaust particles has been suggested to modify the immune microglia cell in the brain, which influences neuronal connections and behaviors. Prenatal exposure to air pollutants, such as diesel exhaust and perchloroethylene, has been reported to be associated with brain functions and behavior. Myeloid progenitors disperse into tissues very early in embryonic development, and as for microglia in the brain, they may be integral to organogenesis in other organs. Thus, pollutants can alter as early as yolk sac derivations. In addition to innate early immune cells seeding into multiple organs affecting their development and later functions, pollutants can induce developmental immunotoxicological modifications that can have long-term consequences on autoimmune diseases, allergies, cancer, and susceptibilities to infections.

The recent Zika virus influence on brain development is evidence documenting the major differences of prenatal and adult exposures. Infected adults have relatively mild flu-like symptoms, whereas prenatal exposure can result in microcephaly or worse. It has been suggested that prenatal Zika pathology be referred to as a congenital Zika syndrome in that microcephaly is but one clinical sign of the disorder. A similar situation exists for congenital rubella syndrome, with prenatal infection leading to a number of different birth defects. Even without Zika-mediated microcephaly, a silent neurotoxicity (i.e., a neural abnormality not obvious at the time of birth) may be unmasked later in life with exposure to another stressor.

David A. Lawrence

See Also: Bisphenol A (BPA); Children's Environmental Health; Endocrine Disruptors; Environmental Toxicology; Heavy Metal Pollution; Phthalates; Zika Virus

Further Reading

Govarts, Eva, et al. "Combined Effects of Prenatal Exposures to Environmental Chemicals on Birth Weight." *International Journal of Environmental Research and Public Health*, vol. 13, no. 5 (May 2016).

Kaneko, Kotaro J. "Metabolism of Preimplantation Embryo Development: A Bystander or an Active Participant?" *Current Topics in Developmental Biology*, vol. 120 (June 2016): 259–310.

Kraft, Andrew D., et al. "Unmasking Silent Neurotoxicity Following Developmental Exposure to Environmental Toxicants." *Neurotoxicology and Teratology*, vol. 55 (May–June 2016): 38–44.

Lenters, Virissa, et al. "Prenatal Phthalate, Perfluoroalkyl Acid, and Organochlorine Exposures and Term Birth Weight in Three Birth Cohorts: Multi-Pollutant Models Based on Elastic Net Regression." *Environmental Health Perspectives*, vol. 124, no. 3 (March 2016): 365–372.

Levy-Marchal, Claire, and Delphine Jaquet. "Long-Term Metabolic Consequences of Being Born Small for Gestational Age." *Pediatric Diabetes*, vol. 5, no. 3 (September 2004): 147–153.

Melo, Adriana, et al. "Congenital Zika Virus Infection: Beyond Neonatal Microcephaly." *JAMA Neurology*, vol. 73, no. 12 (December 2016): 1407–1416.

Puscheck, Elizabeth E., et al. "Molecular Biology of the Stress Response in the Early Embryo and Its Stem Cells." *Advances in Experimental Medicine and Biology*, vol. 843 (May 2015): 77–128.

Russ, Karin, and Sarah Howard. "Developmental Exposure to Environmental Chemicals and Metabolic Changes in Children." *Current Problems in Pediatric and Adolescent Health Care*, vol. 46, no. 8 (August 2016): 255–285.

Stingone, Jeanette A., et al. "Association between Prenatal Exposure to Ambient Diesel Particulate Matter and Perchloroethylene with Children's 3rd Grade Standardized Test Scores." *Environmental Research*, vol. 148 (July 2016): 144–153.

PUBLIC HEALTH SERVICE

The U.S. Public Health Service (PHS) is a federal agency within the Department of Health and Human Services charged with the central mission of protecting the health of the U.S. population. Today's PHS has its roots in the Marine Hospital Service, founded in 1798 to care for ill and disabled seamen. The official journal of the PHS, *Public Health Reports*, has been published since that year.

During the 19th century, the organization's mission expanded to include the public health of all Americans. Accordingly, in 1902, the name was changed to the Public Health and Marine Hospital Service. Major duties included quarantine and medical inspection of immigrants arriving at Ellis Island. In 1912, the name was shortened to the Public Health Service. With this new name came congressional legislation broadening PHS authority to investigate illnesses and address sanitation, water, and sewage. In addition to conducting public health research, the PHS tracked the spread of diseases and imposed quarantines to stem epidemics.

On July 3, 1944, President Franklin D. Roosevelt signed the Public Health Service Act. The act broadened the scope of PHS authority to make research grants-in-aid for any disease, to expand public health programs generally, and to specifically address tuberculosis. Additionally, it provided for the commissioning of nurses and specialists, such as entomologists, chemists, and zoologists. The act has been amended a number of times to address issues as disparate as family planning, cancer research, and health insurance.

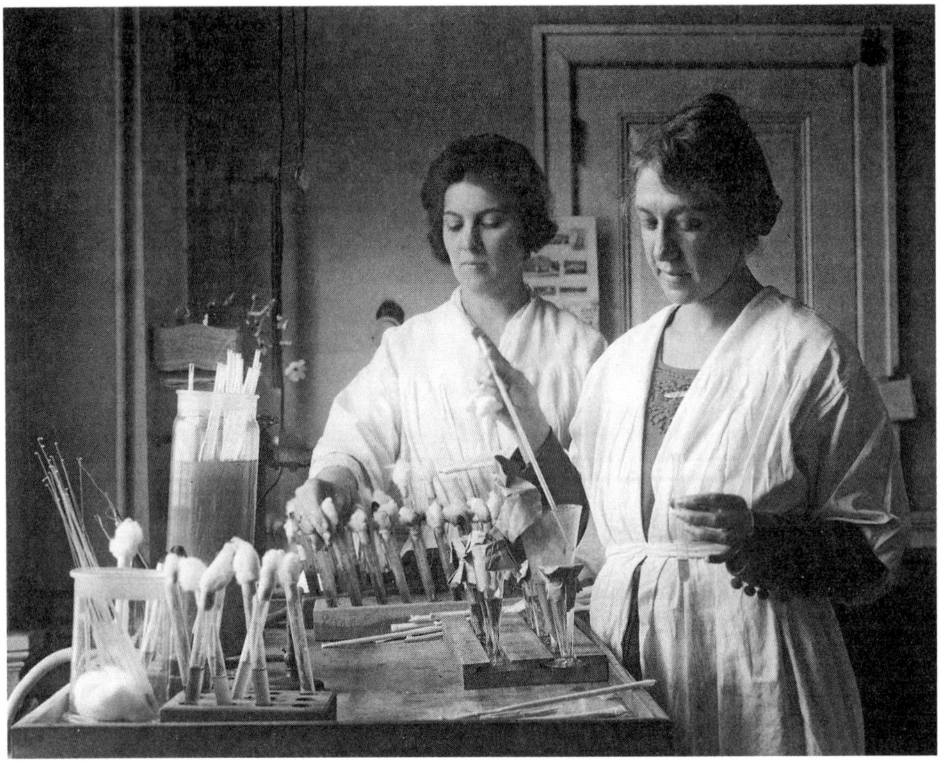

Public Health Service doctor Ella Eulows (right) and laboratory assistant Sadie Carlin test antipneumococcal serum for potency, ca. 1920. Environmental health officers within the Public Health Service have a long history of disease and injury prevention, food safety, emergency preparedness, and public education. (National Archives)

The PHS is one of the uniformed services of the federal government. Officers hold rank and wear uniforms similar to those worn by U.S. Navy personnel. Through the PHS, more than 6,500 public health professionals hold duty stations within over 20 federal departments and agencies, where they respond to public health needs, provide leadership regarding public health practices, and advance public health science. The surgeon general, often called America's Doctor, oversees the PHS and educates the nation on public health matters. In recent years, major surgeon general initiatives have addressed HIV/AIDS, the dangers of tobacco use, and the psychological health of military service members and their families.

The health professionals who comprise the PHS represent a broad range of expertise, including physicians, dentists, nurses, clinical and rehabilitation therapists, pharmacists, dieticians, veterinarians, engineers, researchers, social scientists, allied clinical care providers, health educators, healthcare administrators, and environmental health experts. Among their myriad duties, environmental health officers in the PHS are concerned with epidemiological surveillance, disease prevention, radiological health, industrial hygiene, food safety, injury prevention and education, emergency preparedness, public health emergencies, and natural disasters.

Kathy Stolley

See Also: Disaster Preparedness and Response; Drinking Water Quality and Regulation; Environmental Epidemiology; Environmental Health Profession; Food Safety and Technology; Industrial Hygiene; Natural Disasters; Sewage Treatment and Disposal

Further Reading

McKenzie, James F., R. R. Pinger, and Denise Seabert. *An Introduction to Community and Public Health*. Burlington, MA: Jones and Bartlett Learning, 2016.
Riegelman, Richard K., and Brenda Kirkwood. *Public Health 101: Healthy People—Healthy Populations*. Burlington, MA: Jones and Bartlett Learning, 2015.
U.S. Department of Health and Human Services. *Commissioned Corps of the U.S. Public Health Service*. https://www.usphs.gov (accessed February 18, 2017).

PUBLIC TRANSPORTATION AND ENVIRONMENTAL HEALTH

All over the world, communities in both urban and rural areas are expanding at impressive rates, especially in urban areas. It is expected that approximately two-thirds of the world's population will be living in urban areas by 2050. This is causing traditional infrastructures, especially related to transportation, to be stretched to their limits, resulting in increased delays and inefficiencies. For example, traffic congestion in 2014 caused U.S. drivers to waste more than 4 billion gallons (15 billion liters) of fuel and kept travelers stuck in traffic for nearly 7 billion extra hours. Additionally, the increased traffic congestion leads to deterioration in air quality, which adversely affects public health and the environment.

In addition to building new transportation infrastructure, increasing the use of rides with shared public transportation is being increasingly favored as an option for reducing traffic congestion. However, while public transportation ridership has been increasing, it is still not growing fast enough on average to effectively tackle the problem of congestion. The fundamental problem is uncertainty in the real-time schedule of public transportation services. Additionally, commuters become frustrated finding transportation options to and from the transit network.

Variations in travel and arrival times have been found to have a substantial impact on commuter satisfaction, and commuter tolerance to delays in bus schedules is quite low. To address this concern, some transit agencies have been integrating real-time sensors into public transit systems, and a number of approaches have been developed by academic researchers and commercial companies to process the sensor data. For instance, automatic vehicle location and passenger counter technology can provide real-time data (e.g., vehicle travel time, arrival and departure times, and passenger boarding counts), and these data can be used for traveler information displays, bus time prediction, and schedule planning optimization. The aim of these approaches is to provide real-time information to improve passenger experience and increase ridership. A direct benefit of increased ridership on public transportation is the reduced use of personal vehicles, and hence, reduction in both traffic congestion and vehicle pollution, with concomitant health benefits. Another solution is to use mobile device (e.g., smartphone) applications to provide travelers accurate, real-time information about potential travel options at the moment they are choosing how to get to where they need to go.

To alleviate the problem of first and last mile travel, a new market supported by connected applications and the shared economy has appeared. In this market, private ride-sharing companies, such as Uber and Lyft, have thrived. Recently, with the introduction of pooled services (e.g., uberPOOL and Lyft Line), these companies are helping bridge a gap between required and available services. A number of transit agencies are also focusing on shared rides, realizing that it is important to take the whole mobility problem into consideration, with the goal of reducing solo car trips. Over the long term, this will lead to reduced vehicle pollution, improved air quality, and lower healthcare costs.

Abhishek Dubey

See also: Air Pollution; Ambient Air Quality; Asthma; Automobile and Truck Emissions and Controls; Climate Change and Human Health; Green Space in Urban Environments; Hybrid and Electric Automobiles, Health Benefits from

Further Reading

Americans Took 10.6 Billion Trips on Public Transportation in 2015. American Public Transportation Association, Washington, DC, 2016. http://www.apta.com/mediacenter/pressreleases/2016/Pages/160331_Ridership.aspx.

Bates, John, et al. "The Valuation of Reliability for Personal Travel." *Transportation Research Part E: Logistics and Transportation Review*, vol. 37, no. 2 (April–July 2001): 191–229.

Creating Equitable, Healthy, and Sustainable Communities: Strategies for Advancing Smart Growth, Environmental Justice, and Equitable Development, EPA 231-K-10–005. Washington, DC: U.S. Environmental Protection Agency, 2013.

Dora, Carlos, and Margaret Phillips. *Transport, Environment, and Health*. Copenhagen, Denmark: World Health Organization, 2000.

Frank, Lawrence D., Peter O. Engelke, and Thomas L. Schmid. *Health and Community Design: The Impact of the Built Environment on Physical Activity*. Washington, DC: Island Press, 2003.

Gooze, Aaron, Kari Watkins, and Alan Borning. "Benefits of Real-Time Transit Information and Impacts of Data Accuracy on Rider Experience." *Transportation Research Record: Journal of the Transportation Research Board*, vol. 2351, transit, vol. 2 (December 2013): 95–103.

Levy, Jonathan I., Jonathan J. Buonocore, and Katherine V. Stackelberg. "Evaluation of the Public Health Impacts of Traffic Congestion: A Health Risk Assessment." *Environmental Health*, vol. 9, article 65 (October 2010).

Nicolopoulou-Stamati, P., L. Hens, and C. V. Howard, eds. *Environmental Health Impacts of Transport and Mobility*. Dordrecht, the Netherlands: Springer, 2005.

Ragland, David, R., et al. *Transportation and Health: Policy Interventions for a Safer, Healthier People and Communities*. Berkeley, CA: Safe Transportation Research and Education Center, 2011.

Schrank, David, et al. *2015 Urban Mobility Scorecard*. College Station, TX: Texas A&M Transportation Institute and INRIX, 2015.

Thorsen, Joel. *Land Use, Transportation and Environmental Quality Interactions and Smart Growth Strategies*. New York: Nova Science, 2013.

Q

QUIET, BENEFITS OF

Time spent in quiet environments can be relaxing and restorative, and quiet homes and neighborhoods are highly valued. Quiet areas offer respite from distraction and stress, resulting in an improved mood and a better ability to concentrate. Understanding the value of quiet, manufacturers have developed quieter household appliances, aircraft technology, cars, lawn machinery, and even quieter pavement. "Buy quiet" initiatives encourage the use and purchase of quiet equipment as well as the design and manufacture of quiet products and tools to protect industrial workers and others.

Research typically examines the negative health impacts of noise rather than the positive impacts of quiet. However, a significant body of research focuses on the acoustic environment—the soundscape—and frames sound in neutral terms. This research examines quiet as an amenity in one framework and as benefiting health and well-being in another. Access to quiet may also be considered in studies looking at the restorative value of natural and green areas. Sometimes the health benefits of quiet—or silence—are found by accident. A 2006 study measured cardiac and respiratory responses to the various musical styles, tempo, and structure of 12 musicians and 12 nonmusicians. During the two minutes of silence intended as a pause between segments, researchers observed greater evidence of relaxation in subjects compared to their status during musical segments or at baseline.

Investing in Quieter Choices

Approximately 26 million Americans are affected by high-frequency hearing loss, and more than 45 million Americans suffer from tinnitus, a condition involving a sensation of ringing or other sounds in the ears. Both of these conditions are typically caused by noise exposure. Because hearing loss is usually cumulative, it is often associated with aging, but noise-induced hearing loss is preventable and does not have to be an inevitable part of aging. Investing in quieter choices can result in better hearing as we age and greater enjoyment of the sounds around us. Suggestions for protecting your hearing include limiting your exposure to sounds measuring 70 dBA and above, wearing hearing protection during loud activities, limiting the use of portable audio devices, and keeping the volume down when using such devices.

Structured quiet time in a hospital environment results in patients spending more time asleep or at rest, which is integral to the healing process. Nursing staff report that scheduled quiet time provides an opportunity to catch up on paperwork and offers relief from feeling rushed. Many hospitals feature sanctuaries or meditation rooms where patients, visitors, and staff can benefit from a few minutes alone in a quiet place. In residential buildings with high traffic noise exposure, bedrooms facing away from the street allow people to fall asleep more easily and to awaken less frequently, which can be especially important for people who are sensitive to noise.

In settings where environmental noise is unavoidable, people with access to a natural setting or green space close to home report an improved sense of physical and psychological well-being as well as the ability to recover from stress and feel restored. In some areas, traffic noise may still intrude upon green spaces and natural settings. Urban dwellers with access to this type of area might find an early morning visit to be sufficiently quiet to provide some tranquility before the start of a busy day. Residents in noisy areas with access to quiet courtyards often enjoy an improvement in quality of life that is significant enough to mitigate the annoyance and disruption caused by noise. Acousticians recommend that urban planners consider public health lessons learned from studying "quiet side" bedrooms and quiet courtyards that are shielded from traffic noise. However, they warn that the introduction of quiet side aspects will not completely mitigate the effects of building in noisy areas.

Sound is measured with sound level meters, and the unit of measurement is a decibel, or dB. The human ear is most responsive to frequencies between 500 hertz and 8 kilohertz, and higher and lower sounds are not heard as well. Frequency weighting in sound measurement allows sound level meters to "hear" frequencies in a way similar to the human ear. The most common weighting used is A-weighting, which is most similar to the human ear.

Quiet places are rarely devoid of any sound (see Table 15). A relatively quiet soundscape may include natural sounds and have an average sound level below 50 dBA. In quiet rural settings, there is a region—referred to as a "listening radius"—within which one hears faint sounds from distant homes. This provides a sense of community and reduces feelings of isolation. In noisy rural settings, residents may feel compelled to close windows to reduce noise indoors. Because of this, they lose a subtle but meaningful form of social connectedness.

Although many places and products are becoming quieter, noise is increasing in other ways, and the world just seems to be getting noisier. For example, national parks are increasingly grappling with anthropomorphic noise, from lock-signifying beeps and horn honks in automobile parking lots to helicopter tours circling overhead. The National Park Service provides educational material related to soundscape preservation, including ideas for minimizing your noise footprint in parks and suggestions for being a quiet neighbor. Additionally, the Centers for Disease Control and Prevention provides guidance about safe and unsafe noise levels,

Table 15. Average sound levels.

Sound	dB Level
Auditory threshold	0
Grand Canyon at night	10
Rustling leaves	20
Soft whisper	30
Wind blowing through trees	48
Normal conversation	55
Clothes dryer	60
Surf	70
Blender	80
Lawnmower	90
Drill	98
Rock concert	106
Jet plane taking off	130

Source: Noise Navigator Sound Level Database.

and public health advocates often address the deleterious effects of noise exposure by highlighting the benefits of access to quiet.

Jeanine Botta

See Also: Centers for Disease Control and Prevention; Green Space in Urban Environments; Noise Pollution

Further Reading

American Tinnitus Association. *Home Page*. https://www.ata.org/understanding-facts/demographics (accessed April 9, 2017).

Berger, Elliott H., Rick Neitzel, and Cynthia A. Kladden. *Noise Navigator Sound Level Database with over 1700 Measurement Values*. Indianapolis, IN: 3M E-A-RCAL Laboratory, 2015.

Chepesiuk, Ron. "Decibel Hell: The Effects of Living in a Noisy World." *Environmental Health Perspectives*, vol. 113, no. 1 (January 2005): A35–A41.

Gidlöf-Gunnarsson, Anita, and Evy Öhrström. "Attractive 'Quiet' Courtyards: A Potential Modifier of Urban Residents' Responses to Road Traffic Noise?" *International Journal of Environmental Research and Public Health*, vol. 7, no. 9 (September 2010): 3359–3375.

Gross, Daniel A. "This Is Your Brain on Silence: Contrary to Popular Belief, Peace and Quiet Is All about the Noise in Your Head." *Nautilus*, no. 16 (August 2014). http://nautil.us/issue/16/nothingness/this-is-your-brain-on-silence.

National Institute on Deafness and Other Communication Disorders. *Home Page*. https://www.nidcd.nih.gov (accessed April 9, 2017).
Pollard, Bryan, and Daniel Fink. "What Is a Safe Noise Level?" *Tinnitus Today*, vol. 41, no. 2 (Fall 2016): 12–14.
Shepherd, D., et al. "Do Quiet Areas Afford Greater Health-Related Quality of Life Than Noisy Areas?" *International Journal of Environmental Research and Public Health*, vol. 10, no. 4 (March 2013): 1284–1303.

R

RADIATION, IONIZING AND NONIONIZING

Radiation, which is energy in the form of electromagnetic waves or subatomic particles, is all around us. Radio waves, microwaves, and visible light are examples of radiation, as are X-rays and cosmic particles from outer space. Some radiation occurs naturally, for example, from minerals found in the ground, while other radiation is produced by medical diagnostic equipment and other types of machinery. Radiation exposure can also occur from accidents at nuclear power plants and from nuclear weapons. Radiation is a concern because exposure to some forms of radiation can cause serious health problems and even death. Pregnant women and children are particularly susceptible to radiation exposure.

There are two types of radiation: ionizing and nonionizing. Ionizing radiation is strong enough to dislodge electrons from their atomic orbits, causing the atom to become charged (i.e., ionized). Ionizing radiation can damage tissues, alter the DNA in genes, and sometimes cause cancer. (Because cancers are slow to develop, the effects of chronic exposure to ionizing radiation may not be apparent for 20 years or longer.) Exposure to high levels of ionizing radiation over a short period can cause radiation sickness and even death if there is significant damage to bone marrow, the gastrointestinal tract, or the central nervous system.

Leading Cause of Cancer Deaths

Lung cancer is the leading cause of cancer deaths in the United States among both men and women, accounting for over 150,000 deaths per year in recent years, or one-quarter of all cancer deaths. About 80 percent of lung cancers in men and 90 percent in women are attributed to cigarette smoking, and nonsmokers also have an increased risk of developing lung cancer if they are exposed to secondhand or thirdhand smoke. Lung cancer is also caused by exposure to radon gas (the second-leading cause of lung cancer), air pollution, and occupational exposure to substances such as asbestos, uranium, coke, and certain carcinogenic chemicals. Around two-thirds of all people diagnosed with lung cancer are age 65 or older, with an average diagnosis age of about 70. The five-year survival rate for people with lung cancer is only about 20 percent, and over 50 percent of people diagnosed with lung cancer die within a year. However, when lung cancer is detected early, before it has had time to spread to other organs, the survival rate is significantly improved.

The degree to which ionizing radiation causes adverse health effects depends on the type, strength, and duration of radiation and the organs exposed. The types of ionizing radiation include:

- Alpha Particles: Consisting of two protons and two neutrons from the nucleus of an atom and resulting from the decay of heavy radioactive elements, such as uranium, radium, and polonium. Alpha particles cannot penetrate the skin, but if ingested or inhaled, can severely damage cells and DNA.
- Beta Particles: Small, fast-moving particles emitted by unstable atoms, such as tritium, strontium-90, and carbon-14. Beta particles can penetrate the skin, causing burns, but they are much more dangerous if ingested or inhaled.
- Gamma Rays: Packets of energy called photons that can penetrate the human body, damaging cells and DNA. Gamma rays are so powerful that several inches of lead or several feet of concrete are needed to stop them.
- X-rays: Similar to gamma rays but lower energy and less penetrating. X-rays can occur naturally or be produced by machinery, such as medical diagnostic equipment. Medical X-rays represent the largest source of human created (i.e., nonnatural) radiation exposure.
- Neutrons: Usually resulting from nuclear fission processes, neutrons are the only type of radiation that can make other materials radioactive. Neutrons can travel long distances but can be blocked by concrete or water.

Radioactive decay occurs when radioactive elements called radionuclides release energy in the form of ionizing radiation. As this process of decay occurs, the radionuclide is transformed into a different atom called a decay product. The rate at which decay occurs is called the half-life, which is the time required for half of the radioactive atom to decay. Half-lives can be as short as a few seconds or as long as hundreds or millions of years.

In contrast to ionizing radiation, nonionizing radiation is not powerful enough to dislodge electrons. Nonionizing radiation excites atoms (i.e., causes them to move around and vibrate), resulting in an increase in temperature, for example, in the way a microwave oven thaws a frozen dinner or warms leftovers. The background levels of nonionizing radiation that are always present are generally harmless. However, there is some controversy about whether long-term exposure to some nonionizing radiation sources, including cell phones and high-power transmission lines, represents a health risk. Occupation exposure to high levels of nonionizing radiation (e.g., laser light and high-intensity radio waves and microwaves) can also lead to adverse health effects.

All radiation travels through empty space at the same speed of about 186,000 miles per second (3.0×108 meters per second), but radiation types differ according to their wavelength (which is inversely proportional to frequency) and energy. Ionizing radiation has a shorter wavelength than nonionizing radiation, which means that there is a higher frequency of waves passing a point in space over a given time frame. In contrast, nonionizing radiation has a longer wavelength and lower frequency. Higher frequency waves can impart more energy, which explains why exposure to ionizing radiation represents a greater health risk.

Most of the radiation we receive comes from background sources, for example, cosmic radiation from outer space and naturally occurring radioactive minerals (e.g., uranium and thorium) found in the soil and water and even trace amounts in our bodies. Radon, a radioactive gas that forms naturally from the decay of radioactive elements found in soil and rock, is the second leading cause of lung cancer in the United States. A large fraction of our radiation exposure also comes from medical diagnostic equipment using X-rays and from radiation therapy for treating cancer. Accidental nuclear power plant releases, such as occurred at Chernobyl and Fukushima, can also result in radiation exposure.

Radiation levels are characterized in four different ways (common units followed by SI units):

- Radioactivity: the amount of ionizing radiation coming from a material (i.e., the number of atoms decaying over a given period), measured as the curie (Ci) and becquerel (Bq).
- Exposure: the amount of radiation that travels through the air, measured as the roentgen (R) and coulomb per kilogram (C/kg).
- Absorbed dose: the amount of radiation actually absorbed by an object or person, measured as the radiation absorbed dose (rad) and gray (Gy).
- Dose equivalent (or effective dose): takes into account both the amount of radiation absorbed and the health effects of that type of radiation. The dose equivalent is same as the absorbed dose for beta and gamma radiation, but it is larger than the absorbed dose for alpha and neutron types of radiation, which cause more severe health effects. Dose equivalent is measured as the roentgen equivalent man (rem) and sievert (Sv).

The physical size and weight of a material has little to do with the amount of radiation it emits. For example, a pound of uranium-238 has about 0.00015 curies of radioactivity, whereas a pound of cobalt-60 has about 518,000 curies of radioactivity.

Richard Crume

See Also: Cancer Risk from Environmental Exposure; Chernobyl Incident; Electric Power Generation, Health Implications of; Fukushima Daiichi Incident; Nuclear Safety; Radiation Sickness; Radon

Further Reading

Federal Communications Commission. *Wireless Devices and Health Concerns*. https://www.fcc.gov/consumers/guides/wireless-devices-and-health-concerns (accessed August 22, 2016).

Gale, Robert P., and Eric Lax. *Radiation: What It Is, What You Need to Know*. New York: Alfred A. Knopf, 2013.

Hitchcock, R. Timothy. *Radio-Frequency and Microwave Radiation*. Fairfax, VA: American Industrial Hygiene Association, 2004.

National Cancer Institute. *Electromagnetic Fields and Cancer*. http://www.cancer.gov/about-cancer/causes-prevention/risk/radiation/electromagnetic-fields-fact-sheet#q4 (accessed August 22, 2016).

Prasad, Kedar N. *Radiation Injury Prevention and Mitigation in Humans*. Boca Raton, FL: CRC Press, 2012.
U.S. Environmental Protection Agency. *Radiation Protection*. https://www.epa.gov/radiation (accessed August 22, 2016).
U.S. Environmental Protection Agency. *Radon*. https://www.epa.gov/radon (accessed August 22, 2016).

RADIATION SICKNESS

Radiation sickness (also known as acute radiation sickness and acute radiation syndrome) is a serious and even fatal condition that occurs when people are exposed to a large amount of radiation over a relatively short period. Such exposure is rare and usually caused by an accident at a nuclear power plant or some other industrial facility using radioactive materials. The very small levels of radiation received from common medical diagnostic equipment, for example, a radiograph used to examine a broken bone, are not nearly high enough to cause radiation sickness.

Preparing for a Nuclear Power Plant Incident

Nearly 3 million Americans live within three miles of a nuclear power plant. What would you do if there were an incident at a nearby plant resulting in the release of radiation? Are you prepared? Fortunately, state and local governments, the federal government, and the electric utilities that own nuclear power plants all have emergency response plans for the possibility of a nuclear power plant incident. Additionally, there are steps you can take as an individual to be prepared. For example, you should have an emergency supply kit that contains all the items you will need (including medical prescriptions and supplies and important documents) in case of evacuation. Additionally, you should develop a family emergency plan that includes information on what to do, how to contact family members, and where to meet during an emergency. Knowing the local evacuation routes is also a good idea. Finally, become familiar with the following emergency notification terms so that you will better understand the seriousness of a situation and know what actions to take:

- Notification of Unusual Event: A small problem has occurred at the plant. No radiation leak is expected. No action on your part will be necessary.
- Alert: A small problem has occurred, and small amounts of radiation could leak inside the plant. This will not affect you, and no action is required.
- Site Area Emergency: Area sirens may be sounded. Listen to your radio or television for safety information.
- General Emergency: Radiation could leak outside the plant and off the plant site. The sirens will sound. Tune to your local radio or television station for reports. Be prepared to follow instructions promptly.

You can learn more at the Department of Homeland Security's Ready website (ready.gov).

Radiation is energy in the form of waves or tiny particles that is released from atoms. When people are exposed to high levels of radiation (particularly X-rays and gamma rays), the skin and other organs can be damaged. The intestinal tract and the blood cell-producing cells of bone marrow are most vulnerable to radiation sickness. Additionally, having radiation sickness increases the risk of developing leukemia or some other form of cancer later in life. Children exposed to radiation from nuclear weapons (i.e., Japanese surviving the Hiroshima and Nagasaki attacks during World War II) and power plant accidents are particularly at increased risk of thyroid cancer.

How sick someone becomes depends on the amount of radiation (i.e., the dose) absorbed by their body. The dose of radiation one receives is measured using a unit called the gray, which is the amount of energy absorbed per unit mass of tissue. (1 gray = 1 joule per kilogram.) The symptoms of radiation sickness begin to appear with exposures approaching 1 gray, and doses greater than 10 gray can result in death (see Table 16).

Nausea and vomiting typically appear first (sometimes accompanied by headache, diarrhea, and fever), and the sooner these symptoms appear, the more likely the person has absorbed higher amounts of radiation. Following the initial symptoms, there may be a brief period when no new symptoms appear, followed by the onset of new symptoms that may be more serious (e.g., loss of appetite, fatigue, dizziness, and even seizures and coma). Symptoms may appear within minutes or days after exposure, and they may come and go. With high doses, damage to the skin may be apparent, including swelling, itching, redness, and

Table 16. Symptoms of radiation sickness.

Symptom	**Mild Exposure (1–2 Gray)**	**Moderate Exposure (2–6 Gray)**	**Severe Exposure (6–9 Gray)**	**Very Severe Exposure (≥ 10 Gray)**
Nausea and vomiting	Within 6 hours	Within 2 hours	Within 1 hour	Within 10 minutes
Diarrhea	–	Within 8 hours	Within 3 hours	Within 1 hour
Headache	–	Within 24 hours	Within 4 hours	Within 2 hours
Fever	–	Within 3 hours	Within 1 hour	Within 1 hour
Dizziness and disorientation	–	–	Within 1 week	Immediate
Weakness and fatigue	Within four weeks	Within one to four weeks	Within one week	Immediate
Hair loss, bloody vomit and stools, infections, poor wound healing, and low blood pressure	–	Within one to four weeks	Within one week	Immediate

Source: Mayo Clinic.

even blisters and ulcers. Skin damage may appear within a few hours of exposure or be delayed several days. When death occurs, the cause is typically due to the destruction of bone marrow, which results in infections and internal bleeding.

The way radiation sickness is treated depends on the severity of exposure. The first step is often to remove any clothing that is contaminated with radioactive particles, and the body is washed with soap and water. Any injuries, including serious burns are treated, fevers and infections are addressed, hydration is maintained, and steps are taken to reduce symptoms and manage pain. Medications may be prescribed to counter the effects of radiation on bone marrow, and with severe bone marrow damage, blood transfusions may be needed.

Richard Crume

See Also: Cancer Risk from Environmental Exposure; Chernobyl Incident; Disaster Preparedness and Response; Emergency Planning and Community Right-to-Know Act; Fukushima Daiichi Incident; Nuclear Safety; Radiation, Ionizing and Nonionizing; Three Mile Island Incident

Further Reading

Allman, Toney. *Radiation Sickness*. Detroit, MI: Lucent Books, 2013.

Centers for Disease Control and Prevention. *Acute Radiation Syndrome (ARS): A Fact Sheet for the Public*. http://emergency.cdc.gov/radiation/ars.asp (accessed August 15, 2016).

Gale, Robert P., and Eric Lax. *Radiation: What It Is, What You Need to Know*. New York: Knopf Doubleday, 2013.

Hersey, John. *Hiroshima*. London: Penguin Books, 2015. (Editor's note: This classic book, reprinted in 2015, about the atomic bombing of Hiroshima, Japan, during World War II is worth reading.)

Mayo Clinic. *Diseases and Conditions: Radiation Sickness*. http://www.mayoclinic.org/diseases-conditions/radiation-sickness/basics/definition/con-20022901 (accessed August 15, 2016).

Merck Manual (Professional Version). *Radiation Exposure and Contamination*. http://www.merckmanuals.com/professional/injuries-poisoning/radiation-exposure-and-contamination/radiation-exposure-and-contamination (accessed August 15, 2016).

Southard, Susan. *Nagasaki: Life after Nuclear War*. New York: Viking Press, 2015.

U.S. Department of Homeland Security. *Ready: Prepare, Plan, Stay Informed*. https://www.ready.gov (accessed August 15, 2016).

U.S. Nuclear Regulatory Commission. *Radiation Basics*. http://www.nrc.gov/about-nrc/radiation/health-effects/radiation-basics.html (accessed August 15, 2016).

RADIOACTIVE WASTES

Radioactive waste is waste material that poses a threat to human health due to ionizing radiation. This is the type of radiation that has sufficient energy to displace electrons or break molecular bonds when passing through certain materials, including living tissue. Radioactive waste is a dangerous health hazard because even moderate amounts of radiation exposure can cause cancer, and the waste can

Yucca Mountain—For and Against

The status of the proposed nuclear waste depository at Yucca Mountain, Nevada, remains uncertain due to vigorous opposition and escalating costs. The spent fuel rods at nuclear power facilities are highly radioactive and must be disposed of with the utmost care. The Yucca Mountain site in Nevada is considered by many to be an ideal repository for radioactive waste because of its isolated desert location far away from population centers. Additionally, the wastes can be stored there securely 1,000 feet (305 meters) underground in a closed hydrologic basin, and the site is surrounded by federal lands. However, opponents to the Yucca Mountain project argue that the site is unsuitable given that it is a seismically active region with numerous earthquake faults and nearby volcanic cinder cones. Furthermore, they contend that there are interconnecting faults and fractures that could allow groundwater and radioactive materials to move rapidly through the site, potentially affecting the aquifer beneath and eventually being released to the environment. Finally, opponents are worried about accidents during transportation of large quantities of radioactive materials by rail. If ever approved, the cost to build a transport railroad line in Nevada alone could exceed $3 billion in today's dollars, and the funding required to actually construct and operate the site could reach $100 billion or more.

remain radioactive for tens of thousands of years. Exposure to a large amount of ionizing radiation over a short period (referred to as "acute" exposure) can cause radiation sickness and even death.

The most common form of highly radioactive waste in the United States originates at nuclear electric power plants. The nuclear material in the fuel rods at these plants is composed of either uranium or plutonium, and the disposal of spent fuel rods must be done with great care to avoid radiation exposure. Additionally, other dangerous forms of radioactive waste include uranium mill tailings and "transuranic waste," which is waste generated from the recycling of spent fuel materials or fabrication of nuclear weapons. Radioactive waste products are regulated by the U.S. Nuclear Regulatory Commission (NRC).

As nuclear fuel rods in reactors expend their fissile material, they become highly radioactive waste. Most spent fuel rods are stored in on-site pools, typically 40 feet (12 meters) deep, where the water helps contain the radiation as the rods cool. Because many reactor water pools have reached capacity, older fuel rods must be moved to dry storage, typically after 5 to 10 years. In dry storage, the spent fuel rods are surrounded by inert gas inside a closed steel cylinder called a cask. Each individual cask is encased in more steel, in concrete, or in other materials that can shield workers from radiation. Nationwide, about 78 percent of spent nuclear fuel rods are contained in pools, with the remaining 22 percent in dry casks.

In addition to spent fuel rods, other high-level radioactive wastes must also be disposed of in a manner that protects the public. For example, uranium mill tailings, a by-product of mining and extracting, are stored in special disposal cells licensed by the NRC. Furthermore, in all nuclear power generating facilities, the reactor cores heat water to drive a turbine, and this water at some of these facilities can become radioactive, as does the water used to cool spent fuel rods. Radioactive water is treated on-site until radiation is below federal limits and can be discharged locally.

Since the early 1980s, when the first nuclear plants began to accumulate large numbers of spent fuel rods, the United States has been trying to establish a permanent waste disposal location for this highly radioactive and dangerous material. Geologic burial deep below the earth's surface was determined to be the best option for disposal over several other possibilities. (One proposed disposal option was to shoot the radioactive waste into outer space!) In 1987, the federal government determined that Yucca Mountain in Nevada, about 90 miles northwest of Las Vegas, was a prime location for storing spent fuel rods. However, disagreeing with the assessment that disposal at Yucca Mountain was safe, this plan was strongly opposed by many local residents, environmental advocacy groups, and the state of Nevada. While Yucca Mountain is still a potential long-term site for storing these radioactive wastes, the issue is still being debated, and at present, there is no funding to continue the project. Earlier work was limited to constructing an exploratory rail tunnel, which is now closed.

There are currently no viable alternatives to Yucca Mountain that all interested parties agree on. A small amount of nuclear waste material is housed at the Waste Isolation Pilot Project outside Carlsbad, New Mexico, and some dry fuel rod casks are housed at a facility near Idaho Falls, Idaho, which is only meant as an interim solution. Two locations, one in Andrews County, Texas, and the other in Lea County, New Mexico, are under consideration for becoming interim storage sites. Some nuclear waste can be reprocessed to be used again as reactor fuel, and a number of European countries have reprocessing facilities for their nuclear power plants. These reprocessing facilities produce some radioactive waste themselves, but by reprocessing the waste into fuel, the total amount of radioactive material to be disposed of is reduced.

Not all radioactive waste is as dangerous as spent fuel rods. The U.S. Environmental Protection Agency (EPA) defines "low-activity" radioactive waste as having small enough concentrations of radionuclides that regulation for containment and disposal need not be as stringent. For example, certain medical, research laboratory, and industrial wastes are radioactive but at relatively low levels. Four sites in the United States are licensed to accept low-level radioactive waste, and in some cases, this waste may be allowed to decay until it is safe enough to dispose of in a regular landfill.

To date, the only major accident in the United States involving radioactive waste is the partial meltdown of the Unit No. 2 Reactor at the Three Mile Island nuclear power plant, near Middletown, Pennsylvania, in 1979. A series of mechanical and human errors resulted in coolant water leaking and exposing the fuel rods, causing half of the nuclear core to melt down over a short period. However, the containment building functioned as designed, preventing any radioactive contamination of the surrounding area. This incident prompted a number of regulatory changes to nuclear power facility design and safety.

Recently, radioactive wastewater from hydraulic fracturing operations has become an issue as newer drilling operations come into contact with soil and rock that contain various contaminants, including naturally radioactive materials. Because public wastewater treatment facilities are not designed to treat this type of wastewater discharge, the EPA has developed regulations to ensure this wastewater is not sent to publicly owned treatment works.

Aaron Dorman

See Also: Electric Power Generation, Health Implications of; Environmental Protection Agency; Hydraulic Fracturing; Nuclear Regulatory Commission; Nuclear Safety; Radiation, Ionizing and Nonionizing; Sewage Treatment and Disposal; Three Mile Island Incident

Further Reading

Biello, David. "Spent Nuclear Fuel: A Trash Heap Deadly for 250,000 Years or a Renewable Energy Source?" *Scientific American* (January 2009). https://www.scientificamerican.com/article/nuclear-waste-lethal-trash-or-renewable-energy-source.

Eureka County, Nevada, Nuclear Waste Office. *Frequently Asked Questions*. http://www.yuccamountain.org/faq.htm#status (accessed December 22, 2016).

Lee, William E., Michael Ojovan, and Carol Jantzen, eds. *Radioactive Waste Management and Contaminated Site Clean-Up: Processes, Technologies, and International Experience*. Sawston, UK: Woodhead (Elsevier), 2013.

Meldrum, J., et al. "Life Cycle Water Use for Electricity Generation: A Review and Harmonization of Literature Estimates Unconventional Oil and Gas Extraction Effluent Guidelines." *Environmental Research Letters*, vol. 8, no. 1 (March 2013): 1–18.

Pretreatment Standards for the Oil and Gas Extraction Point Source Category, EPA 821-F-16-001. Washington, DC: U.S. Environmental Protection Agency, 2016.

U.S. Environmental Protection Agency. *Radiation Protection, Radiation Health Effects*. https://www.epa.gov/radiation/radiation-health-effects#tab-3 (accessed December 22, 2016).

U.S. Nuclear Regulatory Commission. *Backgrounder on the Three Mile Island Accident*. https://www.nrc.gov/reading-rm/doc-collections/fact-sheets/3mile-isle.html (accessed December 22, 2016).

U.S. Nuclear Regulatory Commission. *Radioactive Waste*. http://www.nrc.gov/waste.html (accessed December 22, 2016).

RADON

Radon is a radioactive, colorless, tasteless, and odorless gas found naturally in rocks and soil, from which it can escape into buildings, homes, and the environment. Radon is the second-leading cause of lung cancer in the United States after smoking, and it is the leading cause of lung cancer among nonsmokers. Around 21,000 Americans die of radon-related lung cancer each year.

Testing for Radon

If you want to test for radon in your home or business, there are two types of monitors: passive and active. Passive monitors are inexpensive and easy to set up, and they do not require electricity. Active monitors require electric power, but they can provide hourly readings and an average for the entire test period. Information on testing for radon, including the types of testing devices and the ones most appropriate to your situation, can be obtained from your state radon office. Discounted test kits and helpful information are available through the National Radon Program Services office at Kansas State University (http://sosradon.org), and test kits are also available commercially, for example, at home improvement stores and through online retailers.

Radon can readily enter buildings from the ground through basements and crawl spaces, cracks and gaps in floors and walls, construction joints, exhaust fans, and gas appliances. Additionally, certain materials used in the construction of buildings can release radon, such as bricks and mortar, cinder blocks, concrete, gravel, sheet rock, and stone. Well water and groundwater containing radon can be additional sources of exposure when used in sinks and showers and certain home appliances. For example, the heating and agitation of the water in a dishwasher or washing machine can cause radon to become airborne, leading to inhalation exposure.

Radon levels are not uniform across the United States or even in localities. The U.S. Environmental Protection Agency (EPA) estimates that as many as 1 in 15 American homes have radon levels above the EPA-recommended action level of 4 pCi/L. Furthermore, the EPA cautions that levels below 4 pCi/L can still potentially pose adverse health effects. Thus, residents are advised to check radon levels in their homes and to take action to reduce radon exposure when elevated levels are found.

Elevated radon levels across the United States have prompted many states to enact programs to help schools, homeowners, and building owners mitigate the amount of radon in indoor air. The increase in shale gas extraction over the past decade has raised additional concerns in some states because the waste streams from hydraulic fracturing techniques may contain elevated radon concentrations.

Radon emits alpha particles that are deposited deep in the lungs, and lung cancer can result when radon is inhaled over long periods. Small cell carcinoma, adenocarcinoma, and squamous cell carcinoma can develop in response to long-term radon exposure. Some studies suggest that radon is also linked to a higher incidence of leukemia, lymphoma, and multiple myeloma. In addition, elevated indoor air exposure to radon can lead to nonmalignant respiratory diseases.

The only way to know if you are exposed to elevated radon levels is to have your home or building tested. Radon testing is relatively inexpensive, and the testing is easy to do. In cases where elevated levels are found, a certified radon mitigation specialist should be consulted. Many states require that people in the business of radon mitigation be certified, and requirements for testing and disclosure are also common.

There are several methods to mitigate radon in buildings. Mechanical radon reduction systems rely on suction techniques that draw radon away from the interior of the building. One common example of a radon reduction system is sub-slab suction (depressurization), which relies on inserting suction pipes into the bottom floor or concrete slab. The suction pipes are connected to a radon vent fan that discharges the radon to the outside air. Radon levels may also be lowered by improving basement or crawlspace ventilation, sealing cracks or spaces, pressurizing a room or building, and improving basement, crawlspace, or living space ventilation.

In new construction, improved techniques can mitigate radon exposure. For example, a layer of course gravel can be placed below the building foundation, thereby allowing the radon and other naturally occurring gases to move freely beneath the building but not enter the structure. Plastic sheeting or a vapor barrier can be installed on top of the gravel to further prevent radon gases from entering the building. A pipe installed vertically from the gravel layer through cavities in the building can help vent the radon away from the structure, and all openings can be sealed to keep radon from entering the building. Before embarking on radon mitigation project, be sure to consult with an expert to determine the best approach for your situation.

Elizabeth Ann Glass Geltman and Nichole LeClair

See Also: Cancer Risk from Environmental Exposure; Environmental Protection Agency; Hydraulic Fracturing; Indoor Environment; Radiation, Ionizing and Nonionizing

Further Reading

Kansas State University. *National Radon Program Services*. http://sosradon.org (accessed March 7, 2017).

Lantz, Paula M., David Mendez, and Martin Philbert. "Radon, Smoking, and Lung Cancer: The Need to Refocus Radon Control Policy." *American Journal of Public Health*, vol. 103, no. 3 (March 2013): 443–447.

Neri, A., S. L. Stewart, and W. Angell. "Radon Control Activities for Lung Cancer Prevention in National Comprehensive Cancer Control Program Plans, 2005–2011." *Preventing Chronic Disease*, vol. 10, no. 8. (August 2013): E132.

Peckham, E. C., et al. "Residential Radon Exposure and Incidence of Childhood Lymphoma in Texas, 1995–2011." *International Journal of Environmental Research and Public Health*, vol. 12, no. 10 (September 2015): 12110–12126.

Public Health Statement: Radon. Atlanta, GA: Agency for Toxic Substances and Disease Registry, 2012.

U.S. Environmental Protection Agency. *Radon*. https://www.epa.gov/radon (accessed March 7, 2017).

WHO Handbook on Indoor Radon. Geneva, Switzerland: World Health Organization, 2009.

RECYCLING

Recycling has been an important part of maintaining a healthy environment since the early days of the Industrial Revolution. The first recycled paper plant, using discarded cotton and linen rags, was built at the Rittenhouse Mill near Philadelphia in 1690. As early as the Revolutionary War, it was realized that recycling was an essential method of recovering valuable materials that were in short supply. In recent times, supply shortages of some materials, combined with modern environmental consciousness and complex waste disposal requirements, have led to an increase in recycling for all kinds of waste materials.

The U.S. Environmental Protection Agency (EPA) defines "recycling" as "the process of collecting and processing materials that would otherwise be thrown away as trash and turning them into new products." The health benefits of recycling include the avoidance of any negative consequences that would have happened without the recycling process. This includes benefits not only from reducing the waste stream but also from reducing the need to find new resources, which can often be an intensive and environmentally destructive process.

Only about one-third of waste in the United States is recycled or composted (see the following figure), and although that rate has been going up, so has the total amount of garbage produced as well as per capita garbage generation. Also, recycling statistics do not account for trash like electronic waste that is either exported to other countries or stored unused in someone's basement or garage. There is also an increasing amount of discarded plastic material that has become part of

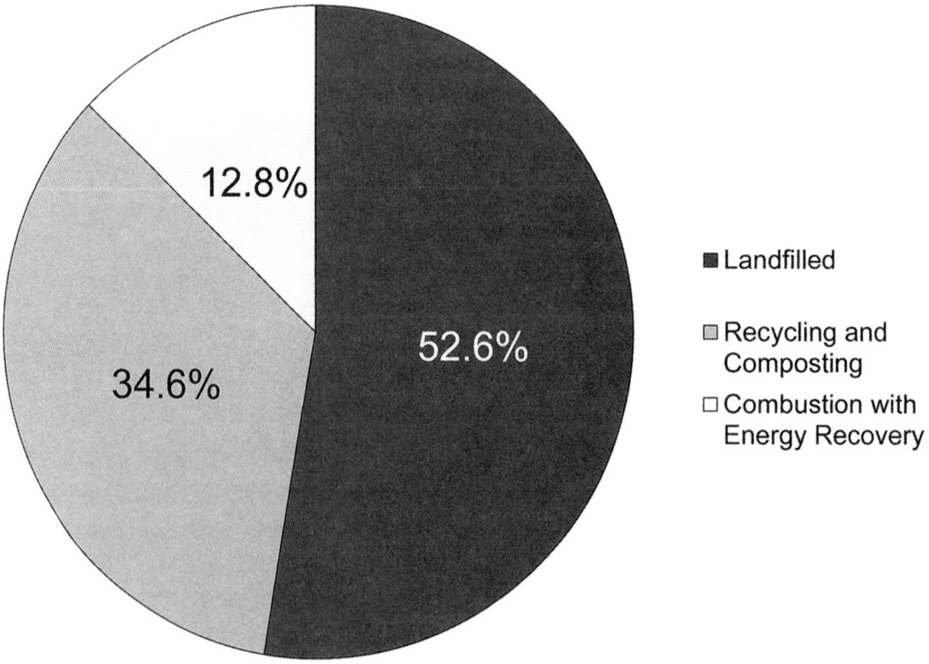

Management of municipal solid waste in the United States, 2014. (U.S. EPA, Advancing Sustainable Materials Management: 2014 Fact Sheet)

the large ocean garbage gyres and may not be accounted for in waste statistics. In the United States, the majority of garbage that is not recycled ends up in a landfill. Additionally, about 13 percent of U.S. garbage is incinerated with energy recovery. Under the Resource Conservation and Recovery Act, landfills cannot simply be holes in the ground where garbage collects and slowly disintegrates. Instead, they are lined with an impervious material like plastic or concrete and equipped to collect leachate (i.e., garbage that breaks down to a liquid form) and methane, a byproduct of anaerobic decomposition.

Several decades ago, there were over 7,500 active landfills in the United States. But since then, many have become filled to capacity and permanently closed, and now less than 2,000 landfills remain in operation. (The decreasing number of landfills is partially offset by an increase in size of remaining landfills.) The main hazards today of garbage disposal are impacts on climate change and disruptive land use. Many areas of the United States no longer have active landfills, and garbage is hauled long distances. For example, the garbage in New York City is transported to Ohio, Pennsylvania, or West Virginia for disposal. Therefore, the environmental effects of garbage must also include the pollution produced during transportation to disposal sites.

Although the odors near landfills can be noxious, the trace amounts of ammonia and hydrogen sulfide that typically cause the stinky smell are generally not high enough to impair human health. Over 90 percent of the gaseous output from landfills is methane or carbon dioxide, neither of which produces an

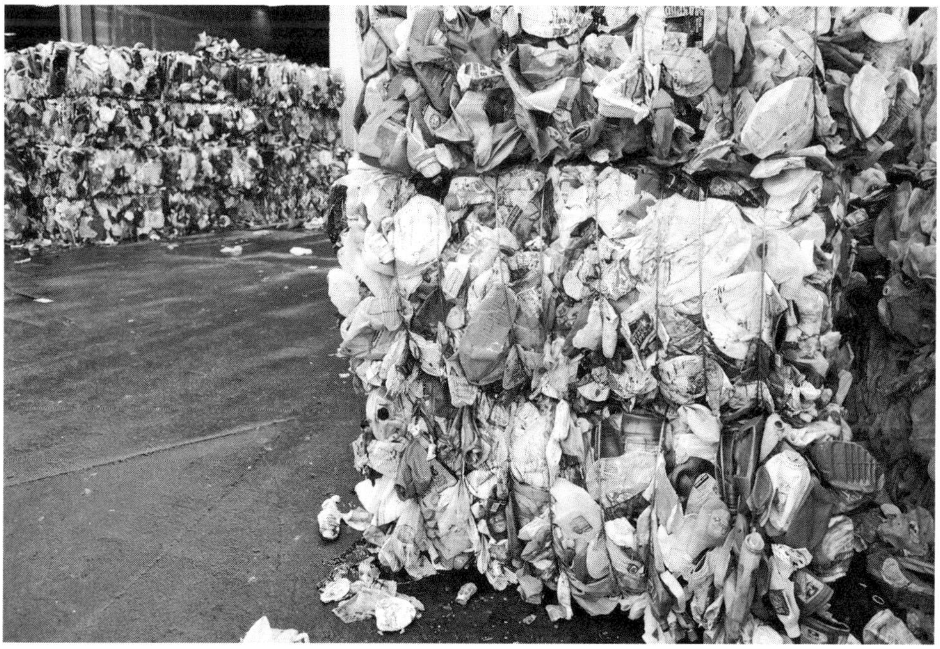

Packaged plastic trash ready to be recycled. Today about one-third of the municipal waste generated in the United States is recycled or composted. (Shutterstock)

odor or directly harms humans, although both are greenhouse gases contributing to climate change. An alternative to landfilling, waste incineration, effectively reduces the volume of wastes but can cause toxic air pollution, including dioxins and mercury.

The mining, extraction, processing, and manufacturing of new materials take a high toll on our health and environment, and the benefits of recycling are typically measured in terms of reducing these impacts. For example, the EPA reports that 89 million tons (81 metric tons) of municipal wastes were recycled or composted in 2014, equivalent to an annual reduction of 200 million tons (181 million metric tons) of carbon dioxide (equivalent) emissions, or the annual emissions from 38 million passenger cars. Recycling rates differ for different materials. For example, in the United States, 99 percent of lead-acid batteries and 90 percent of corrugated boxes are recycled successfully, but only 41 percent of tires, 33 percent of glass containers, and about 30 percent of plastic bottles and jars are recycled.

For some common materials, such as aluminum, recycling saves up to 95 percent of the energy required to mine and extract the same amount of new material, and the recycling of paper goods requires only half the energy needed for fresh pulp. Water conservation is another important benefit from recycling, where recovering 1 ton (0.9 metric ton) of paper is equivalent to saving 7,000 gallons (26,500 liters) of water. The most significant health benefit of recycling may come from efforts to reduce plastics in the environment. Plastics are difficult to break down and can persist in the environment for centuries, and plastic debris and chemical additives can easily enter the food chain. Heart disease and reproductive abnormalities have been linked to the presence of Bisphenol A (BPA), which is found in polycarbonate bottles and can linings. The U.S. Centers for Disease Control and Prevention estimates that at least trace amounts of BPA can be found in the bodies of over 90 percent of Americans.

Despite their intrinsic benefits, most recycling efforts leave something to be desired. Recycling plants themselves require energy input, and at present that nearly always comes in the form of nonrenewable fuels. Furthermore, when oil prices are low, recycled plastic may become more expensive than manufacturing new plastics. Quality can sometimes be an issue when a recycled material is not of the same quality as a newly made material and consumers find this objectionable.

Legislation on recycling varies by state, but some of the more effective practices include curbside recycle bins and small monetary incentives for returning glass and plastics. Also, there are efforts to limit certain kinds of packaging and toxic ingredients, for example, in the manufacture of BPA-free bottles.

Aaron Dorman

See Also: Bisphenol A (BPA); Carbon Dioxide and the Carbon Cycle; Dioxin Pollution; Electronic Waste Disposal; Environmental Protection Agency; Land Disposal of Waste Materials; Mercury Pollution; Municipal Solid Waste Management; Ocean Dumping and the Pacific Garbage Patch; Odor Pollution; Resource Conservation and Recovery Act; Three Rs of Waste Management; Waste Incineration

Further Reading

Advancing Sustainable Materials Management: 2014 Fact Sheet. Washington, DC: U.S. Environmental Protection Agency, 2016.

McDonough, William, and Michael Braungart. *Cradle to Cradle: Remaking the Way We Make Things*. New York: North Point Press, 2002.

Minter, Adam. *Junkyard Planet: Travels in the Billion-Dollar Trash Trade*. New York: Bloomsbury Press, 2013.

New York State Department of Health. *Important Things to Know about Landfill Gas*. https://www.health.ny.gov/environmental/outdoors/air/landfill_gas.htm (accessed December 19, 2016).

Toxic Actions Center. *The Problems with Waste*. http://www.toxicsaction.org/problems-and-solutions/waste (accessed December 19, 2016).

U.S. Environmental Protection Agency. *Advancing Sustainable Materials Management: Facts and Figures*. https://www.epa.gov/smm/advancing-sustainable-materials-management-facts-and-figures (accessed December 19, 2016).

U.S. Environmental Protection Agency. *Reduce, Reuse, Recycle*. https://www.epa.gov/recycle (accessed December 19, 2016).

Worrell, Ernst, and M.A. Reuter. *Handbook of Recycling: State-of-the-Art for Practitioners, Analysts, and Scientists*. Amsterdam, the Netherlands: Elsevier, 2014.

REGIONAL HAZE POLLUTION

Many Americans travel to national parks to enjoy nature and take in the view, often of distant mountains or sunrise over the ocean. However, sometimes the view is obscured by white or brownish haze. Some haze is natural, but most is caused by air pollution present over a wide region. Some of the pollutants causing haze are associated with serious health conditions and environmental damage.

When sunlight strikes small pollution particles in the atmosphere, some of the light is absorbed by the particles and other light is scattered in all directions. This absorption and scattering of light reduces the visibility of distant objects and makes the sky appear hazy. In the eastern United States, haze often reduces the visibility to just 15 to 25 miles (24 to 40 kilometers), down from the 90-mile (145-kilometer) visibility expected on a perfectly clear day. In the western United States, where visibilities tend to be higher because humidity is lower and air pollution is less, haze often reduces visibility from 140 miles (225 kilometers) on a clear day to between 35 and 90 miles (56 and 145 kilometers). Reduced visibility is particularly bothersome to more than 300 million annual visitors to U.S. national parks, many of whom are hoping to escape urban smog and experience pristine conditions.

The small particles that cause haze can either be emitted directly into the atmosphere or form from gases (e.g., the formation of sulfate and nitrate particles from sulfur dioxide and nitrogen oxide gases). The sources of haze-forming particles and gases include coal-burning electric utility power plants, motor vehicles, and various manufacturing operations. These particles can also originate with natural events, such as forest fires and wind-entrained dust (e.g., the dust storms prevalent in the western United States). These pollutants can travel hundreds of miles, causing haze far away from the original sources of pollution.

Some of the haze-forming pollutants can also cause adverse health effects. For example, sulfur dioxide and nitrogen oxides can result in a variety of respiratory problems, including increased asthma symptoms, and elevated levels have been associated with an increase in emergency room and hospital admissions. The inhalation of small particles has been linked to increased respiratory illness, decreased lung function, and premature death. Small particles, such as the sulfate and nitrate particles common in haze, can also contribute to acid rain formation, which makes lakes and streams unsuitable for many aquatic species and can damage building and automobile surfaces.

While it is tempting to characterize haze and visibility in terms of how far we can see, it is actually much more complicated than that. For example, while admiring a distant mountain range, any haze that is present in the atmosphere may affect our perception of colors, forms, contrasts, and details. For some observers, this may be bothersome, whereas others may not even notice a perception difference. Furthermore, how we are affected by haze may depend on personality factors such as our interest in a particular view or what value we place on the object being observed. Time of day is also an important factor because our perception of haze is usually more acute during the early morning and late afternoon hours, when the sun is lower in the sky. The result is that haze is a controversial topic, often with unclear solutions. In the case of haze, beauty is truly in the eye of the beholder!

Richard Crume

See Also: Air Pollution; Asthma; Automobile and Truck Emissions and Controls; Electric Power Generation, Health Implications of; Fugitive Dust; Particulate Matter and Bioaerosols Pollution; Respiratory Disease and Air Pollution

Further Reading

Friedlander, Sheldon K. *Smoke, Dust, and Haze: Fundamentals of Aerosol Dynamics*. New York: Oxford University Press, 2000.

Malm, William C. *Visibility: The Seeing of Near and Distant Landscape Features*. Amsterdam, the Netherlands: Elsevier, 2016.

National Park Service. *Visibility Effects of Air Pollution*. https://www.nature.nps.gov/air/aqbasics/visibility.cfm (accessed March 28, 2017).

National Park Service. *Visibility Monitoring Overview*. https://www.nature.nps.gov/air/monitoring/vismon.cfm (accessed March 28, 2017).

U.S. Environmental Protection Agency. *Visibility and Regional Haze*. https://www.epa.gov/visibility (accessed March 28, 2017).

RENEWABLE ENERGY, HEALTH IMPLICATIONS OF

Fossil fuels, such as coal, oil, and gas, and nuclear power are used to produce much of the electricity the United States depends on. The transition from fossil fuels and nuclear power to renewable energy can greatly improve public health while helping to protect the environment. This transition is currently underway.

Greensburg Rebuilds with Renewable Energy

In 2007, Greensburg, Kansas, was mostly destroyed by a massive tornado—hardly a building was left standing throughout the town. Rather than rebuilding the city the way it was before the tornado, the residents viewed their misfortune as an opportunity to become a model for energy efficiency and renewable energy. This vision became a reality with the installation of a large wind farm and a number of smaller solar and biogas installations and with building codes designed to conserve energy. Green corridors and a walkable downtown were also part of the city's redevelopment plan. Today, the city is powered by 100 percent renewable energy.

Can Renewable Energy Make Us a Healthier Nation?

Technological innovations and volume sales have helped make renewable energy more affordable than ever.

An Interview with Carly Rixham

Executive Director, American Solar Energy Society

Carly Rixham is executive director of the American Solar Energy Society, the world's leading association of solar professionals and advocates. Rixham has a diverse background in solar power, biofuels, and wastewater management, and she has taught biology and ecology at the university and high school levels. As solar energy becomes more popular in the United States and throughout the world, Rixham is interested in promoting solar energy at the grassroots level and connecting science with the greater community of solar advocates.

By now, most people are familiar with the concepts of solar energy and a sustainable energy economy, but there has been little discussion in the press about how solar and sustainable energy benefit people's health. Can you comment on how replacing fossil fuel energy sources with innovative technologies, such as solar power, will help make us a healthier nation?

There are several ways in which solar and other renewable energy technologies improve public health. By replacing conventional fossil fuel-fired power plants, renewable energy is playing an increasing important role in the fight against climate change by cutting greenhouse gas emissions. We know that climate change will cause more severe heat waves and droughts, increase urban smog, and enhance the spread of diseases by ticks and mosquitoes. Thus, by replacing the sources of climate change gases, renewables help make the earth a healthier place to live. Fossil-fuel power plants also contribute significantly to air pollution in our major cities. Did you know that over 120 million Americans live in areas where federal air quality standards are exceeded? Again, clean renewable energy is obviously a better choice than fossil fuels!

Interest in renewable energy has been growing as evidence of climate change begins to emerge. Yet, proponents of traditional energy sources, like coal,

oil, natural gas, and nuclear power, argue that the required renewable energy infrastructure will take many more years to develop. Is there still time for renewable energy to play a major role in combating climate change?

Not replacing fossil fuel power plants with solar and other renewable energy sources is *not* an option. Technological innovations and volume sales have helped make renewable energy more affordable than ever. As proof of this, almost two-thirds of new electrical generation placed in service in the United States in 2015 comprised renewable energy—solar, wind, geothermal, biomass, and hydropower. That's an impressive accomplishment for an industry that some experts thought could not compete much longer with cheap coal and natural gas. While much must be accomplished to improve our power infrastructure and install sufficient renewable energy capacity, natural gas and possibly nuclear power can serve as a bridge, weaning us off of fossil fuels as we more fully develop renewable sources.

The American Solar Energy Society organizes the National Solar Tour, which provides an annual opportunity for Americans to tour innovative green homes and buildings and to see how solar energy can be used efficiently. These homes are not only environmentally friendly, but they also provide a healthy indoor environment. Do you see green buildings playing a complementary role with renewable energy in reducing the nation's dependence on fossil fuels and creating a healthy environment?

Reducing the energy consumption of buildings is essential to solving the climate change problem. This is because buildings in the United States account for almost 40 percent of total energy use and almost 70 percent of total electricity consumption. Because much of this energy comes from fossil fuel-powered power plants that are the leading source of climate changes gases, reducing building energy use can help fight climate change in a really big way. New buildings can be constructed so that they are much more energy efficient than in the past, and existing buildings can be retrofitted with energy-saving features. How we live and work in buildings makes a difference too. For example, simple actions like turning the lights out when we leave a room, washing clothes in warm water, and setting the thermostat back a few degrees in the winter can help a lot, especially if every American can be convinced to save energy. Passive solar houses that incorporate large south-facing windows and thermal mass for storing daytime heating can be especially effective in reducing heating costs in cold climates.

What is a good career path for a recent college or university graduate who is interested in addressing climate change and environmental pollution by promoting renewable energy and green buildings?

This is a tough question because there are so many fields someone might go into to develop and install renewable energy systems and promote green building practices—engineering, architecture, physics, materials science, and various trade professions, to name a few. The important thing is to find what you are good at and be the best you can be. Gaining practical experience through an internship or entry-level position is especially important.

For transportation fuels, ethanol (made from corn and other plant materials) and biodiesel (made from vegetable oils, animal fats, or recycled restaurant grease) are generally considered renewable energy. However, significant amounts of fossil fuels are used in growing the feedstock for these biofuels, refining and processing the feedstock, and transporting the feedstock and biofuels. In addition, combustion of biofuels in vehicles produces similar amounts of air pollution to fossil fuels. Thus, the health benefits of biofuels over fossil fuels may not be significant when the entire life cycle is taken into account.

Generating electricity from renewable sources rather than fossil fuels, however, does present the opportunity for significant public health improvements. The major sources of renewable energy include hydroelectric, wind, biomass (wood and waste), solar, and geothermal power. Table 17 lists the percent that each of these sources contributes to total electricity generation in the United States. While these percentages are currently small, wind and solar power, in particular, have experienced rapid growth, which is expected to continue well into the future. (Renewable energy makes up about 13 percent of total U.S. electricity generation. Nuclear power contributes 20 percent, coal 33 percent, natural gas 33 percent, and petroleum just 1 percent.)

Life cycle analysis demonstrates that renewable energy generally has substantial health benefits over fossil fuel and nuclear power sources. This is to be expected because renewables depend on clean, natural energy sources like sunlight and the

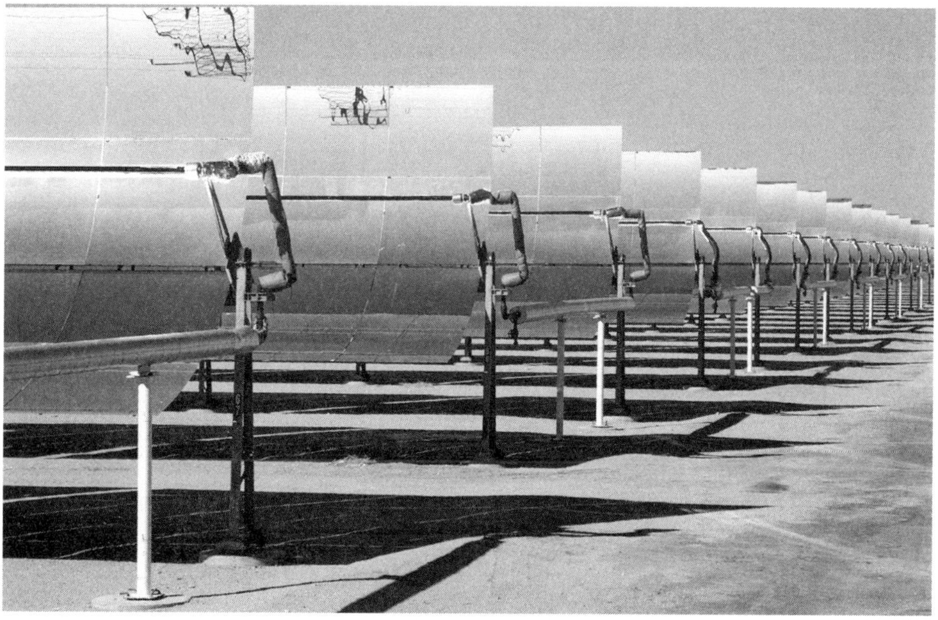

A solar energy generating facility in California's Mojave Desert. Renewable energy, including solar, wind, hydroelectric, biomass, and geothermal power, makes up only about 13 percent of U.S. energy production, but the percentage is growing every year. (iStockphoto.com)

Table 17. Contribution of renewable energy sources to total U.S. electricity generation in 2015.

Source	Contribution to Total U.S. Electricity Generation (Percentage)
Hydroelectric	6.0
Wind	4.6
Biomass wood	1.0
Solar	0.7
Biomass waste	0.4
Geothermal	0.4

wind. In contrast, the extraction, processing, and transportation of coal, oil, natural gas, and uranium (for nuclear fuel) produce copious amounts of air and water pollution and solid waste. Although concentrating solar power (CSP) facilities can cause some thermal pollution (i.e., the discharge of warm water into nearby lakes and streams), these facilities are rare, and the thermal pollution can be mitigated or eliminated through the use of technologies such as dry cooling.

Whereas renewable energy sources are generally clean, fossil-fuel and nuclear plants create large volumes of air, water, and solid waste pollution, including greenhouse gases, other common air pollutants, heavy metals, dioxins and furans, and high-level radioactive wastes. These pollutants cause adverse health consequences leading to thousands of premature deaths per year, tens of thousands of nonfatal illnesses, and resultant missed days at work and school. In 2015, reductions in sulfur dioxide and nitrogen oxides associated with the consumption of more wind power (at the expense of fossil fuels) saved $7.3 billion in public health costs.

In addition, fossil fuel and nuclear power plants are major sources of water use, second only to agriculture in many states. In comparison, wind and solar power facilities (except for some CSP plants) use practically no water. This leaves extra water for other purposes, such as agriculture, municipal uses, and maintaining healthy aquatic ecosystems.

Many misconceptions exist about renewable energy and its health implications. For example, claims have been made about the pollution that is created during the manufacturing of solar photovoltaic (PV) panels because of the amount of energy needed to make silicon, a basic building block of more than half of the PV panels manufactured today. These claims are based on out-of-date data that do not reflect the current manufacturing processes, which have become much more efficient in the past few years. Such claims also ignore that many silicon manufacturing facilities are now powered themselves by renewable energy and that fossil fuel and nuclear power plants also require energy-intense materials during manufacturing and construction (e.g., concrete and highly specialized metals). In addition, some solar PV panel manufacturers offer recycling programs for their products. Laws and regulations mandating the recycling of solar panels are not currently common but could be enacted in the future.

Misconceptions about health impacts from wind power largely focus on two issues: noise (caused by the wind turbine blades rotating through the air) and shadow flicker (a flickering on the ground as sunlight passes between the blades). While these issues can be annoying to some people, there is no credible evidence that wind turbines directly cause health (including mental health) problems or disease. Opposition to wind power also often focuses on bird deaths, although bird advocacy groups like the Audubon Society strongly support properly sited wind power facilities. Furthermore, many conservation biologists believe wind power's contribution to reducing greenhouse gases is important in the fight against climate change, which threatens wildlife on a global scale.

Switching to 100 percent renewable electricity through on-site generation or purchasing programs is already achievable, as evidenced by the hundreds of cities, states, countries, homes, and industries that have already achieved this level of renewables or have made serious commitments to do so in the future. Cities already achieving 100 percent renewable electricity include Aspen, Colorado; Georgetown, Texas; Burlington, Vermont; Kodiak, Alaska; and Greensburg, Kansas. Larger cities, such as Vancouver, Canada, and San Francisco, California, have committed to achieving 100 percent renewables in the next decade. Hawaii is on track to generate 100 percent of its electricity from renewable sources by 2045, and in Vermont, 75 percent of the electricity sold by its electric companies will come from renewables by 2032. The U.S. operations of technology giants Apple and Google are powered with 100 percent renewable energy.

Not only are solar, wind, and hydroelectric facilities nonpolluting, but they are often the lowest-cost source of electricity generation. For example, wind power is so inexpensive and plentiful in Texas that at times it has driven wholesale electricity rates into negative territory (i.e., electric generators have had to pay utilities to put their electricity on the grid). This has prompted some retail electric utilities, such as Amigo Energy in Texas, to offer free electricity at night when wind generation tends to be strongest and electricity demand lowest. Similarly, regulators in California and other states have chosen solar power plants over natural gas power plants, based on cost alone. While adequate long-distance transmission lines and electric storage continue presenting obstacles to renewable energy in some situations, the main obstacle to increased use of renewable energy is political inertia.

Robert Ukeiley

See Also: Climate Change and Human Health; Dioxin Pollution; Electric Power Generation, Health Implications of; Heavy Metal Pollution; Life Cycle Assessment; Noise Pollution; Nuclear Safety; Radioactive Wastes; Recycling

Further Reading

American Solar Energy Society. *About ASES*. www.ases.org (accessed May 16, 2016).

American Wind Energy Association. *Home Page*. www.awea.org (accessed May 16, 2016).

Biomass Power Association. *Home Page*. www.biomasspowerassociation.com (accessed May 16, 2016).

Brown, Lester R. *The Great Transition: Shifting from Fossil Fuels to Solar and Wind Energy*. New York: W.W. Norton and Company, 2015.
Geothermal Energy Association. *Home Page*. http://geo-energy.org/Default.aspx (accessed May 16, 2016).
National Hydropower Association. *Home Page*. www.hydro.org (accessed May 16, 2016).
National Renewable Energy Laboratory. *Home Page*. http://www.nrel.gov (accessed May 16, 2016).
Solar Energy Industries Association. *Issues and Policies, PV Recycling*. http://www.seia.org/policy/environment/pv-recycling (accessed May 16, 2016).
Sørensen, Brent. *Renewable Energy, Fourth Edition: Physics, Engineering, Environmental Impacts, Economics, and Planning*. Amsterdam, the Netherlands: Academic Press, 2010.
U.S. Department of Energy, Office of Energy Efficiency and Renewable Energy. *Alternative Fuels Data Center*. www.afdc.energy.gov/fuels (accessed May 16, 2016).
U.S. Energy Information Administration. *Energy in Brief: How Much U.S. Electricity Is Generated from Renewable Energy?* www.eia.gov/energy_in_brief/article/renewable_electricity.cfm (accessed May 16, 2016).
U.S. Renewable Energy Association. *Home Page*. https://usrea.org (accessed May 16, 2016).

REPRODUCTIVE HEALTH AND ENVIRONMENTAL EXPOSURES

Environmental pollutants interfere with reproductive function in experimental models, with corroborating evidence provided by observational human epidemiology studies. Synthetic, geogenic, and biogenic agents pollute air, water, and food from anthropogenic activities, including manufacturing and energy recovery, and these pollutants are also liberated by natural processes, such as volcanic eruptions and forest fires. Many pollutants alter endocrine function, changing gene expression and modifying cell communications, with resulting dysfunction. Additionally, pollutants can increase oxidative stress and inflammation, leading to tissue damage and death, and they can modify the acquired pattern of epigenetic molecules that bind to deoxyribonucleic acid (DNA) and regulate gene expression.

With the substantial growth of industry and manufacturing since World War II, exposure to toxic trace elements and synthetic organic compounds has become nearly ubiquitous. Toxic trace elements, such as arsenic (As), cadmium (Cd), lead (Pb), and mercury (Hg), are widespread contaminants of air, water, and food and have been shown to diminish semen quality, increase pregnancy loss and stillbirth, and foster developmental delays in offspring. Persistent organic pollutants (POPs), polychlorinated biphenyls (PCBs), and polybrominated diphenyl ethers (PBDEs), for instance, biomagnify in food chains, leading to dietary exposure through consumption of animal fats or ingestion of dust liberated from household furniture and carpeting. These agents accumulate over time and may interfere with estrogen and androgen (testosterone) signaling, raising risks for endometriosis, uterine fibroids, and infertility, and they may also impact intelligence and behavior in offspring.

Other, nonpersistent organic pollutants, such as bisphenol A (BPA), phthalate diesters, and paraben esters, tend to be rapidly metabolized and eliminated from the human body. Yet, populations are continually exposed to these pollutants through the use of consumer goods, personal care products, and pharmaceuticals, including ingestion from food and beverage packaging and containers, inhalation from air fresheners and building materials, and absorption from lotions and cosmetics. Nonpersistent organic compounds have been associated with a spectrum of adverse reproductive outcomes in animal and human research. BPA, for example, appears to be an ovarian toxicant and raises oxidative stress levels, whereas phthalates are implicated as testicular toxicants and may cause increased inflammation.

Various pollutants with suspected reproductive toxicity, including toxic trace elements, POPs, and nonpersistent organic pollutants, were detected in most blood and urine specimens collected from pregnant women during a 2003–2004 Centers for Disease Control and Prevention biomonitoring study. Many pollutants, including As, Cd, Pb, Hg, PCBs, PBDEs, BPA, phthalates, and parabens, cross the placenta, placing a developing fetus at risk. Even at low levels, fetal exposures within limited critical developmental windows (e.g., during gonadal differentiation starting around the seventh week of gestation) may lead to a spectrum of adverse effects that manifest after delivery or even in adulthood. The structural malformations, infertility, and reproductive cancers postulated by testicular and ovarian dysgenesis syndromes (i.e., defective development of the gonads) are examples of "fetal programming" impacts that may result from maternal pollutant exposure.

Despite growing evidence, the reproductive effects of low-level, background exposures to environmental pollutants experienced by most people remain controversial. Additional investigation, coupled with a precautionary approach to exposure, is recommended by many doctors and scientists.

Michael S. Bloom

See Also: Arsenic Pollution; Biomonitoring and Biomarkers; Bisphenol A (BPA); Centers for Disease Control and Prevention; Endocrine Disruptors; Environmental Epidemiology; Environmental Toxicology; Heavy Metal Pollution; Lead Poisoning Prevention; Mercury Pollution; Personal Care Products, Health Issues with; Pharmaceuticals in the Environment; Phthalates; Polychlorinated Biphenyls; Toxicogenomics

Further Reading

American College of Obstetricians and Gynecologists and American Society for Reproductive Medicine. "Committee Opinion No. 575: Exposure to Toxic Environmental Agents." *Obstetrics and Gynecology*, vol. 122, no. 4 (March 2013): 931–935.

Buck Louis, Germaine M., Maureen A. Cooney, and Matthew C. Peterson. "The Ovarian Dysgenesis Syndrome." *Journal of Developmental Origins of Health and Disease*, vol. 2, no. 1 (February 2011): 25–35.

Di Renzo, Gian Carlo, et al. "International Federation of Gynecology and Obstetrics Opinion on Reproductive Health Impacts of Exposure to Toxic Environmental Chemicals." *International Journal of Gynecology and Obstetrics*, vol. 131, no. 3 (December 2015): 219–225. https://www.journals.elsevier.com/international-journal-of-gynecology-and-obstetrics/.

Kay, Vanessa R., Michael S. Bloom, and Warren G. Foster. "Reproductive and Developmental Effects of Phthalate Diesters in Males." *Critical Reviews in Toxicology*, vol. 44, no. 6 (July 2014): 467–498.

Skakkebaek, Niels E., et al. "Male Reproductive Disorders and Fertility Trends: Influences of Environment and Genetic Susceptibility." *Physiological Reviews*, vol. 96, no. 1 (January 2016): 55–97.

Sutton, Patrice, Linda C. Giudice, and Tracey J. Woodruff. "Reproductive Environmental Health." *Current Opinions in Obstetrics and Gynecology*, vol. 22, no. 6 (December 2010): 517–524.

Woodruff, Tracey J., Ami R. Zota, and Jackie M. Schwartz. "Environmental Chemicals in Pregnant Women in the United States: NHANES 2003–2004." *Environmental Health Perspectives*, vol. 119, no. 6 (June 2011): 878–885.

RESOURCE CONSERVATION AND RECOVERY ACT

The Resource Conservation and Recovery Act (RCRA) was established in 1976 as a national waste management program that protects communities and resources from inappropriate waste disposal. The RCRA allows the U.S. Environmental Protection Agency (EPA) to control the creation, transportation, treatment, storage, and disposal of hazardous waste, and it also provides a structure for disposing of nonhazardous waste. Put into practice, the RCRA is a set of regulations, guidance, and policies developed by the EPA to safely manage and clean up both solid and hazardous waste and to encourage reuse and source reduction.

The RCRA is often described as cradle-to-grave legislation because it provides authority to control hazardous waste from when it is first generated to when it is ultimately disposed of and all the steps in between (e.g., moving the waste from one location to another and treating the waste to make it less hazardous or more stable). Amendments to the RCRA in 1984 addressed waste minimization, the phasing out of land disposal of hazardous waste, and corrective actions for releases. The 1986 amendments addressed environmental contamination problems specifically resulting from the storage of petroleum and other hazardous substances in underground tanks.

Examples of the impact the RCRA has had on the United States include (1) contamination prevention programs that reduce the potential for future Superfund sites that negatively affect communities; (2) programs that reward companies that adjust manufacturing processes to reduce waste and promote safe reuse of materials; and (3) improvements to the country's recycling infrastructure. These improvements have resulted in an increase to the municipal solid waste recycling/composting rate from 7 to 35 percent.

Hana Elliott

See Also: Composting, Health Benefits of; Environmental Protection Agency; Hazardous Waste Disposal; Recycling; Three Rs of Waste Management; Underground Storage Tanks, Health Concerns with

Further Reading

Caccavale, Salvatore. *A Basic Guide to RCRA: Understanding Solid and Hazardous Waste Management*. Des Plaines, IL: American Society of Safety Engineers, 2016.

RCRA Orientation Manual. Washington, DC: U.S. Environmental Protection Agency, 2014.

U.S. Environmental Protection Agency. *Resource Conservation and Recovery Act (RCRA) Laws and Regulations*. https://www.epa.gov/rcra (accessed May 4, 2017).

U.S. Environmental Protection Agency. *Summary of the Resource Conservation and Recovery Act*. https://www.epa.gov/laws-regulations/summary-resource-conservation-and-recovery-act (accessed May 4, 2017).

U.S. Environmental Protection Agency. *Sustainable Materials Management*. https://www.epa.gov/smm (accessed May 4, 2017).

RESPIRATORY DISEASE AND AIR POLLUTION

Air pollution has been recognized as a public health problem for several thousand years, adversely affecting human health and contributing to respiratory diseases. From early humans using fire for cooking and heating to the concentration of urban home chimneys and industry smokestacks, humankind has contributed significantly to air pollution. Over 2,500 years ago, the Greek physician Hippocrates (c. 460–c. 370 BCE), considered the father of medicine, described how health could be compromised by the quality of air.

Air pollution can be found in both outdoor and indoor environments and comes from both anthropogenic (human) and natural sources. Major air pollutants include emissions from automobiles and industries that burn fossil fuels and from natural events such as forest fires. Widespread air pollution can have a significant impact on climate change. For example, carbon dioxide, a by-product of fossil fuel combustion, contributes to global warming, which can affect air quality by increasing ground-level ozone and extending the length of the growing season for plants that produce allergens. This can lead to damaged lungs from ozone exposure and allergic reactions from pollens in the air.

Anthropogenic sources of outdoor air pollution are associated with mobile and stationary sources. Mobile sources include on-road vehicles such as cars, trucks, and buses and nonroad vehicles such as trains, ships, and planes. Pollution from these mobile sources involve the combustion of fossil fuels, causing gases to be emitted into the atmosphere from the engine exhaust. Stationary sources of anthropogenic pollution include facilities such as power plants, manufacturing operations, and oil refineries. These types of pollution sources can emit a variety of pollutants, including carbon monoxide, nitrogen oxides, particulate matter, sulfur dioxide, volatile organic compounds, and various toxic compounds. Many of these pollutants contribute to the smog common in many large cities. Natural sources of air pollution emit gases and particulate matter that can be dispersed over wide areas by the wind. This includes dust clouds, smoke and ash from forest fires and volcanic eruptions, and various types of allergens like ragweed pollen, animal dander, and mold.

Inhaling air pollution often results in irritation to the upper respiratory tract, breathing difficulties, allergic reactions, and eye irritation. Additionally, air pollution can trigger asthma attacks and lead to a general decline in lung function. Long-term exposure to some air pollutants, often termed "air toxics," can cause serious health issues, including cancer and cardiovascular problems. Older adults, children, and people with existing health conditions are particularly susceptible to air pollution. Because humans spend more than 90 percent of their time indoors, exposure to indoor pollutants can also be a serious problem. Sources of indoor pollution includes household chemicals, molds, dust mites, pests, environmental tobacco smoke, and lead paint dust, many of which are considered asthma triggers. Indoor air pollution has also been linked to sick building syndrome and Legionnaires' disease.

Recognizing the significant health and environmental problems associated with air pollution, the U.S. Congress passed the Clean Air Act in 1970, with major amendments in 1977 and 1990. This law regulated air emissions from mobile and stationary sources and authorized the U.S. Environmental Protection Agency (EPA) to develop national ambient air quality standards (NAAQS) that protect the health and welfare of the public, in addition to regulating toxic air pollutants. The EPA set primary NAAQS for carbon monoxide, lead, nitrogen dioxide, ozone, particulate matter, and sulfur dioxide, and it set secondary standards for the same pollutants (except for carbon monoxide). Primary standards establish regulatory emission limits to protect public health, including the health of sensitive populations such as asthmatics, children, and the elderly. Secondary standards establish limits to protect the welfare of the public, including protections for crops, vegetation, visibility, animals, and buildings. The 1990 Clean Air Act Amendments incorporated provisions to address acid rain, urban air pollution, and toxic air emissions. The EPA established AirNow and the Air Quality Index to quickly inform the public about poor air quality days, potential adverse health effects, and actions to reduce exposure.

R. Christopher Rustin

See Also: AirNow and the Air Quality Index; Allergens in the Environment; Ambient Air Quality and Health; Asthma; Automobile and Truck Emissions and Controls; Cancer Risk from Environmental Exposure; Carbon Dioxide and the Carbon Cycle; Children's Environmental Health; Clean Air Act; Climate Change and Human Health; Crops and Vegetation, Air Pollution Damage to; Electric Power Generation, Health Implications of; Environmental Protection Agency; Fugitive Dust; Hazardous Air Pollutants; Indoor Environment; Lead Poisoning Prevention; Legionnaires' Disease; Ozone and Smog in the Urban Environment; Particulate Matter and Bioaerosols Pollution; Sick Building Syndrome; Tobacco Smoke, Secondhand and Thirdhand; Volatile Organic Compound Pollution

Further Reading

Friis, Robert H. *Essentials of Environmental Health*. Sudbury, MA: Jones and Bartlett, 2012.

Frumkin, Howard, ed. *Environmental Health, From Global to Local*. San Francisco, CA: Jossey-Bass, 2016.

Godish, Thad, Wayne T. Davis, and Joshua S. Fu. *Air Quality*. Boca Raton, FL: CRC Press, 2014.
Phalen, Robert N., and Robert F. Phalen. *Introduction to Air Pollution Science: A Public Health Perspective*. Burlington, MA: Jones and Bartlett, 2013.
U.S. Centers for Disease Control and Prevention. *Air Pollution and Respiratory Health*. https://www.cdc.gov/nceh/airpollution (accessed February 1, 2017).
U.S. Environmental Protection Agency. *AirNow*. https://www.airnow.gov (accessed June 23, 2016).
U.S. Environmental Protection Agency. *Criteria Air Pollutants*. https://www.epa.gov/criteria-air-pollutants (accessed June 23, 2016).

RIVER BLINDNESS

River blindness, or Onchocerciasis, is an infection caused by the nematode *Onchocerca volvulus* that leads to skin disease and possible blindness. Most commonly found in sub-Saharan Africa, this disease has been estimated to have infected 37 million people worldwide. More than 99 percent of infections occur across 30 African countries. It is the second leading infectious cause of blindness, affecting 500,000 people throughout the world.

Black flies are the disease vector for *Onchocerca volvulus*, and humans are the only definitive host. Humans contract the disease when an infected black fly bites and deposits third-stage larvae into the skin. The larvae mature into adults over the next 6 to 12 months, after which the females start producing offspring called microfilariae. *Onchocerca volvulus* is a prolific reproducer and can make 1,000 to 3,000 microfilariae per day, leading to a total microfilaria load in heavily infected humans of more than 100 million. Once another black fly bites an infected person, microfilariae are transferred back to the fly, where they mature into infectious third-stage larvae over one to three weeks. This completes the infectious cycle.

Over their 3- to 15-year life span, female *Onchocerca volvulus* can grow to 20 inches (50.8 centimeters) long, and males typically grow to 5 inches (12.7 centimeters) long. The females burrow into subcutaneous and deeper muscle tissue and become encapsulated by fibrous tissue, forming hard nodules. The males move through subcutaneous, dermal, and ocular tissues as well as the lymphatic system.

As the worms die, they release antigens that activate the body's immune system, causing corneal inflammation and leading to anterior and posterior segment onchocercal eye disease as well as a variety of onchocercal skin diseases. Virtually no deaths are directly attributed to *Onchocerca volvulus* itself. However, infection reduces immunity and resistance to other diseases, which leads to an estimated reduction in life expectancy of 13 years.

The first signs of infection are intensely pruritic skin eruptions and rashes, followed by swelling of the lymph nodes. Patients may also complain of generalized symptoms like back and joint pain and weight loss. The first sign of ocular disease is the presence of microfilariae in the anterior segment of the eye on slit-lamp examination. With chronic exposure, corneal lesions occur, along with optic nerve atrophy, retinal death, and loss of the underlying choroid.

Diagnosis of the disease is primarily made via microscopic analysis of skin snip biopsies. Additionally, a more sensitive patch test has been developed as a noninvasive and cheaper alternative to skin snips and is widely used in endemic areas of Africa. Ultrasound may also be useful in identifying deeper nodules filled with adult worms.

Treatment for onchocerciasis is by a single dose of ivermectin repeated every 3 to 6 months until the patient is asymptomatic. There have also been very successful mass drug treatment programs in hyperendemic areas by the African Program for Onchocerciasis Control and the Onchocerciasis Elimination Program for the Americas. These programs rely on ivermectin dosing every 6 to 12 months for up to 10 to 16 years in symptomatic individuals.

Timothy J. Sutton

See Also: Environmental Toxicology; Infectious Diseases; Insect-Borne Diseases

Further Reading

Boatin, Boakye A., and Frank O. Richards Jr. "Control of Onchocerciasis." *Advances in Parasitology*, vol. 61 (May 2006): 349–394.

Centers for Disease Control and Prevention. *Parasites—Onchocerciasis (Also Known as River Blindness)*. https://www.cdc.gov/parasites/onchocerciasis.

Cupp, E. W., M. Sauerbrey, and F. Richards. "Elimination of Human Onchocerciasis: History of Progress and Current Feasibility Using Ivermectin (Mectizan (®)) Monotherapy." *Acta Tropica*, vol. 120, sup. 1 (September 2011): S100–S108.

Dunn, Caitlin, et al. "The Contributions of Onchocerciasis Control and Elimination Programs toward the Achievement of the Millennium Development Goals." *PLOS Neglected Tropical Diseases*, vol. 9, no. 5 (May 2015).

Fenwick, A. "The Global Burden of Neglected Tropical Diseases." *Public Health*, vol. 126, no. 3 (March 2012): 233–236.

Keating, Joseph, et al. "Lymphatic Filariasis and Onchocerciasis Prevention, Treatment, and Control Costs across Diverse Settings: A Systematic Review." *Acta Tropica*, vol. 135 (July 2014): 86–95.

Onchocerciasis Fact Sheet. World Health Organization, Geneva, Switzerland, 2017. http://www.who.int/mediacentre/factsheets/fs374/en.

ROCKY MOUNTAIN SPOTTED FEVER

Rocky Mountain spotted fever (RMSF) is a serious, potentially fatal tick-borne disease caused by the intracellular bacterium *Rickettsii rickettsii*. It was first described in Idaho in 1906 by Howard Ricketts and is found natively throughout the United States, Canada, Mexico, Central America, and parts of South America. Historically, fatality rates were as high 65 to 80 percent, but today mortality ranges from about 0.3 to 3 percent in areas where the disease is established. RMSF is the most common rickettsial infection in the United States, with 4,470 cases of presumed infection in 2012 reported by the Centers for Disease Control and Prevention.

Rickettsii rickettsii gains entrance into its host through the saliva of a tick bite. The primary vector for infection in the United States is the American dog tick (*Dermacentor variabilis*) and Rocky Mountain wood tick (*Dermacentor andersoni*).

The bacteria quickly make their way into the intracellular space of local cells and begin replication in both the nucleus and cytoplasm. The bacteria then hijack host-cell filopodia for locomotion as well as stealing ATP and glutamine for energy. These adaptations allow the bacteria to move between cells at the incredible rate of over 3 inches (8 centimeters) per second!

The incubation period for infected patients to become symptomatic is 2 to 14 days after being bitten by the tick. The early symptoms of RMSF are nonspecific and include fever, headache, muscle and joint pain, nausea, abdominal pain, and overall flu-like symptoms. After a few days, a characteristic skin rash develops, which consists of red blotches that turn white when pressed and usually begin on the ankles and wrists and spread centrally. Over time, the red blotches form tiny bruises. *Rickettsii rickettsii* has no direct exotoxin to explain its morbidity and mortality. Instead, its tropism for vascular endothelial cells leads to direct vascular injury, which, when combined with host immune response, can lead to interstitial pneumonitis, myocarditis, and encephalitis.

When clinical symptoms are consistent with RMSF, the presence of the disease may be presumed by a medical professional, who may prescribe antibiotics and other treatments, even before a skin rash develops. Diagnosis is complicated because *Rickettsii rickettsii* is an obligate intracellular bacterium that cannot be cultured in most laboratories. Thus, serologic testing or skin biopsy staining is needed for definitive diagnosis.

Host factors influencing the severity of RMSF include (1) age 10 and younger or age 60 and older, (2) male gender, (3) glucose-6-phosphate dehydrogenase deficiency, (4) African-American, and (5) chronic alcohol abuse. Additionally, delay in treatment of five or more days after symptoms first appear is associated with an increased risk of mortality.

The virulence of *Rickettsii rickettsii* remains one of its most puzzling attributes. Historically, RMSF has had greater than 80 percent mortality in Bitteroot Valley, Montana, but only 3 percent mortality in the adjacent Snake River Valley. Bacterial isolates from both areas proved to be essentially identical. Thus, studies continue into the virulence of this bacterium.

The best prevention strategy is to avoid tick bites by wearing close-toed shoes, long-sleeve shirts, and long pants when out of doors. Additionally, wearing light colors can aid in identifying ticks on clothing. Using DEET bug spray on skin and permethrin-based bug repellents on clothing and gear is recommended.

Timothy J. Sutton

See Also: Environmental Toxicology; Infectious Diseases; Insect-Borne Diseases

Further Reading

Centers for Disease Control and Prevention. *Rocky Mountain Spotted Fever (RMSF)*. https://www.cdc.gov/rmsf (accessed February 6, 2017).

Chapman, Alice S., et al. *Diagnosis and Management of Tickborne Rickettsial Diseases: Rocky Mountain Spotted Fever, Ehrlichioses, and Anaplasmosis—United States: A Practical Guide for Physicians and Other Health-Care and Public Health Professionals*. Atlanta, GA: Centers for Disease Control and Prevention, 2006.

Drexler, N.A., et al. "National Surveillance of Spotted Fever Group Rickettsioses in the United States, 2008–2012." *The American Journal of Tropical Medicine and Hygiene*, vol. 94, no. 1 (January 2016): 26–34.

Openshaw, J.J., et al. "Rocky Mountain Spotted Fever in the United States, 2000–2007: Interpreting Contemporary Increases in Incidence." *American Journal of Tropical Medicine and Hygiene*, vol. 83, no. 1 (July 2010): 174–182.

Regan, J.J., et al. "Risk Factors for Fatal Outcome from Rocky Mountain Spotted Fever in a Highly Endemic Area—Arizona, 2002–2011." *Clinical Infectious Diseases*, vol. 60, no. 11 (June 2015): 1659–1666.

Walker, D.H. "Rickettsiae and Rickettsial Infections: The Current State of Knowledge." *Clinical Infectious Diseases*, vol. 45, sup. 1 (July 2007): S39–S44.

S

SAFE DRINKING WATER ACT

The Safe Drinking Water Act (SDWA) is a federal law enacted by the U.S. Congress in 1974 (with amendments in 1986 and in 1996) in response to serious concerns relating to the quality of the nation's drinking water. The rise of industry and agriculture in the middle of the 20th century led to an increase in chemicals and contaminants in drinking water sources in the United States. Several studies in the late 1960s revealed major problems at water treatment facilities and contaminants in drinking water across the country, and this ultimately prompted passage of the SDWA.

The SDWA directs the U.S. Environmental Protection Agency (EPA) to develop national, minimum health-based standards to ensure a safe drinking water supply for the American public. These standards are called the National Primary Drinking Water Regulations, and they apply to any public water system serving at least 25 people from any source (well or municipal water). Public water systems can be publicly or privately owned, but they must serve over 25 people to be covered by the SDWA. (Private wells that serve fewer than 25 people are not subject to the requirements of the SDWA). Commercial passenger services, such as passenger trains and airlines, are also subject to the SDWA if they meet the threshold of 25 users on average. More than 250 million Americans receive their water from public water systems subject to the SDWA.

The EPA's drinking water standards are aimed at contaminants that cause, or are likely to cause, adverse human health effects. The contaminants of concern may

The Water We Drink

The SDWA is a major contributor to human health, protecting our drinking water from contaminants that are natural or occur from human activities and making it easier for Americans to access information about the quality of their local drinking water. The United States arguably has the safest drinking water supply in the world, and the overwhelming majority of Americans get their water from supplies regulated by the act. Because what we pay for clean drinking water rarely covers the costs of preserving surface water quality and protecting groundwater from contamination, consumers are often misled into thinking that clean, safe drinking water is cheap and plentiful.

be naturally occurring (e.g., bacteria from animal waste) or result from human activities (e.g., industrial chemical waste). Even treatment chemicals used to purify water, including chlorine, can break down over time into other chemicals that pose a health hazard. For each identified contaminant, the EPA sets two limits: (1) a Maximum Contaminant Level Goal (MCLG), which represents the level of the contaminant below which there is no known human health risk; and (2) a Maximum Contaminant Level (MCL), which is as close as one can get to the MCLG, taking into account costs, benefits, detection ability, and best available treatment technologies. The MCLGs are nonenforceable goals that inform the MCLs, which are legally enforceable standards. The EPA has established MCLs for approximately 90 different contaminants.

The MCLs are established based on conservative estimates of risk of prolonged water consumption over a lifetime, such as a person drinking 2 liters (about 2 quarts) of water every day from the same source for 70 years. For example, the MCLG for arsenic is zero, whereas the MCL for arsenic is 0.010 milligrams per liter, or 10 parts per billion. Every six years the EPA must review each primary drinking water standard and determine if revisions are necessary to incorporate any new science, data, information, or advancements in analysis or treatment technologies.

Public water suppliers subject to the SDWA must routinely sample and analyze their water at specific locations and times to ensure compliance with the primary drinking water regulations. If a violation of any of these standards is confirmed, the supplier must provide notice (usually in the form of a letter sent by mail) to its customers, the state, and the EPA about the violation and potential health effects, given the contaminant and the extent of noncompliance.

The EPA sets the standards under the SDWA, but the states generally have primary responsibility for developing SDWA programs and enforcing the federal limits. States also must provide quarterly reports of any violations and other information to the EPA. These data from the states are stored in the Safe Drinking Water Information System, a database that helps the EPA monitor the success of the SDWA and serves to inform the public about the quality of its drinking water.

The SDWA originally focused on treatment technologies to remove contaminants, but later amendments broadened the focus to include the protection of drinking water sources, such as underground aquifers, rivers, lakes, and streams. Because the majority of community water systems in the United States obtain drinking water from underground sources, a major component of the SDWA is the Underground Injection Control (UIC) program. Injecting wastewater into deep underground wells for purposes of disposal has long been a practice used by agriculture, industry, and in some cases, cities. The SDWA, however, prohibits all underground injection of fluids unless done pursuant to a permit. The states can submit a UIC program to EPA and apply to become the primary enforcement authority (i.e., achieving "primacy" status) over their UIC program. Currently, 34 states have EPA-approved UIC programs, and the EPA shares enforcement authority or directly implements programs in the remaining states. State-run, EPA-approved UIC programs must meet the minimum federal standards established by the SDWA and the EPA. Whether by the EPA or a state with primacy, no permit for underground injection may be issued unless the state or the EPA determines that the underground injection "will not endanger drinking water sources."

It is well recognized that the number of water-related disease outbreaks has greatly decreased since the early 1900s. However, the EPA and the Centers for Disease Control and Prevention have recognized that many waterborne illnesses go unreported because they generally create symptoms similar to other illnesses or are not widespread and thus are not directly traceable to drinking water. Moreover, gathering data and statistics on waterborne diseases and reporting these data are voluntary efforts that not all states undertake. The largest waterborne disease outbreak in the United States occurred in 1993, when over 400,000 people became ill and 50 people died after drinking water contaminated with a parasite in the water supply of Milwaukee, Wisconsin.

In response to concerns regarding waterborne diseases, the EPA has implemented several programs aimed at reducing microbe and bacteria contamination. The Total Coliform Rule imposes additional monitoring and mitigation requirements (beyond the MCL for total coliform) for pathogens such as *E. coli* that are common to the feces of many animals, including humans. Additionally, the Surface Water Treatment Rule applies to water supply systems that use surface water, and the rule specifically targets reductions in viruses and giardia through treatment or filtration.

Surprisingly, what most people pay for their water rarely covers the costs of the protection, collection, treatment, and distribution of that water. While water rates may cover the expenses of operating a water utility, the additional costs of treatment to preserve surface water quality and to protect groundwater from contamination are not captured in consumer water bills. Some believe that this hidden subsidy shields consumers from an appreciation of the complex task of preserving and delivering healthful drinking water, and it reduces what otherwise would be public pressure on pollutant sources to better protect drinking water supplies.

The primary aim of the SDWA is to protect public health, and by that measure, it has been an important foundation in providing safe drinking water to nearly all Americans. The United States is one of the few countries in the world, if not the only country, where you can turn on a tap virtually anywhere across the entire nation and expect water safe for consumption. The SDWA not only sets minimum safety standards for contaminants in drinking water but also provides funding for research and programs to protect drinking water at its source. Together with the Clean Water Act, the SDWA is an important component to protecting the health and safety of the nation.

Leah A. Dundon and Richard S. Davis

See Also: Clean Water Act; Cyanobacteria Toxins; Drinking Water Quality and Regulation; Environmental Protection Agency; *Escherichia coli* (*E. coli*) Infection; Fluoridation of Water; Groundwater Pollution and Depletion; Industrial Effluents; Water Pollution; Waterborne Diseases

Further Reading

25 Years of the Safe Drinking Water Act: History and Trends (EPA 816-R-99–007). Washington, DC: U.S. Environmental Protection Agency, 1999.

U.S. Environmental Protection Agency. *Drinking Water Contaminants—Standards and Regulations*. http://www.epa.gov/dwstandardsregulations (accessed January 2, 2016).

U.S. Environmental Protection Agency. *Federal Water Pollution Control Act, 33 U.S.C. §1251 et seq. (1972)*. (Also known as the Clean Water Act.) http://www.epa.gov/laws-regulations/summary-clean-water-act (accessed January 2, 2016)

U.S. Environmental Protection Agency. *Summary of the Safe Drinking Water Act, 42 U.S.C. §300f et seq. (1974)*. http://www.epa.gov/laws-regulations/summary-safe-drinking-water-act (accessed January 2, 2016).

SAFETY DATA SHEET

Safety Data Sheets (SDSs) are documents that contain information on specific hazardous chemicals or chemical mixtures. The primary purpose of these documents is to help protect human health and the environment by ensuring the proper use, storage, handling, and cleanup of hazardous chemicals. SDSs, formerly called Material Safety Data Sheets (MSDSs), have been required in the United States since 1985 for every hazardous chemical manufactured, imported, or used in the country. MSDSs were renamed SDSs in 2013 to better align the information available in the data sheets with international requirements and to facilitate international trade in chemicals.

The U.S. Occupational Safety and Health Administration (OSHA) defines hazardous chemicals or chemical mixtures as those that pose a physical or health hazard. A chemical presenting a physical hazard may be combustible, explosive, flammable, or unstable, whereas a chemical can be classified as a health hazard if there is evidence that it can cause adverse health effects, such as cancer, reproductive problems, skin or mucous membrane irritation, or other toxic effects involving the human body.

The information provided in SDSs include (1) the chemical composition of the product; (2) its physical and chemical properties (e.g., melting point, boiling point, pH, and solubility); (3) stability and reactivity; (4) toxicity and health effects; (5) proper uses and handling procedures (e.g., transport, storage, disposal, cleanup, and the use of protective equipment); (6) ecological information (e.g., ecotoxicity, persistence, bioaccumulation potential, and mobility); and (7) emergency phone numbers, first-aid protocols, and fire-fighting measures in the event of an accident.

Manufacturers or distributors of hazardous chemicals or chemical mixtures are required to prepare SDSs for their chemicals, and worksites are required to ensure that SDSs on hazardous chemicals used, manufactured, or warehoused at the worksite are readily available to workers. OSHA is responsible for ensuring worksites comply with the requirement to post SDS records at locations available to all workers.

Research to evaluate the information and data presented in SDSs has found inaccuracies or gaps in some SDSs. Manufacturers of hazardous chemicals can be subject to citations or even "failure to warn" lawsuits if any information or data in these documents are inaccurate or missing. Another potential problem with some SDSs is the difficulty some workers with limited formal education have in understanding the information and data. Efforts to improve the way information and data are presented in SDSs are ongoing.

Adrienne L. Katner

See Also: National Institute for Occupational Safety and Health; Occupational Safety and Health Administration; Persistent, Bioaccumulating, and Toxic Chemicals

Further Reading

Occupational Safety and Health Administration. *OSHA Brief: Hazard Communication Standard: Safety Data Sheets.* https://www.osha.gov/Publications/OSHA3514.html (accessed April 17, 2016).

U.S. Department of Labor. *OSHA Occupational Chemical Database.* https://www.osha.gov/chemicaldata/ (accessed April 17, 2016).

U.S. Department of Labor. *OSHA Standards: Hazard Communication.* https://www.osha.gov/dsg/hazcom/standards.html#interpretations (accessed April 17, 2016).

SCHISTOSOMIASIS

Schistosomiasis, also known as bilharzia or snail fever, is a waterborne parasitic infection. Caused by blood flukes (trematode worms), known as schistosomes, it is one of the most common parasitic diseases worldwide. The number of deaths due to schistosomiasis are difficult to pinpoint, but estimates range up to well over 200,000 per year.

Schistosomiasis is not found in the United States. However, it is endemic in more than 70 countries, affecting well over 200 million people. Schistosomiasis occurs in parts of Asia, the Middle East, South America, and the Caribbean, with the majority of cases occurring in Africa. It is considered a neglected tropical disease, which are diseases found primarily in tropical and subtropical locations, particularly areas with high rates of poverty and inadequate sanitation or access to clean water. These types of diseases cost billions of dollars in economic loses and untold human suffering. Migration and the movement of refugees from endemic areas, population growth patterns that tax environments and infrastructures, and the growth of tourism, including ecotourism, all contribute to the spread of infection.

Transmission occurs when an infected person's urine or feces contaminate fresh water with schistosoma eggs. The eggs hatch, becoming larvae that infect a particular kind of snail. The larvae multiply in the snails and are then released back into the water as parasites, which can penetrate the skin of people in contact with the water, for example, while bathing, doing laundry, fishing, fetching water, swimming, or caring for livestock. Inside the body, the parasites mature within the blood vessels, where they mate and produce thousands of eggs that can be excreted in the urine and feces, potentially perpetuating transmission.

There are two major forms of schistosomiasis. Urinary schistosomiasis mainly affects the urinary system and can lead to bladder cancer if the infection is long-term. It is also considered an HIV risk factor, particularly for women. Intestinal schistosomiasis can cause intestinal damage, hypertension of the abdominal blood vessels, and abdominal bleeding. The intestinal form of the disease also affects the liver, spleen, and lungs. Seizures, spinal cord inflammation, or paralysis can result in the rare cases when eggs migrate to the spinal cord or brain.

In children, a group especially at risk for contracting the disease, schistosomiasis can result in poor growth, malnutrition, cognitive impairment, and anemia. Early stage infections are often asymptomatic, with fever, chills, coughs, or muscle aches beginning within a month or two. The body's immune system reaction to the parasites causes scarring and other internal damage.

The anthelminthic drug, praziquantel, has been used for several decades to treat schistosomiasis. For maximum benefit and cost-efficiency, schistosomiasis treatment can simultaneously tackle several conditions, including river blindness and various kinds of intestinal worms. Development of a schistosomiasis vaccine is also underway. Health education campaigns emphasize the importance of not urinating or defecating in water and encourage people to take praziquantel when available. Environmental approaches to controlling schistosomiasis focus on establishing clean water and sanitation systems and vector control of snails.

Kathy Stolley

See Also: Drinking Water Quality and Regulation; Infectious Diseases; River Blindness; Sewage Treatment and Disposal; Waterborne Diseases

Further Reading

Ahmed, Shadab H. *Schistosomiasis*. Medscape, New York, 2016. http://emedicine.medscape.com/article/228392-overview.

Centers for Disease Control and Prevention. *Parasites—Schistosomiasis*. http://www.cdc.gov/parasites/schistosomiasis (accessed February 18, 2017).

National Institute of Allergy and Infectious Diseases. *Schistosomiasis (Bilharzia)*. https://www.niaid.nih.gov/topics/schistosomiasis/Pages/default.aspx (accessed February 18, 2017).

Secor, W. Evan, and Daniel G. Colley. *World Class Parasites: Volume 10. Schistosomiasis*. New York: Springer, 2005.

Wei, Grant, and Tanya Shevavesh. *Emergent Management of Acute Schistosomiasis*. Medscape, New York, 2016. http://emedicine.medscape.com/article/788867-overview.

World Health Organization. *Neglected Tropical Diseases*. http://www.who.int/neglected_diseases/en (accessed February 18, 2017).

World Health Organization. *Schistosomiasis*. http://www.who.int/topics/schistosomiasis/en (accessed February 18, 2017).

SEA ICE, GLOBAL WARMING IMPLICATIONS FOR

Sea ice is found almost exclusively in the remote polar oceans, specifically, in the Arctic Ocean and around Antarctica. On average, sea ice makes up roughly 9.7 million square miles (25 million square kilometers) of the earth's surface (an area more than twice the size of Canada). Over the past century, due to the changing global climate, the amount of sea ice has been steadily decreasing at an alarming rate (e.g., 13.3 percent per decade over the past 30 years). By allowing global temperatures to rise, melting sea ice can indirectly affect human health by making heat waves and droughts worse and by increasing urban air pollution and the spread of disease.

Sea ice is ocean water that is frozen. Glaciers, icebergs, ice shelves, and ice sheets are different from sea ice because they are formed on land from precipitation. While the melting of glaciers and ice shelves poses significant issues, such as sea level rise and depleted freshwater sources, sea ice presents a different set of problems. Sea ice melts during the summer months and grows during the winter, and some areas of sea ice remain throughout the year, mainly in the Arctic Ocean. Arctic sea ice tends to be thicker and melt more slowly than Antarctic sea ice. This is because the Arctic Ocean is surrounded by land, which restricts the movement of ice and allows it to thicken during the winter months, whereas the sea ice surrounding Antarctica is exposed to open water, which allows more melting during the summer because the ice can more easily break away from the main ice pack. In contrast to Arctic sea ice, the extent of Antarctic sea ice has actually been increasing, by about 1.1 percent per decade. Scientists attribute this growth, which is relatively small compared with the rapid sea ice decrease in the Arctic Ocean, to a combination of winds and ocean circulation that have made the ice more compact and rigid and less susceptible to melting.

The Albedo of Sea Ice

Albedo is a scientific measure used to indicate how well a surface reflects sunlight. The albedo value of a surface can vary from 0 to 1. A value of 0 means that the surface is black and *absorbs* all incoming solar energy, whereas a value of 1 means that the surface is white and *reflects* all incoming solar energy back into space. Values between 0 and 1 indicate different gradations between black and white. Albedo is important in predicting how much the earth's climate may warm as a result of losing sea ice and other bright surfaces (e.g., glaciers, icebergs, ice shelves, ice sheets, and snow) that help regulate global temperatures by reflecting sunlight. Sea ice (with no snow cover) typically has an albedo of 0.5 to 0.7, indicating that sea ice reflects 50 to 70 percent of the incoming solar energy. The albedo of ocean water, in the absence of any ice, is 0.06, and the albedo of snow can be as high as 0.9.

The particular danger posed by the melting of sea ice involves the albedo effect, which describes the degree to which sunlight is reflected back into space—the more sunlight is reflected, the less the earth heats up, and conversely, with less sunlight reflected, the earth gets warmer. As the extent of sea ice declines, less sunlight is reflected into space, and the earth gets warmer. As the earth gets warmer, even more sea ice melts, even less sunlight is reflected, and the earth gets warmer still. This cycle of repeated warming and melting, described by scientists as a positive feedback loop, tends to accelerate the overall warming of the earth. Additionally, as the extent of sea ice has declined, its thickness has also decreased.

There are a number of ways melting of sea ice can affect human health. For example, many local indigenous communities, such as the Inuit (indigenous people of northern Canada and parts of Greenland and Alaska), depend on sea ice for hunting in the spring. If the sea ice melts too quickly, the hunting season is shortened as transportation becomes more difficult due to unsafe ice. As a result, indigenous communities that were once able to sustainably hunt are now forced to eat store-bought food to survive, and this has led to an increased prevalence of diabetes and obesity. Additionally, unemployment has reached up to 80 percent in some communities, forcing many residents to relocate to other towns.

Warming oceans and melting sea ice have also introduced new species and diseases. For example, there is a concern that the phocine distemper virus present in eastern Arctic seals will soon reach western Arctic seals because sea ice no longer presents the same physical barrier. Also, nonnative predators, like herons, have increased competition for already scarce resources.

On a global level, melting sea ice has the potential to disrupt the thermohaline circulation, which is a cycle of ocean currents that stabilize and regulate the earth's temperature. Warm ocean water travels from the equator around the African and European coasts north to the pole, where it then sinks as it cools. This cold water then travels back down the North American coast toward South America. When sea ice melts, it leaves a layer of fresh water on the surface because the fresh water is less dense than ocean water. This layer has the effect of slowing down the warm water moving north from the equator, thereby disrupting atmospheric temperatures and changing climate.

Anthony G. Papetti

See Also: Climate Change and Human Health; Drought and Desertification, Health Consequences of; Greenhouse Effect and Global Warming; Intergovernmental Panel on Climate Change

Further Reading

Climate Change 2014: Synthesis Report. Geneva, Switzerland: Intergovernmental Panel on Climate Change, 2014.

Gass, Henry. "As Ice Sheets Melt, Communities Worry That Health Effects Are Overlooked." *Climatewire*, May 2014, http://www.eenews.net/climatewire/2014/05/29/stories/1060000353.

Marshall, Christa. "Arctic Ice Close to Record Lows, with Major Ripple Effects." *Climatewire*, August 2013, http://www.eenews.net/climatewire/2013/08/05/stories/1059985599.
National Aeronautics and Space Administration. *Impacts of a Warming Arctic*. http://climate.nasa.gov/resources/education/pbs_modules/lesson2Engage/ (accessed March 14, 2016).
National Snow and Ice Data Center. *All about Sea Ice, Introduction*. https://nsidc.org/cryosphere/seaice/index.html (accessed March 14, 2016).

SEPTEMBER 11 WORLD TRADE CENTER ATTACK

Tuesday, September 11, 2001—an unforgettable date in American history when terrorists flew two planes into the former World Trade Center (WTC) in New York City. A third plane flew into the Pentagon, and a fourth plane crashed in a field in Pennsylvania. In all, 2,977 people lost their lives that day. Local New York residents and rescue/recovery workers witnessed horrific events and experienced stress, fear, and uncertainty as many lost relatives, friends, and colleagues.

The collapse of the WTC towers exposed local people to many hazardous substances and complex chemical mixtures, including "WTC dust," which mainly consisted of inhalable particulate matter. The WTC dust and debris contained pulverized cement, gypsum, glass fibers, chrysotile asbestos, polycyclic aromatic hydrocarbons, polychlorinated biphenyls (PCBs), polychlorinated dioxins and furans, and metals. The dust was highly alkaline, which caused respiratory irritation and persistent upper airway disorders.

The earliest residential study conducted after the event found that affected-area residents reported more lower respiratory symptoms (LRS) and upper respiratory symptoms (URS) three months post–9/11 compared with control-area residents, and both LRS and URS in the affected areas were three times more persistent one year after 9/11. A pilot study indicated the possibility of an increase in bronchial hyperresponsiveness in exposed residents. Furthermore, in studies among first responders, LRS and URS were reported by nearly half of participants. Both respiratory and posttraumatic stress disorder (PTSD) symptoms were associated with being in the dust cloud, but smoke exposure may have had a greater impact than resuspended dust on LRS. "WTC cough" was a major complaint for both residents and responders, and chronic bronchitis was identified as a persistent problem five years post–9/11.

Regarding mental health, PTSD and depression in New York City after 9/11 were reported at twice the national baseline rate, and researchers found significantly higher rates of PTSD and depression among rescue workers than other workers. Significantly higher rates of PTSD and depression were also observed among lower Manhattan office workers. (Lower Manhattan is in the immediate area of the WTC attack.)

Birth outcomes have also been examined. Proximity to the WTC site after 9/11 did not indicate an increased risk of preterm birth or low birth weight. However, researchers found a 5.3 ounce (149 gram) reduction of birth weight in babies born to mothers within 2 miles (3.2 kilometers) of the WTC site and an increased risk of intrauterine growth restriction in the affected area. Studies examining umbilical cord blood samples did not show a clear relationship between 9/11 exposures and birth outcomes.

While respiratory hospitalizations immediately increased post–9/11, delayed increases in cardiovascular and cerebrovascular admissions after 9/11 also occurred. An analysis using New York City emergency department data found that 790 people with injuries sought medical care within 48 hours post–9/11. Inhalation and ocular injuries were the most common causes. In addition, prevalence of gastroesophageal reflux symptoms was elevated among firefighters and WTC rescue workers and within the WTC Health Registry (a registry used to track the health effects of the disaster), and these symptoms were more prevalent in those who arrived at the WTC site within 48 hours. By examining the WTF Health Registry, an increase in comorbidity (the presence of two or more health conditions) of depression was found among one-third of those with PTSD post–9/11.

Concern about medium- and long-term effects of the 9/11 disaster continues to this day. While a follow-up study showed a decline in symptoms approximately two to four years post–9/11, there still remained a higher rate of persistent symptoms among affected-area residents. Residents with multiple sources of 9/11 exposures were at the greatest health risk at follow-up, and psychological stress, dust/odors, and moisture were all important contributors. Among 3,271 workers who evacuated the WTC towers, 15 percent still had probable PTSD two to three years after 9/11. More importantly, the prevalence of PTSD in the WTC Health Registry

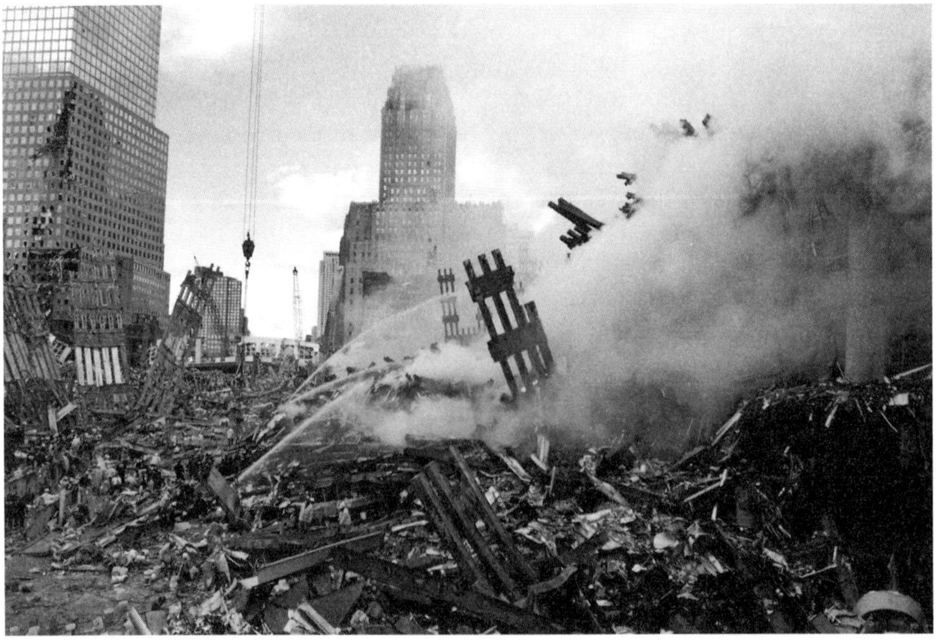

Aftermath of the World Trade Center terrorist attack on September 11, 2001. Many first responders, office workers, and visitors died, and survivors suffered from respiratory disease, posttraumatic stress disorder, and depression. (U.S. Department of Defense)

remained high (19 percent) five to six years after 9/11, with the highest prevalence noted among rescue and recovery workers. Late-emerging health problems may include cancers with long latency periods and premature death.

In conclusion, the most commonly reported health effects in the aftermath of this horrific event were respiratory and mental health consequences, with substantial short- and medium-term effects. Comparing residential with occupational exposures, adverse health effects were slightly higher in responders than residents.

Shao Lin

See Also: Asbestos; Dioxin Pollution; Heavy Metal Pollution; Occupational Safety and Health; Particulate Matter and Bioaerosols Pollution; Polychlorinated Biphenyls; Polycyclic Aromatic Hydrocarbons; Respiratory Disease and Air Pollution

Further Reading

Brackbill, R. M., et al. "Asthma and Posttraumatic Stress Symptoms 5 to 6 Years Following Exposure to the World Trade Center Terrorist Attack." *Journal of the American Medical Association*, vol. 302, no. 5 (August 2009): 502–516.

Brackbill, R. M., et al. "Surveillance for World Trade Center Disaster Health Effects among Survivors of Collapsed and Damaged Buildings." *MMWR Surveillance Summaries*, vol. 55, no. 2 (April 2006): 1–18.

Lin, S., et al. "Lessons Learned from the September 11th Disaster: A State Health Agency Perspective." *Environmental Health Insights*, vol. 6 (April 2012): 27–31.

Lin, S., et al. "Low Respiratory Health Symptoms among Residents Living Near the World Trade Center, Two and Four Years after 9/11." *International Journal of Occupational and Environmental Health*, vol. 16, no. 1 (January–March 2010): 44–52.

Lin, S., et al. "Respiratory and Cardiovascular Hospitalizations after the World Trade Center Disaster." *Archives of Environmental and Occupational Health*, vol. 65, no. 1 (January–March 2010): 12–20.

Lin, S., et al. "Upper Respiratory Symptoms and Other Health Effects among Residents Living Near the World Trade Center Site after September 11, 2001." *American Journal of Epidemiology*, vol. 162, no. 6 (September 2005): 499–507.

Mauer, M. P., K. R. Cummings, and R. Hoen. "Long-Term Respiratory Symptoms in World Trade Center Responders." *Occupational Medicine*, vol. 60, no. 2 (March 2010): 145–151.

Moline, J., R. Herbert, and N. Nguyen. "Health Consequences of the September 11 World Trade Center Attacks: A Review." *Cancer Investigation*, vol. 24, no. 3 (April–May 2006): 294–301.

Perlman, S. E., et al. "Short-Term and Medium-Term Health Effects of 9/11." *Lancet*, vol. 378, no. 9794 (September 2011): 925–934.

Reibman, J., et al. "The World Trade Center Residents' Respiratory Health Study: New Onset Respiratory Symptoms and Pulmonary Function." *Environmental Health Perspectives*, vol. 113, no. 4 (April 2005): 406–411.

SEVESO DIOXIN INCIDENT

On July 10, 1976, a reactor in a chemical plant near Seveso, Italy, exploded, sending a plume of tetrachlorodibenzo-p-dioxin, known more simply as dioxin, into the air. Seveso is a small, middle-class town about 18 miles (29 kilometers) outside of Milan. Years later, studies indicated that more than 270,000 individuals were affected by the incident, either because they lived in nearby areas at the time of the exposure or were born in contaminated zones the decade following the incident.

Industrie Chimiche Media Societa Anonima (ICMESA), which was owned by Givaudin, a Swiss company, operated the Seveso plant. Givaudin manufactured perfumes and other cosmetic ingredients, and this particular plant developed a component of the bacteriostatic agent hexachlorophene, called trichlorophenol (TCP), which is used in soaps and disinfectants. In the early 1970s, 20 infants died after being treated with talcum powder consisting of large amounts of hexachlorophene, and the United States used an herbicide derivative of TCP, called Agent Orange, during the Vietnam War.

Although the plant was shut down during the incident, chemicals continued to react, increasing the temperature in the plant's reactor and causing dioxin to form. Soon after, the reactor exploded, sending contaminants into the air in a foggy cloud. Immediately after the incident, a worker fed water into the reactor's cooling system to prevent more gases from seeping into the air, and reports indicate the leak was contained in about 30 minutes. During that time, the cloud moved over the town of Seveso, spanning an area 4 miles (6.4 kilometers) long and one-third mile (one-half kilometer) wide. Residents reported the cloud's foul smell and white, foggy consistency, and people exposed to the cloud began coughing, experiencing burning eyes, and generally feeling ill.

The director of production for ICMESA, Paolo Paoletti, told residents they had been exposed to an aerosol mixture, noting that some toxic chemicals could have been included in the mix. The company advised residents of nearby towns to stay away from foods grown outdoors, but the police were unable to enforce the advisory due to insufficient information. On the night of the second day of the cloud, Seveso experienced a strong wind that dispersed the fog.

A local health inspector received information from the company that chlorinated phenol was the main ingredient in the cloud mixture and that no additional substances could be identified. A week later, workers at the plant went on strike, having suspicions that crucial information about the cloud had been hidden from the public. Later examinations found that there were high dioxin levels present in the soil, and 10 days after the incident, Paoletti was arrested and charged with causing the disaster.

During the second week following the incident, exclusion zones were created. Zone A residents were evacuated immediately. Zone B residents were allowed to continue living in their homes, but children and pregnant woman were evacuated each day to reduce their exposure. Later, Zone A was expanded and an additional Zone R was created, where residents would be monitored but not evacuated. Some reports suggest the dioxin distribution levels were so irregular throughout the area that the zone boundaries were arbitrarily drawn only to alleviate public concern. In the immediate aftermath, at least 30 people were hospitalized due to the incident, and over 200 cases of chloracne, a skin condition of pustules and sores, were reported.

In following years, studies indicated that exposure resulted in more cases of heart disease, chronic obstructive pulmonary disease, and diabetes, all conditions that stress from the disaster may have contributed to. Cases of gastrointestinal, lymphatic, and hematopoietic tissue cancer also increased, although they have not been directly linked to the dioxin exposure. Later studies found that exposed women were five times more likely to suffer from gallbladder cancer and multiple myeloma, a cancer of bone marrow, and exposed men were twice as likely to develop these cancers. Dioxin exposure is known to have a wide range of adverse effects on human health, including affecting the endocrine, immune, and central nervous systems and the development of fetal tissue.

The ICMESA plant was closed one month after the incident, and cleanup of the hazardous materials took about six years. In 1982, the most toxic chemicals remaining at the plant were put into 41 lead drums and transferred off-site for disposal. Later that year, the drums, which were being improperly stored in an abandoned warehouse outside of Paris, were sent to an incinerator in Switzerland for proper disposal.

The Seveso incident resulted in passage of the Seveso Directive by the European Union (then called the European Common Market), which led to more transparency and accountability in the chemical industry. The chemical companies involved in the incident financed the resettlement of families in Zone A, and they settled out of court around 7,000 individual lawsuits. In total, the estimated cleanup cost for the disaster was $162 million.

Mallory L. Daily

See Also: Air Pollution; Dioxin Pollution; Hazardous Air Pollutants; Hazardous Waste Disposal; Particulate Matter and Bioaerosols Pollution; Respiratory Disease and Air Pollution; Waste Incineration

Further Reading

Bernucci, L., et al. "The Seveso Studies on Early and Long-Term Effects of Dioxin Exposure: A Review." *Environmental Health Perspectives*, vol. 106, no. 2 (April 1998): 625–633.

Consonni, D., et al. "Mortality in a Population Exposed to Dioxin after the Seveso, Italy, Accident in 1976: 25 Years of Follow-Up." *American Journal of Epidemiology*, vol. 167, no. 7 (April 2008): 847–858.

Hernan, Robert E. *This Borrowed Earth: Lessons from the Fifteen Worst Environmental Disasters around the World*. New York: St. Martin's Press, 2010.

Wesselink, A., et al. "Maternal Dioxin Exposure and Pregnancy Outcomes over 30 Years of Follow-Up in Seveso." *Environment International*, vol. 63 (February 2014): 143–148.

SEWAGE TREATMENT AND DISPOSAL

Since the beginning of human settlements, water has been essential for drinking, sanitation, and irrigation. As population centers have grown, so too has the need for more and more water for these same purposes. Adequate water resources, and the ability to remove and clean the water of impurities for repeated use, are essential to a healthy and vibrant society. Wastewater treatment is particularly important so that we can use rivers, streams, and lakes for fishing, swimming, and drinking water—these same waters often serve the dual purposes of supply *and* disposal.

It is common for communities to have a system of sewers and wastewater treatment plants to collect wastewater from homes, businesses, and industries and convey it to publicly owned treatment works (POTWs) for treatment before it is discharged to receiving water bodies or land, or in some cases, before it is reused. Prior to POTWs, the organic matter in collected waste was largely assimilated in the receiving stream, and consequently, waterways serving large population centers experienced frequent occurrences of low dissolved oxygen, fish kills, algal blooms, and bacterial contamination. Over time, the natural environment was having trouble keeping up with the increased amounts of discharges, and something had to be done. Thus, the POTW came into use.

Wastewater and sanitary engineers have harnessed, emulated, and expedited natural treatment processes in what is commonly termed "secondary treatment." This involves the physical separation of solids heavy enough to settle out and a biological process that converts dissolved and suspended organic matter into biomass and carbon dioxide. Following secondary treatment, the converted biosolids are settled and retained/recirculated in the treatment plant (or extricated from the system), and the less potent treated wastewater is discharged. The biochemistry and operation of such processes, whether aerobic or anaerobic, is well understood and readily implemented. This type of system is the basis of the majority of POTWs across the United States. Note that POTWs must meet permitted levels of pollutants in the discharge prior to releasing it to the receiving body of water.

The strength of domestic sewage is often measured in terms of its oxygen-demanding characteristic, or more specifically, the biochemical oxygen demand. Organic waste is decomposed by bacteria, which use oxygen in the process of respiration to extract energy, grow, generate new biomass, and break down the organic matter. During the respiration process, carbon dioxide and water are generated (along with energy and biomass). As the organic matter passes through the treatment plant, care must be taken to ensure that the bacteria have an adequate supply of dissolved oxygen, a means for remaining in the treatment process (so they do not get discharged with the treated wastewater), and adequate nutrients (especially nitrogen, phosphorous, and trace elements) to sustain the bacterial process. As the biomass is grown to the optimal concentration, it must be settled out in a clarifier and some returned back into the process to repeat the cycle. Biomass that is not returned to the activated sludge basin to sustain the biodegradation becomes waste sludge, which is typically dewatered and pressed to remove excess moisture. The remaining sludge cake can normally be disposed of in a landfill or sometimes applied to land as a fertilizer.

An important feature and characteristic of the activated sludge system described previously is the growth, age, retention, and return of the biomass (i.e., the activated sludge). A gravity clarifier or quiescent zone is often used to allow the biomass to settle out, from where it is wasted or recirculated with the clarified supernatant discharged into the receiving stream. This process, however, can require a large area when dealing with large volumes or other design constraints. An alternate technique to retaining the activated biomass population is to provide a medium upon which it can grow, thus eliminating the need for a clarifier. Such attached growth systems can be implemented using packed vessels, rotating biocontactors, floating media, or other engineered substrates for an attachment surface. Yet another alternative is the membrane bioreactor, in which a semipermeable membrane is used for biomass retention.

A less sophisticated method of sewage treatment that may be suitable in some circumstances (e.g., highway rest stops and rural communities) is land treatment/application of the wastewater. This method involves the controlled application of wastewater directly to the land, where physical, chemical, and biological processes treat the wastewater as it passes across or through the soil. Land treatment systems may be designed as slow-rate, overland flow, or rapid-infiltration systems. It may be desirable to provide some treatment prior to land application. For example, in arid western states, pretreated municipal wastewater is regularly used to irrigate crops. Land treatment options are gaining popularity in the United States.

Another land treatment option that is becoming popular is the concept of a constructed wetland. Wetlands are areas where the water saturates the ground long enough each year to develop hydric soils and wetland vegetation. Thus, a constructed wetlands treatment system is where wastewater is treated by passing it through an intentionally designed wetland. Similar to the emulation of natural aerobic biodegradation in activated sludge systems, constructed wetland treatment uses enhanced natural physical, chemical, and biological wetland processes to treat domestic wastewater.

There is a growing concern about pharmaceuticals (i.e., prescription and nonprescription medications) and health and beauty care (HBC) products in wastewater. Modern-day medicines, shampoos, perfumes, and other exotic healthcare and beautification products are routinely being flushed into sewer systems and have recently been detected in wide-ranging samples of the nation's waters. For example, in a recent study of effluents from 50 large POTWs, trace amounts of hydrochlorothiazide and valsartan were found in every sample, and metoprolol, atenolol, and carbamazepine were found in over 90 percent of the samples. Other studies have found in surface waters endocrine disruptors, antibiotics (e.g., erythromycin), hormones (e.g., 17ß-estradiol and 17ß-ethinylestradiol), steroids (e.g., coprostanol), and over-the-counter medications such as ibuprofen and acetaminophen. And regarding HBC products, various studies have found parabens, synthetic fragrances, triclosan, triclocarban, and ultraviolet-filtering compounds in wastewater discharges. Conventional treatment plants often do not degrade or remove these constituents to a large degree. Just as industrial effluents with new and exotic constituents presented new challenges to industrial wastewater engineers in the 20th century, pharmaceuticals and HBC products promise to present the next big challenge for the 21st century.

John K. Borén

See Also: Bioremediation for Waste Treatment; Industrial Effluents; Land Disposal of Waste Materials; Municipal Solid Waste Management; Water Pollution

Further Reading

Benjamin, Mark M., and Desmond F. Lawler. *Water Quality Engineering: Physical/Chemical Treatment Processes*. Hoboken, NJ: John Wiley and Sons, 2013.

Howe, Kerry J., et al. *Principles of Water Treatment*. Hoboken, NJ: John Wiley and Sons, 2012.

Primer for Municipal Wastewater Treatment Systems (EPA 832-R-04–001). Washington, DC: U.S. Environmental Protection Agency, 2004.

Spellman, Frank R. *Handbook of Water and Wastewater Treatment Plant Operations*. Boca Raton, FL: CRC Press, 2014.

Tchobanoglous, George, et al. *Wastewater Engineering: Treatment and Resource Recovery*. New York: McGraw-Hill Education, 2014.

U.S. Environmental Protection Agency. *National Pollutant Discharge Elimination System (NPDES): Municipal Wastewater*. https://www.epa.gov/npdes/municipal-wastewater (accessed May 1, 2017).

SICK BUILDING SYNDROME

Sick building syndrome (SBS) describes the discomfort building occupants sometimes experience while inside the building. SBS is most common in office buildings, but it can also occur in apartments, schools, and other buildings with multiple occupants. To be considered SBS, health professionals typically look for symptoms among a group of occupants rather than one or two isolated cases.

Common SBS symptoms include headache, cough, dry and itchy skin, dizziness, nausea, loss of concentration, fatigue, odor sensitivity, and irritation of the eye, nose, or throat. The cause of these symptoms is often unknown, but because the symptoms typically subside, if not completely disappear, after occupants leave the building, the cause of the discomfort is assumed to be something inside. The symptoms may be limited to a specific room or area of the building, or they may be reported throughout the building, and they may or may not occur seasonally. (SBS is different from the condition known as building-related illness, which

Is Your Carpeting Toxic?

A surprising number of chemicals are used in carpeting. For example, there are chemicals in glues, dyes, backing materials, and flame retardants, and these chemicals are often volatile (i.e., they vaporize into the surrounding air). Some of these chemicals are capable of causing adverse reactions in sensitive individuals, including irritation, breathing difficulty, and even neurological symptoms. Additionally, some chemicals are believed to be carcinogenic. Fortunately, a number of carpets on the market today are specifically designed to minimize the release of toxic gases into the surrounding air. Environmentally conscious consumers may also be interested in carpets made of natural fibers and recycled materials.

covers diagnosable illnesses like Legionnaires' disease that can be directly attributed to specific agents in the building.)

Inadequate building ventilation is thought to contribute to many cases of SBS because without enough ventilation, air contaminants can increase to levels that adversely affect health. Air contaminants may originate inside the building, for example, from carpeting, wall paint, particle board, pesticides, office machines, air fresheners, dust mites, and even marking pens, or the air contaminants may be associated with outside air pollution and pollen drawn into the building by the ventilation system. Occupant health can also be affected by mold and other microbial contaminants, particularly when the contaminants build up in air-handling equipment and in water-damaged wallboard, ceiling tile, carpeting, and insulation. Odors, stagnant air, thermal gradients, high humidity, poor lighting, office noise, and inadequate sanitary and cleaning practices may also contribute to occupant discomfort.

Some examples of indoor air contaminants and their sources include the following:

- Acetic Acid: X-ray equipment, caulking compounds
- Formaldehyde: insulation, plywood, particle board, paneling, carpeting, fabric adhesives, tobacco smoke
- Inorganic Gases: window cleaners, acid drain cleaners, tobacco smoke, blueprint equipment, gas furnaces and appliances, engine exhausts. (Inorganic gas examples include ammonia, hydrogen sulfide, and sulfur dioxide.)
- Microbials: air-handling systems, cooling towers, humidifiers, water-damaged materials, plants, food and food products. (Microbials are microorganisms and other biological contaminants, including viruses, fungi, mold, bacteria, pollen, dander, and mites.)
- Nitrogen Oxides: gas furnaces and appliances, welding, engine exhausts, tobacco smoke
- Ozone: copy machines, electrostatic air cleaners, outside air
- Volatile Organic Compounds—paint, cleaning products and disinfectants, mothballs, glues, photocopiers, caulking materials, pesticides, cosmetics, and other personal products. (Volatile organic compound examples include trichloroethylene, benzene, toluene, methyl ethyl ketone, alcohols, and acrolein.)

Investigations of SBS complaints can be difficult because the symptoms are often subjective and nonspecific, and sometimes the symptoms are mistaken for other health conditions like asthma or the flu. In some cases, SBS may affect only a few individuals who are unusually sensitive to the offensive agents, and in other cases the entire workforce may be affected, causing the facility to be evacuated.

What can be done to remediate SBS? It is often difficult to identify the exact cause of the symptoms experienced by building occupants. Nevertheless, poor ventilation is suspected about half the time. Ventilation can be improved by adjusting or replacing mechanical systems, adding air treatment (e.g., carbon filters), locating air intakes away from potential air pollution sources (e.g., garages and roadways), regularly performing preventive maintenance (e.g., cleaning ducts and dampers and changing air filters), and ensuring temperature and humidity standards are consistently maintained. (Humidity should generally be below 60 percent to discourage microbial growth.) Standing water should be removed, for example, from humidifier reservoirs and drain pans, and any water-damaged materials should be replaced, including wallboard, ceiling tile, carpeting, and insulation. Carpeting and other materials that give off offensive gases can be replaced with more environmentally friendly materials, and nonporous surfaces can be cleaned with a disinfectant. Of course, cigarette smoking should always be banned indoors. You should consult with an indoor air quality professional to determine the steps most appropriate for your situation.

Occasionally a building occupant may exhibit hypersensitivity to something in the indoor environment that does not cause symptoms in other people. The occupant should be evaluated by a health professional, and if the problem persists despite all possible steps to remove what may be causing the symptoms, the occupant should be relocated to another part of the building where the symptoms do not occur.

While researchers believe SBS is mainly an air quality issue, research suggests that synergistic effects involving occupational stress may result in symptoms that otherwise may not be present. Thus, stress management programs might be considered along with other measures to address the problem. A number of conditions might lead to occupational stress, including tight deadlines, a noisy work environment, poor work area lighting and temperature control, eye strain and ergonomic problems from computer work, work/life balance issues, and communication problems with coworkers or supervisors.

Workers reporting SBS symptoms were once dismissed as complainers, but today these complaints are taken seriously as researchers find that even modern buildings can have indoor air quality problems. While significant advances in the manufacture of low-vapor carpets, wall paints, and other building materials have helped reduced the number of indoor air quality complaints, issues with microbial contaminants may be increasing. This could be related to the proliferation of energy-efficient buildings, where ventilation rates may not be ideal for discouraging the growth of molds, fungi, bacteria, and other biological contaminants.

Richard Crume

See Also: Air Pollution; Cancer Risk from Environmental Exposure; Environmental Toxicology; Formaldehyde; Hazardous Air Pollutants; Indoor Environment; Legionnaires' Disease; Mold and Dampness; Noise Pollution; Occupational Safety and Health; Odor Pollution; Ozone and Smog in the Urban Environment; Particulate Matter and Bioaerosols Pollution; Personal Care Products, Health Issues with; Pesticides and Herbicides; Quiet, Benefits of; Volatile Organic Compound Pollution

Further Reading

Goldstein, Walter E. *Sick Building Syndrome and Related Illness: Prevention and Remediation of Mold Contamination*. Boca Raton, FL: Taylor and Francis, 2011.

National Institute for Occupational Safety and Health. *Indoor Environmental Quality*. https://www.cdc.gov/niosh/topics/indoorenv (accessed November 3, 2016).

OSHA Technical Manual (OTM), Instruction TED 01–00–015 (Update). Washington, DC: Occupational Safety and Health Administration, 2016. https://www.osha.gov/dts/osta/otm/index.html.

Straus, David C. *Sick Building Syndrome*. Amsterdam, the Netherlands: Elsevier Academic Press, 2004.

U.S. Environmental Protection Agency. *Indoor Air Quality (IAQ)*. https://www.epa.gov/indoor-air-quality-iaq (accessed November 4, 2016).

Yanagisawa, Yukio, et al. *Chemical Sensitivity and Sick-Building Syndrome*. Boca Raton, FL: CRC Press, 2017.

SILICA

Silica is a chemical compound made of silicon and oxygen atoms, chemically known as silicon dioxide. It can exist in either a crystalline or noncrystalline (also called amorphous) state. The crystalline state is the primary cause of environmental concerns because it has long been recognized as an occupational inhalation hazard in several industries, where it has caused many disabilities and deaths. In contrast to the adverse health effects of inhalable silica, silica in the diet has been linked by some research to health benefits for bones, joints, collagen, and teeth.

Crystalline silica can occur in any of several forms, including quartz (the most common natural form), cristobalite, tridymite, and tripoli. These forms differ from each other in the arrangements of the tetrahedron structures that make up the crystals. The basic silica tetrahedron consists of one silicon atom surrounded by four oxygen atoms. Pure crystalline silica is also called free silica. When other elements are combined with silica, such as sodium, potassium, calcium, or magnesium, the compound is called a silicate. Among the many types of silicates are vermiculite, kaolin, talc, micas, and feldspar. Noncrystalline silica is found naturally in diatomaceous earth and other sediments and rocks as well as in synthetic materials such as silica gel.

According to the National Institute for Occupational Safety and Health (NIOSH), more than 2 million U.S. workers in the mining and construction industries are exposed to inhalable silica every year, and hundreds of these workers die annually from exposure to silica dust. Mining and quarrying activities involving sand, gravel, metal ore, and coal are the main sources of silica exposure. Increasingly, hydraulic fracturing is another major source. Construction activities that generate inhalable silica include both indoor and outdoor work, such as sandblasting and drilling, concrete mixing and pouring, and drywall installation.

Other industries where workers may be exposed to large amounts of inhalable silica are brick and clay, glass and ceramic, and metal manufacturing. The crushing and processing of raw materials, preparation of sand casts, and cleaning of residue are some of the manufacturing steps that generate silica dust. Silica is also used in the electronics, pharmaceutical, and food industries, although workers in those industries are generally exposed to little inhalable silica.

Outside of occupational exposures, the general public is at some risk of exposure to inhalable silica in the particulate matter of air pollution. This ambient air pollution is produced by various sources, including power plant emissions from the combustion of coal, airborne particles generated by vehicular traffic on paved and unpaved roads, tilling of soil in agriculture, and natural sources such as forest fires and wind erosion of soil. Children, the elderly, and individuals with weakened immune systems are most vulnerable to silica exposure.

The primary health hazards associated with silica are respiratory in nature. The tiny silica particles are inhaled into the respiratory tract and lungs, where they get carried into the deepest and smallest tissues—the alveoli—where oxygen is exchanged with the blood. Typical symptoms initially include respiratory irritation and dry coughing. However, during continued exposure over time, the silica particles can accumulate in the respiratory tract and lungs, causing severe inflammation that can lead to or aggravate other respiratory conditions, including bronchitis, emphysema, and chronic obstructive pulmonary disease.

The most common serious health problem caused by inhaling silica dust is silicosis, an acute or chronic inflammation of the lungs that is a type of pulmonary fibrosis. This condition, which is potentially fatal, may include bloody sputum production, shortness of breath, lung scarring, and reduced lung function. It may also lead to heart enlargement and damage as the heart pumps harder to compensate for the weakened pulmonary system.

In some cases, the silica particles are transported to the kidneys, lymph nodes, or other tissues of the body, resulting in renal failure or other serious problems outside the respiratory system. Still other possible diseases associated with silica inhalation include autoimmune disorders, such as rheumatoid arthritis and systemic lupus erythematosus, and lung cancer. The risk of severe disorders increases with the intensity and duration of exposure.

Numerous regulations and guidelines have been established by the U.S. government, as well as the governments of other nations, to minimize human exposure to inhalable silica. However, not all companies in the mining, construction, and other industries regularly perform surveillance of employee silica exposure to generate data sufficient for guideline compliance evaluation. Government researchers and regulators from NIOSH and the Occupational Safety and Health Administration (OSHA) sometimes detect unsafe worker exposure levels, in which case OSHA may issue a hazard alert to warn workers of the risk and to warn the company of the need to rectify the problem.

In 2016, OSHA enacted stricter rules for occupational exposure to silica, estimating that the rules will save more than 600 lives and prevent more than 900 cases of silicosis each year. Industries were given one to five years to comply with the new standards. While there are no federal standards for ambient air exposure to silica outside the workplace, several states have enacted such standards.

A. J. Smuskiewicz

See Also: Cancer Risk from Environmental Exposure; Fugitive Dust; Hydraulic Fracturing; Industrial Hygiene; National Institute for Occupational Safety and Health; Occupational Safety and Health; Occupational Safety and Health Administration; Particulate Matter and Bioaerosols Pollution; Respiratory Disease and Air Pollution

Further Reading

Bhagia, L. "Non-Occupational Exposure to Silica Dust." *Indian Journal of Occupational and Environmental Medicine*, vol. 16, no. 3 (September 2012): 95–100.

Danger in the Air: Health Concerns for Silica in Outdoor Air. Environmental Working Group, Washington, DC, 2014. http://www.ewg.org/research/sandstorm/health-concerns-silica-outdoor-air.

National Institute for Occupational Safety and Health. *Silica*. https://www.cdc.gov/niosh/topics/silica (accessed April 7, 2017).

Steenland, Kyle, and Elizabeth Ward. "Silica: A Lung Carcinogen." *CA: A Cancer Journal for Clinicians*, vol. 64, no. 1 (January–February 2014): 63–69.

U.S. Department of Labor. *OSHA's Final Rule to Protect Workers from Exposure to Respirable Crystalline Silica*. https://www.osha.gov/silica (accessed March 24, 2017).

SNOW, JOHN

John Snow (1813–1858) was an English physician who did pioneering work spanning public health, anesthesia, intensive care medicine, and medical cartography. He is also hailed as a father of modern epidemiology for his scientific and systematic approach to mapping cholera transmission through contaminated water.

Born in York, England, on March 15, 1813, Snow was the oldest of nine children. As a young man, he became a vegetarian for some years, and he was also a teetotaler who advocated for the temperance movement. Snow's medical training began as an apprenticeship when he was 14. By age 23, when he went to London for formal medical education, Snow had apprenticed with three practitioners. He qualified as a surgeon-apothecary (a general practitioner) in 1838, and after additional study culminating at the University of London, he qualified as a physician in 1844. In 1850, Snow passed the exam to become a member of the elite Licentiate of the Royal College of Physicians of London. He practiced medicine in London's Soho neighborhood, developed a reputation as an excellent diagnostician, and was an active member of several professional organizations, including the Westminster Medical Society.

Snow became London's foremost anesthesiologist, making anesthesia safer by developing an inhaler to control the concentration of gases a surgical patient received. He also invented a device for resuscitating newborns. Snow regularly treated both poor and wealthy, famously administering chloroform to Queen Victoria for the births of both Prince Leopold and Princess Beatrice.

When cholera struck London, Snow conducted investigations that refuted the widely held miasmatic theory of cholera, which is the idea that the disease is spread by bad quality air, polluted by noxious odors from rotting organic matter. Snow disagreed with airborne theories, holding that the cause of cholera was a contagion passed by ingesting water contaminated by a cholera victim's bodily eliminations. The miasmatists (i.e., people who believed in miasmatic theory) advocated for sanitation reform projects that flushed sewage and trash away from homes and into waterways serving municipal water supplies. However, if Snow was correct, this approach actually spread disease such as cholera, which could be stopped with proper hygiene and sanitary water supplies.

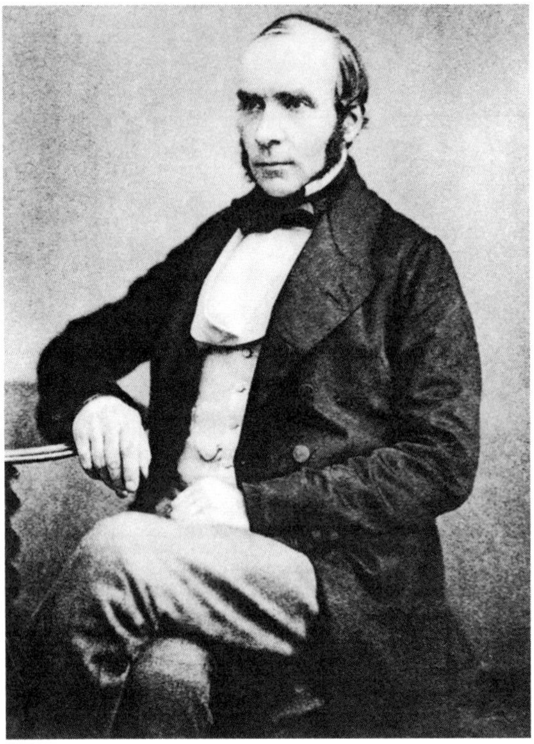

John Snow, considered the father of modern epidemiology. Snow is recognized for his scientific and systematic approach to mapping cholera transmission through contaminated water. (National Library of Medicine)

Two consecutive cholera outbreaks afforded him the opportunity to conduct his "grand experiment," which involved comparing cholera deaths in households supplied by two different water companies. During the earlier epidemic, both companies had originally drawn water from the same polluted area of the Thames River. However, between outbreaks, one water company had changed its supply to a cleaner part of the river. Those customers showed a lower risk for cholera in the next epidemic. Snow combed available data on cholera and conducted his own investigations, including plotting a map of cholera deaths that led him to the public Broad Street water pump as the source of the outbreak. The pump handle was removed, and cholera cases quickly diminished.

Snow died of a stroke and kidney failure on June 16, 1858. It is speculated that Snow's propensity to experiment on himself with anesthetic agents having unknown health effects at the time may have contributed to his early demise. Within a decade of his death, there was another cholera outbreak in London. Drawing from Snow's work, the connection between contaminated water and disease outbreak was more firmly established for those who had remained skeptical. With improved knowledge and better engineering of water systems, large-scale cholera outbreaks in Britain were finally put to an end.

Kathy Stolley

See Also: Cholera; Drinking Water Quality and Regulation; Environmental Epidemiology; Sewage Treatment and Disposal; Waterborne Diseases

Further Reading

Hempel, Sandra. *The Strange Case of the Broad Street Pump: John Snow and the Mystery of Cholera*. Berkeley: University of California Press, 2007.

Johnson, Steven. *The Ghost Map: The Story of London's Most Terrifying Epidemic—and How It Changed Science, Cities, and the Modern World.* New York: Riverhead Books, 2006.

Morris, Robert D. *The Blue Death: The Intriguing Past and Present Danger of the Water You Drink*. New York: HarperCollins, 2007.
Snow, Stephanie J. *Operations without Pain: The Practice and Science of Anaesthesia in Victorian Britain*. New York: Palgrave MacMillan, 2006.
University of California, Los Angeles. *John Snow*. http://www.ph.ucla.edu/epi/snow.html (accessed February 18, 2017).
Vinten-Johansen, Peter, et al. *Cholera, Chloroform, and the Science of Medicine*. New York: Oxford University Press, 2003.

SOCIOECONOMIC STATUS AND HEALTH

Socioeconomic status plays a major role in creating health disparities. Socioeconomic status refers to an individual's level of education and income as well as the occupation that person holds. Each of these three factors can impact various health outcomes. Generally, high socioeconomic status is associated with good health outcomes, and low socioeconomic status is associated with poor health outcomes. Health problems often associated with low socioeconomic status include heart disease, high blood pressure, diabetes, cancer, and low birth weight.

Although education, income, and occupation may be powerful determinants of an individual's overall health, they often do not create health outcomes directly. Instead, these factors underlie an individual's exposure to conditions and situations that have a more direct and immediate impact on health. A person's socioeconomic status is closely associated with their access to and quality of health care, their environmental exposure to harmful substances, and their health behaviors. These three factors combined account for approximately 80 percent of premature mortality, with 50 percent attributed to lifestyle and behavior, 20 percent attributed to environmental exposure, and 10 percent associated with health care.

Tobacco use is the single largest behavioral risk factor for premature death, and those with lower socioeconomic status are more likely to smoke. Those with less education and less income are also more likely to lead a sedentary lifestyle and eat a diet that is low in fresh produce and fiber. The same population may be less informed about how to lead a healthy lifestyle and may live in neighborhoods without recreational facilities (and where it may be unsafe to walk or play outdoors), with fewer stores selling healthy foods, and with more tobacco and alcohol advertising.

Socioeconomic status also impacts exposure to harmful environmental pollutants such as asbestos, mercury, lead, and industrial wastes. Those with lower socioeconomic status are more likely to live and work in unhealthy, contaminated environments. Poorer neighborhoods are more likely to be found in close proximity to highways, industrial business zones, and toxic waste sites because the land in these areas is less desirable and, thus, cheaper. Housing in these neighborhoods is also more likely to be of poorer quality. In the case of lead exposure, high levels of lead in the blood are six times more common in children and adults from poorer families when compared with children and adults from high-income families. (By comparison, middle-class children and adults showed a twofold increase in high blood lead levels.) Rates of childhood asthma are on the rise, and this is especially true in poor, urban neighborhoods. The severity of asthma symptoms also tends to be greater among children of low socioeconomic status.

The impact of an individual's social environment may be even more important than the physical surroundings. Those with low socioeconomic status are more likely to be isolated and not a part of a social network. Those who are socially isolated have increased rates of mortality—between 1.9 and 5 times greater than those who are more socially connected and engaged. The quality and patterns of social interaction can also impact health. For example, sexually transmitted diseases spread more rapidly within high-risk networks (e.g., those who are more likely to engage in unprotected sex with multiple partners), and these high-risk networks are often found in poorer areas.

Lastly, socioeconomic status also has a significant impact on healthcare access and quality. For instance, approximately 40 percent of individuals who did not graduate from high school do not have health insurance, compared to only 10 percent of college graduates. Among uninsured Americans, 60 percent come from low-income families. Uninsured individuals receive less medical care, including preventative screenings and treatment for diseases and conditions. It is important to note, however, that there are programs, such as Medicare, designed to provide health insurance coverage to low-income individuals and families. As such, when it comes to healthcare access and quality, the link between socioeconomic status and poor health outcomes is not as strong as it is for health behaviors and environmental exposure.

Jyotsna S. Jagai

See Also: Asthma; Environmental Justice; Vulnerable Populations, Environmental Threats to

Further Reading

American Psychological Association. *Work, Stress, and Health and Socioeconomic Status*. http://www.apa.org/pi/ses/resources/publications/work-stress-health.aspx (accessed April 10, 2017).

Kronenfeld, Jennie J., ed. *Social Determinants, Health Disparities, and Linkages to Health and Health Care (Volume 31: Research in the Sociology of Health Care)*. Bingley, UK: Emerald Group, 2013.

Reibert, Sarah, and Alice Jannings, eds. *Socioeconomic Status and Health Implications*. New York: Nova Science, 2012.

U.S. Environmental Protection Agency. *Environmental Justice*. https://www.epa.gov/environmentaljustice (accessed April 10, 2017).

SOIL CONTAMINATION AND REMEDIATION

Soil is a natural body on the earth's surface composed of mineral and organic materials, water, and air. In the ecosystem, soil serves as a medium for plant growth, a regulator of water supplies, a recycler of raw materials, a habitat for organisms, and an engineering medium. Soils are said to be contaminated when they cannot perform one or more of these functions.

Soil contamination, a widespread problem in many parts of the world, is the result of the undesirable entry of chemicals into vulnerable ecosystems. These chemicals can be naturally occurring or manufactured by humans (i.e., xenobiotic). Regardless of origin, their undesirable entry into the environment is due to their production, use, and improper disposals during human activities, including agriculture, mining, manufacturing, medical practice, and military defense operations.

The most common contaminants in soil are petroleum hydrocarbons, polynuclear aromatic hydrocarbons (e.g., naphthalene and benzo(a)pyrene), solvents, pesticides, and lead and other heavy metals. Soil contamination can adversely affect human and ecosystem health. For example, human exposure to lead in soil can result in neurological impairment, and exposure to other chemicals is linked to cancers and congenital disorders. Infiltration of soil contaminants into groundwater aquifers can threaten the health of communities that depend on the aquifers for their water supplies. Because soil contaminants can pass into vegetation and enter food chains, the consumption of food crops grown in contaminated soil has become a major health risk in certain regions of the world.

Plants and soil microbes are equally impacted by soil contamination. For example, high levels of certain soil contaminants can be toxic to plant growth, and some contaminants can impair the abilities of soil microbes to conduct life-sustaining biological cycles.

The U.S. Environmental Protection Agency (EPA) is the major federal agency regulating soil contamination. Once EPA finds those responsible for contamination, it requires the contaminants to be cleaned up or the responsible party to pay the cost of cleanup. Cleaning contaminated soil, called soil remediation, involves removing contaminants and restoring the soil to its natural, pollution-free state. Scientists have studied a variety of treatment methods to remediate soil contamination. Depending on the type of contamination, the concentrations of the contaminants in the soil, and the available time frame and funding, different remediation methods have been used, including soil removal or washing, soil vapor extraction, thermal desorption, bioremediation or phytoremediation, and natural attenuation.

Soil removal and washing are simple methods for soil remediation. Soil removal can be used for contamination that covers a small area or is otherwise unresponsive to other in situ remediation technologies. Using buckets, drums, or roll-offs, the removed soil can be moved to landfills that accept contaminated soil or to treatment facilities that can clean contaminated soil, making it usable again. Soil washing, a process that uses surfactants and water to remove contaminants from the soil, involves either dissolving or suspending pollutants in the wash solution and separating the soil by particle size. Soil washing can be applied to soil contaminated with a wide variety of heavy metal, radionuclide, and organic contaminants. (The contaminated water must later be decontaminated.)

Vapor extraction is used to treat volatile and semivolatile organic contaminants in soil. This method uses a series of vacuum extraction wells placed throughout the contaminated zone, and a vacuum pump pulls air through the contaminated area. This method works well in permeable soil with a high sand content.

Thermal desorption is an efficient, environmentally beneficial process that uses heat to increase the volatility of contaminants so that they can be removed from the soil. This method typically consists of two main processes: (1) contaminated soil is heated to the boiling point of the contaminants and (2) the volatized contaminants are then captured and destroyed in a thermal oxidizer or condensed in a vapor recovery unit.

Bioremediation involves the use of living microorganisms, such as bacteria and fungi, to break down organic pollutants in the soil. This method is based on the common practice in microbiology of using microbes to break down organic compounds and other toxic materials in household and industrial wastes. Bioremediation has proved to be a very effective and inexpensive method to treat soils contaminated with toxic chemicals. This method can be used either in situ or ex situ (i.e., off-site). In situ bioremediation techniques are normally applied to soil that is lightly contaminated, difficult to remove, or has contaminants that are volatile. Ex situ bioremediation involves moving the contaminated soil to another location, where it can be processed using bioremediation.

If plants are used to remove contamination from the soil, the process is called phytoremediation. This is an emerging and proven strategy that may involve several processes broadly classified as (1) plant uptake and storage of metal contaminants that can then be harvested and recovered with a technique known as phytomining; (2) plant uptake and metabolizing of organic contaminants; and (3) interactions between soil microbes and plant root exudates that promote contaminant degradation, transformation, or stabilization, or a combination of these.

Many plant species have been used in phytoremediation, including shrubs, trees, flowers, and highly specialized species that can take up and tolerate toxic concentrations of elements (i.e., hyperaccumulators). Sometimes special planting techniques are applied to promote the various means by which contaminants can be removed or destroyed by plants or plant-microbe complexes.

Phytoremediation can be applied to both small and large areas, and compared with other soil decontamination methods, phytoremediation costs are much less and can be implemented with relatively little environmental disturbance. In addition, compared with landfilling, phytoremediation is considered a permanent solution to the cleanup and removal of many soil contaminants, including the most prevalent petroleum hydrocarbons resulting from leaking petroleum storage tanks.

Natural attenuation is a remedial method where contaminants naturally degrade without intervention. This method works well for organic contamination, such as fuels and solvents, which are readily degradable. To facilitate the breakdown of contaminants, microorganisms that feed on the contaminants may be added, or aerobic conditions can be created in the soil to increase microorganism activity. This is the most cost-effective soil remediation method, but it may not be satisfactory for high concentrations of certain contaminants, and routine monitoring is necessary to ensure that proper remediation is proceeding. Natural attenuation may be used in combination with other remedial methods, such as soil vapor extraction and excavation.

Dafeng Hui and E. Kudjo Dzantor

See Also: Bioremediation for Waste Treatment; Drinking Water Quality and Regulation; Ecosystems, Importance of; Environmental Protection Agency; Groundwater Pollution and Depletion; Hexavalent Chromium; Land Disposal of Waste Materials; Lead Poisoning Prevention; Oil Spills, Health Consequences of; Pesticides and Herbicides; Radioactive Wastes; Underground Storage Tanks, Health Concerns with

Further Reading

Cunningham, Scott D., William R. Berti, and Jianwei W. Huang. "Phytoremediation of Contaminated Soils." *Trends in Biotechnology*, vol. 13, no. 9 (September 1995): 393–397.

de Albergaria, Jose T. V. S., and Hendrikus P. A. Nouws, eds. *Soil Remediation: Applications and New Technologies*. Boca Raton, FL: CRC Press, 2016.

Hakeem, Khalid, et al., eds. *Soil Remediation and Plants: Prospects and Challenges*. Waltham, MA: Academic Press, 2015.

Markus, Julie, and Alex B. McBratney. "A Review of the Contamination of Soil with Lead: II. Spatial Distribution and Risk Assessment of Soil Lead." *Environmental International*, vol. 27, no. 5 (November 2001): 399–411.

U.S. Environmental Protection Agency. *Remediation Technologies for Cleaning up Contaminated Sites*. https://www.epa.gov/remedytech/remediation-technologies-cleaning-contaminated-sites (accessed May 28, 2016).

Wilcke, Wolfgang. "Polycyclic Aromatic Hydrocarbons (PAHs) in Soil—A Review." *Journal of Plant Nutrition and Soil Science*, vol. 163, no. 3 (June 2000): 229–248.

STORMWATER RUNOFF

Stormwater runoff results when precipitation flows over the ground instead of infiltrating into the ground. Runoff may occur during a rain event or during snowmelt and can occur in a variety of environments, including urban, residential, agricultural, industrial, commercial, and construction areas. Stormwater can flow off paved streets, lawns, and rooftops, posing a threat to human health by contaminating water used for drinking and recreation.

Stormwater runoff contributes to what is known as nonpoint source pollution, which is different from point source pollution. Point source pollution, which is a single identifiable source of pollution discharge like a smokestack of a factory, is easy to treat because there is a single source of pollution. On the other hand,

Green Cities Are Seeing Green

Many cities have taken the initiative to reduce stormwater runoff from urban landscapes. For example, Philadelphia launched Green City, Clean Waters, which recreates living landscapes to keep water out of city sewers, promotes rain barrel use, and encourages architects and builders to include green roofs and landscaping in their designs. By employing a green approach to reduce stormwater pollution rather than relying on the traditional infrastructure, the Green City is saving an estimated $5.6 billion.

nonpoint source pollution, like stormwater runoff, is much more difficult to identify and treat because the pollution comes from multiple sources and directions. Consider the case of a farmer who spreads a chemical fertilizer on a plot of land just before a big rainstorm. If the rain is heavy enough, water will begin to drain in various directions, carrying the fertilizer with it. It will be difficult to predict where this chemical-laden runoff water will go, and consequently, cleanup will be complicated, if not impossible. Stormwater runoff can carry many different pollutants that can potentially affect human and environmental health.

The types of pollution carried with stormwater runoff depend on the environment in which the runoff is occurring. Urban environments typically have a large amount of stormwater runoff because there tends to be many impervious surfaces in a city and relatively little green space. (Impervious surfaces like concrete or asphalt prevent water from infiltrating into the ground below.) Cities also have considerable automobile and truck traffic, leading to oil and dust deposition on the streets, which can end up in stormwater runoff, as can litter on streets and sidewalks. If the stormwater runoff enters a combined sewer system, where sanitary water and stormwater are combined, there is the potential for a combined sewer overflow (CSO) event. CSOs result in untreated wastewater being released into water bodies that may provide drinking water or be used for recreation. Cities throughout the United States are working to minimize the number of CSO events, and reducing the amount of stormwater runoff from urban landscapes is an important factor in this mission.

Pollution in stormwater runoff is an issue not only with urban streets and sidewalks but also with residential lawns and parks, farms, commercial and industrial facilities, and construction sites. Residential lawns and parks can contribute to stormwater pollution when they are treated with fertilizers and pesticides. Farms and other agricultural operations are a particular problem when heavy amounts of fertilizer are applied and when pet and animal wastes are not appropriately managed. Commercial and industrial facilities may engage in practices that lead to grease and oil spills that will be picked up in stormwater runoff. Construction sites, which often disturb a large area of land, can lead to sediments running off into waterways.

There are various effects of pollutants occurring in stormwater runoff. According to the U.S. Environmental Protection Agency, sediment (sand, clay, or silt) is the most common pollutant in rivers, streams, lakes, and reservoirs. Sediment can cause water to become turbid (cloudy), clog fish gills, and prevent aquatic vegetation from growing. Sediment-rich runoff can also carry nutrients that trigger blue-green algae growth, which then releases cyanotoxins that are harmful to humans. Bacteria and pathogens, which may be present in runoff from land grazed by livestock, can make people extremely ill and have been linked to deaths in vulnerable populations, such as children, the elderly, and those lacking healthy immune systems. Pollutants found in stormwater runoff from agricultural lands may contain unhealthy levels of pesticides and fertilizers. Plastic bags and bottles, food wrappers, and other types of trash that end up on stormwater runoff can harm wildlife. Oils, paints, and soaps used for commercial and industrial purposes can make people sick and harm the environment.

With so many potential sources of harmful pollution in stormwater runoff, it is important to find ways to reduce the pollutant sources as well as the quantity of stormwater runoff. In urban environments, green infrastructure can help reduce runoff by mimicking the natural environment. Some examples of green infrastructure include green roofs (roofs covered with grasses and shrubs instead of an impervious material), permeable pavement (pavement that water can pass through), rain barrels and cisterns (systems that collect rainwater for use in gardens and landscaping), and vegetated swales (large vegetated areas where water is taken up by the plants). In agricultural areas, a vegetated buffer next to a water body can reduce stormwater runoff, as can the rotation of crops and animal grazing areas. Procedures should be in place at commercial and industrial areas that allow chemical spills to be cleaned up immediately. At construction sites, installing silt fences, using silt bags (e.g., at sewer openings), and applying mulch or hay to disturbed areas can help prevent sediments from be carried away with stormwater.

Elise C. Hunter

See Also: Combined Sewer Overflow; Cyanobacteria Toxins; Drinking Water Quality and Regulation; Environmental Protection Agency; Green Space in Urban Environments; Pesticides and Herbicides; Water Pollution; Watershed Management, Health Implications of; Wetlands and Healthy Waterways

Further Reading

Foderaro, Lisa W. "A New Playground in the Bronx Soaks Up the City's Problematic Storm Water." *New York Times*, June 24, 2015, https://www.nytimes.com/2015/06/25/nyregion/a-new-playground-in-the-bronx-soaks-up-the-citys-problematic-storm-water.html.

McRandle, Paul. *Philadelphia Cleans Up Storm Water with Innovative Program.* National Geographic Society, Washington, DC, 2012. http://news.nationalgeographic.com/news/2012/06/120606/philadelphia-storm-water-runoff/.

Philadelphia Water Department. *Green City, Clean Waters.* http://www.phillywatersheds.org/what_were_doing/documents_and_data/cso_long_term_control_plan (accessed September 19, 2015).

Thurston, Hale W., ed. *Economic Incentives for Stormwater Control.* Boca Raton, FL: CRC Press/Taylor and Francis Group, 2011.

U.S. Environmental Protection Agency. *Stormwater Management.* http://www.epa.gov/greeningepa/stormwater-management (accessed December 31, 2015).

STRATOSPHERIC OZONE DEPLETION

Ozone is a naturally occurring molecule made up of three oxygen atoms. The molecules combine to form a stratified gaseous layer in the earth's upper atmosphere known as the stratosphere. This gaseous layer is called the ozonosphere. The ozonosphere sits roughly 9 to 22 miles (14 to 35 kilometers) above the earth's surface, with variations in its thickness based on the season and geographic location. (It is important not to confuse stratospheric ozone with ground-level ozone, which is a major component of smog in large cities and can cause respiratory distress and illness.)

The highest concentrations of ozone occur in the tropics at altitudes of 16 to 17 miles (26 to 27 kilometers) and toward the poles from 7 to 12 miles (11 to 19 kilometers). By encapsulating the planet Earth, the ozone layer protects the earth and hence plants, animals, and humans from the harmful effects of the sun's radiation. The ozone layer, which was discovered in 1913 by two French physicists—Charles Fabry (1867–1945) and Henri Buisson (1873–1944)—can absorb 97 to 99 percent of the ultraviolet (UV) radiation emitted by the sun. The UV rays, if left unchecked, can produce harmful effects on the earth and its habitation.

The ozone molecules of the ozonosphere have the ability to block solar radiation of wavelengths below 290 nanometers from reaching the ground surface. The ozone layer does so by absorbing UV rays, which are damaging to all living things on the earth. If the amount of UV radiation that strikes the earth's surface became truly excessive, the ground organic matter could be destroyed by the radiation, including plants and plankton/phytoplankton (small and microscopic organisms, such as protozoans, diatoms, eggs, and larvae). Phytoplankton acts as food and energy sources for other animals and humans. Phytoplankton productivity is limited to the upper layer of the water column, where there is sufficient sunlight, thus exposing them to increased UV radiation exposure. UV radiation has been noted to cause damage in the early developments of fish, shrimp, crab, amphibians, and other marine animals, resulting in the decreased capacity for natural reproductive processes and an impaired development of larvae.

Recent findings established that excessive exposure to UV radiation increases the chances of developing skin cancer and cataracts (thickening of the lens) in humans. For example, studies show that for every 1 percent decrease in the ozone protective layer, there is a 2 to 5 percent chance of people developing skin cancer. Other problems associated with ozone depletion include sunburns and depression of the immune system.

There are two regions in the world where ozone layer depletion has been apparent. Over Australia, where there is a 5 to 9 percent reduction in the thickness of the ozone layer, there has been an increase in human susceptibility to the effects of UV radiation during outdoor activities. Additionally, studies show there is a significant reduction of the ozone layer in the atmospheric regions over Antarctica, leading to the formation of "ozone holes" through which UV rays can strike the earth's surface. Ozone holes are often noticeable annually in Antarctica during the spring season (between September and November).

Some human-made gases, such as the chlorofluorocarbons (CFCs) used in spray can propellants, refrigerants, and cleaning agents, can survive for one to two years when released into the atmosphere. When CFCs reach the stratosphere, the UV radiation converts them to halogen atoms, which react with the ozone layer. The ongoing destruction of the ozone layer by the reactive products of CFCs results in ozone depletion and reduction in its ability to protect the earth's surface against UV rays. In 1987, the international community created the Montreal Protocol on Substances that Deplete the Ozone Layer. In this agreement and the subsequent Kigali amendment, 197 nations agreed to phase out the production and consumption of ozone-depleting substances, including CFCs and two other classes of ozone-depleting chemicals, hydrochlorofluorocarbons and hydrofluorocarbons. Recent studies indicate that this phaseout strategy is working—there has been a significant reduction in the holes in the ozone layer.

Ifeanyi Abuachi

See Also: Air Pollution; Chlorofluorocarbons; Environmental Protection Agency; Ultraviolet Radiation and the UV Index

Further Reading

Anderson, S. O., M. L. Haberstadt, and N. Borgford-Parnell. "Stratospheric Ozone, Global Warming, and the Principle of Unintended Consequences—An Ongoing Science and Policy Success Story." *Journal of the Air and Waste Management Association*, vol. 63, no. 6 (June 2013): 607–647.

McKenzie, R. L., et al. "Ozone Depletion and Climate Change: Impacts on UV Radiation." *Photochemical and Photobiological Sciences*, vol. 10, no. 2 (February 2011): 182–198.

National Oceanic and Atmospheric Administration. *Research—Ozone Depletion*. https://www.esrl.noaa.gov/gmd/about/ozone.html (accessed May 8, 2017).

U.S. Department of State. *The Montreal Protocol on Substances That Deplete the Ozone Layer*. https://www.state.gov/e/oes/eqt/chemicalpollution/83007.htm (accessed May 8, 2017).

STYRENE

Styrene, consisting of a 2-carbon ethane molecule attached to a benzene ring, is used to make many consumer items, such as plastic packaging, consumer cups and plates, boats, shower stalls, automobile parts, corrosion resistant tanks, and synthetic rubber. Styrene is found outdoors primarily from vehicle exhausts and industrial emissions and indoors primarily from cigarette smoke and outgassing from consumer products, and it occurs naturally in foods such as strawberries, coffee, legumes, and spices. While its association with adverse health effects is controversial, some researchers believe styrene is a possible human carcinogen.

Styrene is consistently among the top 25 manufactured chemicals in the United States. Industrial manufacturing of styrene began just before World War II and has increased steadily since then. More than 12 billion pounds (5.4 billion kilograms) of styrene were manufactured in 2010, with over 10 million pounds (4.5 million kilograms) released to the atmosphere as fugitive emissions (i.e., escaping from various points in the manufacturing process without being captured). Just over 4,000 pounds (1,814 kilograms) of styrene were released into surface waters in 2008.

Reaction with light and microbial activity are the primary means of removing styrene from the environment. The half-life of styrene in air is between 2 and 17 hours. It is slightly soluble in water and volatizes quickly, with a half-life of about 6 hours in shallow water. However, the half-life can be more than 13 days in deeper water, and styrene can take up to 100 times longer to degrade in groundwater. Up to 16 weeks are required for 95 percent of styrene to degrade in soil, although it can persist for up to two years in some soils.

Humans readily absorb styrene through ingestion, inhalation, and to a lesser degree, skin absorption. The highest exposures occur in workplaces where styrene is manufactured or processed, in proximity to fugitive styrene sources, and through exposure to cigarette smoke. In general, occupational exposures are significantly higher than environmental exposures, and styrene exposure from smoking is almost 10 times higher than background exposures.

In the human body, styrene is metabolized to styrene-7,8-oxide, which is genotoxic (i.e., having the ability to damage genetic information within a cell). Most styrene is eliminated from the human body within hours, although some may remain in fatty tissues for a few days. According to the Centers for Disease Control and Prevention's latest National Health and Nutrition Examination Survey, 88 percent of Americans evaluated between 1988 and 1994 had styrene in their blood at concentrations up to 4 ug/L.

There are hundreds of peer-reviewed publications on the health effects of styrene, but they often reach different conclusions. The Styrene Information and Research Center, established in 1987 by styrene manufacturers, has raised more than 20 million dollars to study the effects of styrene on human health and the environment, and it has concluded that styrene is not carcinogenic. Furthermore, the American Conference of Governmental Industrial Hygienists finds that styrene is not classifiable as a human carcinogen. On the other hand, the National Toxicology Program at the National Institute of Environmental Health Sciences reports that styrene is reasonably anticipated to be a human carcinogen and, depending on dose, is associated with increased risk for leukemia, lymphoma, and all lymphohematopoietic cancers (i.e., cancers related to the production of lymphocytes and cells of the blood, bone marrow, lymph nodes, spleen, and thymus). Furthermore, the World Health Organization has classified styrene as a possible human carcinogen. Other research on the noncarcinogenic effects of styrene has found decreased balance, slowed reaction time, tiredness, and the sensation of feeling drunk at high-enough concentrations. Styrene can also be irritating to the nose and mouth.

Mary V. O'Reilly

See Also: Centers for Disease Control and Prevention; Indoor Environment; Integrated Risk Information System; National Institute of Environmental Health Sciences; National Toxicology Program; Occupational Safety and Health; Tobacco Smoke, Secondhand and Thirdhand; World Health Organization

Further Reading

Centers for Disease Control and Prevention (National Center for Health Statistics). *National Health and Nutrition Examination Survey*. https://www.cdc.gov/nchs/nhanes (accessed January 8, 2017).

14th Report on Carcinogens. Research Triangle Park, NC: National Institute of Environmental Health Sciences, 2016.

Health and Environmental Effects Profile for Styrene, EPA/600/X-84/325. Cincinnati, OH: U.S. Environmental Protection Agency, 1984.

Integrated Risk Information System, Chemical Assessment Summary, Styrene, CASRN 100–42–5. Arlington, VA: U.S. Environmental Protection Agency (National Center for Environmental Assessment), 1992.

Styrene in Drinking-Water. Background Document for Preparation of WHO Guidelines for Drinking-Water Quality. Geneva, Switzerland: World Health Organization, 2003.
Summary of the Scientific Research Supported by the Styrene Information Research Center, 1988–2013. Washington, DC: Styrene Information and Research Center, 2013.
Toxicological Profile for Styrene. Atlanta, GA: Agency for Toxic Substances and Disease Registry, 2010.

SUPERFUND ACT

In 1980, the U.S. Congress passed the Comprehensive Environmental Response, Compensation, and Liability Act, which came to be known as Superfund. The goal of Superfund was to address the health and environmental hazards presented by a large number of abandoned or uncontrolled waste sites containing hazardous materials. Under Superfund, a national program was established for emergency response, information collection and analysis, responsible party liability, and site cleanup. Additionally, a trust fund was created (i.e., a "Superfund") to finance emergency response and cleanup operations.

Passage of the Superfund Act was preceded by several environmental disasters that caught the public's attention and eventually demanded action by Congress. These disasters included (1) a large fire at a chemical waste treatment facility in New Jersey that resulted in six deaths; (2) a state of emergency at the Love Canal dump site in New York due to a dramatic increase in skin rashes, miscarriages,

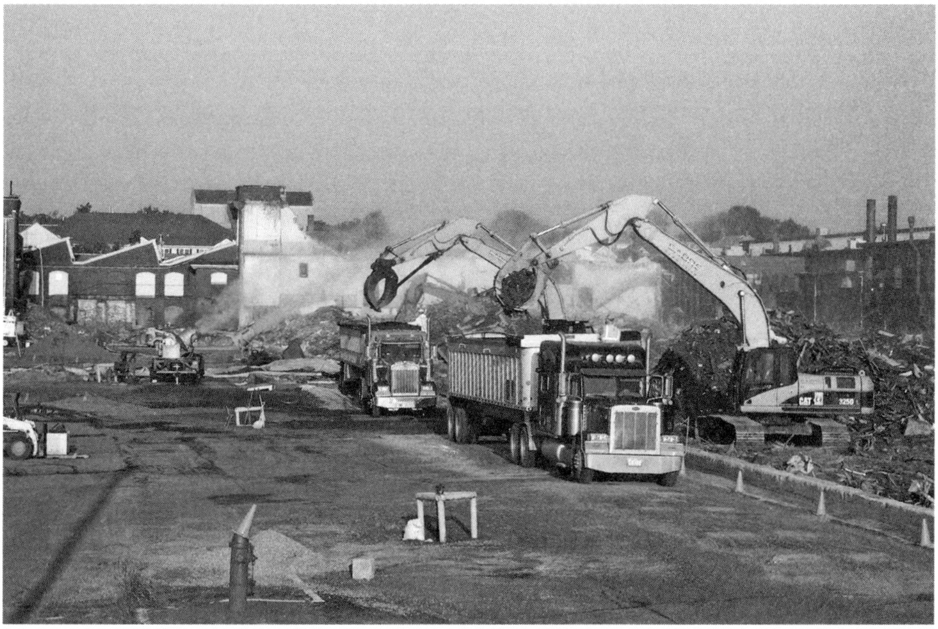

Trucks loaded with debris contaminated with polychlorinated biphenyls at the Aerovox Mill Superfund site in New Bedford, Massachusetts. The Comprehensive Environmental Response, Compensation, and Liability Act (Superfund) established a national program to address the large number of abandoned or uncontrolled waste sites across the United States containing hazardous materials. (Environmental Protection Agency)

and birth defects among local residents; and (3) another big fire in New Jersey, this time at a waste storage facility, causing schools to close and residents over a wide area to remain indoors.

There can be a wide variety of contaminants at Superfund sites, with varying degrees of toxicity. Four of the more common contaminants are lead, asbestos, dioxin, and radioactive waste materials. Some Superfund contaminants may present an immediate hazard, while other hazards may be more long-term, for example, in the case of carcinogens, which typically have long latency periods before cancer develops.

The health benefits from the Superfund program include a reduction of hazardous substances in communities, where sensitive groups like children, pregnant women, and older adults may be particularly vulnerable to exposure. Additionally, Superfund site cleanup helps protect habitats, farmland, and forests from environmental contamination. By restoring hazardous waste sites in urban areas, Superfund encourages economic growth in areas that might otherwise be subject to dumping of trash, vandalism, and trespassing. In this regard, many Superfund cleanup sites have become valuable local assets.

Over the years since passage of Superfund, several important developments related to hazardous waste site cleanup have occurred. These include:

1982: Establishing the Hazard Ranking System for evaluating the environmental hazards of a site
1983: Creating the National Priorities List to prioritize sites for cleanup using Superfund financing
1986: Passing the Superfund Amendments and Reauthorization Act (SARA) to, among other provisions, strengthen enforcement, increase state involvement, focus more on health issues, and encourage citizen participation
1986: Establishing under SARA the first emergency planning and community right-to-know law
1993: Beginning the Brownfields Initiative to redevelop abandoned or underused industrial and commercial sites where environmental contamination is a concern

The U.S. Environmental Protection Agency (EPA), the lead agency for implementing Superfund, typically responds to Superfund sites in one of two ways:

- Removal Actions: for emergency spills or releases requiring quick response
- Remedial Actions: for sites requiring long-term solutions and not presenting immediate threats to public health

Remedial actions often require substantial investigation and planning before cleanup can begin. Several of the most important steps involve conducting a preliminary assessment and site investigation, preparing a remedial investigation and feasibility study, issuing a record of decision, and developing a remedial design/remedial action plan.

Richard Crume

See Also: Asbestos; Brownfields; Dioxin Pollution; Emergency Planning and Community Right-to-Know Act; Environmental Protection Agency; Hazard Ranking System; Hazardous Waste Disposal; Lead Poisoning Prevention; Love Canal Incident

Further Reading

Brooks, David. *Restoring the Shining Waters: Superfund Success at Milltown, Montana*. Norman: University of Oklahoma Press, 2015.

Rumsey, Allison, and Michael Daneker. *Superfund Deskbook*. Washington, DC: Environmental Law Institute, 2014.

This Is Superfund: A Community Guide to EPA's Superfund Program (EPA-540-R-11–021). Washington, DC: U.S. Environmental Protection Agency, 2011.

U.S. Environmental Protection Agency. *Superfund*. https://www.epa.gov/superfund (accessed March 21, 2017).

SUSTAINABLE DEVELOPMENT AND HEALTH

In 1987, the United Nations defined "sustainable development" in the *Brundtland Report* as "development that meets the needs of the present without compromising the ability of future generations to meet their own needs." This is understood to include improving and promoting both environmental and human health as well as economic development.

Health is a critical component of sustainable development, being both affected by and contributing to it. For example, poor health contributes to days lost from work and decreased productivity for adults as well as days missed in school for children, factors resulting in decreased economic development. Conversely, development can impact health when, for example, infrastructure such as roads improve, allowing more people to access health care. The connection between health and sustainable development can also be made clear by considering the costs to environmental protection and sustainability that are often associated with economic development. For example, expanding coal-fired energy production has resulted in air pollution in cities around the world, and extractive industries like mining have caused widespread water pollution. This pollution can expose populations to disease-causing environmental toxicants, such as heavy metals, polychlorinated biphenyls, and pesticides.

Some economic development activities themselves, like clearing forests for building roads, can also have negative environmental and human health impacts. For example, forest clearing introduces local populations to the forest edges, where they may be exposed to insects that are vectors of diseases like malaria, resulting in increased vector-borne disease transmission occurring locally or regionally. Also, the building of roads increases forest fragmentation, which negatively impacts biodiversity. We currently face land-use and land-cover changes, such as the development of monoculture agriculture (e.g., soy or palm oil plantations in tropical forest areas), that are degrading the environment and changing the climate globally. It is imperative that increased attention is paid to carrying out development activities in a more sustainable way than in the past so as to ensure the health of present and future generations.

Addressing global poverty is also key to addressing health. This was first considered at the 1972 Stockholm Convention (i.e., the UN Conference on Human Environment), which led to the founding of the UN Environment Programme. The 1992 Earth Summit in Rio de Janeiro marked the 20th anniversary of the Stockholm Convention, and it is where the Rio Declaration on the Environment and Development and a sustainable development plan called Agenda 21 were signed by 178 countries. These documents outline the ways populations can take control of development in their countries and their responsibilities to protect the environment in doing so. The Rio Declaration states in its 27 guiding principles that the only way to have lasting global economic development is to ensure that such development adheres to the principles of environmental protection.

In September 2000, world leaders adopted the UN Millennium Declaration, which describes a new global partnership to reduce extreme poverty and sets out a series of time-bound targets (with a deadline of 2015) that have become known as the Millennium Development Goals (MDGs). Three of the goals are specifically related to health: Reduce Child Mortality (Goal 4), Improve Maternal Health (Goal 5), and Combat HIV/AIDS, Malaria, and Other Diseases (Goal 6). Other MDGs also address health, such as Ensure Environmental Sustainability (Goal 7), which recognizes that poverty, environmental degradation, and poor health are inherently interlinked. The MDGs galvanized support for and awareness of development issues in low- and middle-income countries, and as such, great progress was made toward reducing poverty and disease globally. However, progress has varied across regions and especially within countries, where some of the most vulnerable populations (the most remote and the poorest) did not experience gains as significant as some less vulnerable populations. For example, Target 7.C of Goal 7 was to halve by 2015 (compared to a 1990 baseline) the proportion of people without sustainable access to safe drinking water. While globally there was a 62 percent reduction in the population without access to improved drinking water resources, thereby meeting this goal, the African and the Eastern Mediterranean regions only saw 38 and 39 percent reductions in this metric, respectively.

Building off of the MDGs, the United Nations introduced Sustainable Development Goals (SDGs) in 2015 to further the goals of the MDGs while addressing some of their limitations. The SDGs follow on the heels of the MDGs, with 17 goals and 169 targets within those goals to be achieved by 2030. These goals integrate the three dimensions of sustainable development (i.e., economic, social, and environmental) around the themes of people, planet, prosperity, peace, and partnership. Goal 3 is specifically directed at ensuring healthy lives and promoting well-being for all ages. The Goal 3 targets include the following:

- Reducing maternal mortality
- Ending preventable deaths for children under age five
- Ending global epidemics (including aids and malaria)
- Reducing noncommunicable diseases and substance abuse through prevention and treatment
- Promoting mental health and well-being

- Reducing deaths and injuries from road accidents
- Increasing family planning and sexual and reproductive healthcare services
- Achieving universal health coverage and medicine and vaccine access for all
- Reducing illness and deaths from environmental pollution
- Increasing tobacco control
- Supporting research and development for medicines and vaccines for diseases that primarily affect developing countries
- Increasing the sustainability of the health workforce in developing countries
- Strengthening all countries' capacities for implementing early warning systems for global health risks

Notably, there are many other health-related SDGs, such as those focused on labor and sustainability. This reflects a recognition that multisectoral policies that have co-benefits for human health, the environment, and economic development are central to promoting public health through sustainable development.

Beth J. Feingold

See Also: Communicable Diseases; Deforestation; Drinking Water Quality and Regulation; Electric Power Generation, Health Implications of; Green Space in Urban Environments; Pesticides and Herbicides; Polychlorinated Biphenyls; Renewable Energy, Health Implications of; United Nations Environmental Programme

Further Reading

Boerma, Ties, et al. *Health in 2015: From MDGs, Millennium Development Goals, to SDGs, Sustainable Development Goals*. Geneva, Switzerland: World Health Organization, 2015.

"Chapter 2: Towards Sustainable Development." In *Our Common Future (also known as the Brundtland Report)*. Oxford, UK: Oxford University Press, 2009 (reprint).

Corvalan, C. F., T. Kjellstrom, and K. R. Smith. "Health, Environment, and Sustainable Development: Identifying Links and Interactions to Promote Action." *Epidemiology*, vol. 10, no. 5 (September 1999): 656–660.

The Rio Declaration on Environment and Development. Nairobi, Kenya: UN Environment Programme, 1992.

UN Environment Programme. *The Rio Declaration on Environment and Development/The Earth Summit and Agenda 21*. http://www.unesco.org/education/nfsunesco/pdf/RIO_E.PDF (accessed January 28, 2017).

United Nations. *Sustainable Development Knowledge Platform*. https://sustainabledevelopment.un.org/sdgs (accessed January 28, 2017).

T

TERRY, LUTHER L.

Luther L. Terry, MD (1911–1985)—a physician and the ninth surgeon general of the United States (serving from 1961 to 1965)—is known for his groundbreaking work in warning the public about the dangers of tobacco use. Dr. Terry was charged by President Kennedy to head a committee of prominent scientists in preparing a 1964 report on tobacco use. The report found that smoking cigarettes contributed substantially to the country's death rate and that "appropriate remedial action" should be taken. Primarily as a result of this report, the percentage of Americans smoking dropped from 43 percent in 1964 to 23 percent in 2001. Dr. Terry was a former cigarette smoker himself, but he switched to a pipe before the report was issued.

During his tenure as surgeon general, Dr. Terry worked tirelessly to eliminate television tobacco advertising, to ensure that health warnings were placed on cigarette packaging and advertising, and to stop the sale of cigarettes to minors. His efforts led to the Federal Cigarette Labeling and Advertising Act of 1965, which required a warning label on each cigarette package.

Dr. Terry's passion for medicine began in Red Level, Alabama, where he helped his father, the town doctor, by working in his clinic and driving him around the countryside for emergency appointments. Dr. Terry earned his medical degree at Tulane University in 1935. After an internship at Hillman Hospital in Birmingham, Alabama, a residency at Cleveland (Ohio) Hospitals, and an internship at Washington University in St. Louis, Missouri, Dr. Terry became an associate professor of preventive medicine and public health at the University of Texas in Galveston in 1940. This is when his consciousness was raised about the disastrous impact of smoking.

The Leading Cause of Death and Disease

What is the leading preventable cause of death and disease in the United States? According to the U.S. Surgeon General's office, it is tobacco smoking. Tobacco smoke contains over 7,000 chemicals that can (1) damage DNA, blood vessels, and lungs; (2) cause blood vessel clotting, heart attacks and strokes, asthma attacks, emphysema, and chronic bronchitis; and (3) result in lung and other cancer. (One of every three cancer deaths in the United States is linked to smoking.) Additionally, the nicotine in tobacco smoke is addictive, which makes it hard to quit. There is no safe exposure to tobacco smoke, and even an occasional cigarette or exposure to secondhand smoke can be harmful. The surgeon general warns there is no safe cigarette.

Is It Safe to Be around Others Who Smoke?

When you breathe tobacco smoke from cigarettes, cigars, or pipes that other people are smoking and from the air they exhale (breathe out), you are breathing secondhand smoke. Similar to smoking, people exposed to secondhand smoke are at higher risk for heart disease, stroke, and lung cancer, and children are at particular risk for ear infections, asthma attacks, respiratory symptoms (e.g., shortness of breath), respiratory infections, and sudden infant death syndrome. Since 1964, about 2.5 million nonsmokers have died from health problems associated with secondhand smoke. There is no safe level of exposure to secondhand smoke, and even exposure of brief duration can be harmful.

Dr. Terry was called to active duty in the Public Health Service in 1942 and became the chief of medical service in 1943 at the U.S. Marine Hospital in Baltimore, Maryland. He was concurrently a teacher and researcher at Johns Hopkins University. In 1950, he became a researcher and later assistant director at the National Heart Institute, where his research focused on the causes and prevention of hypertension.

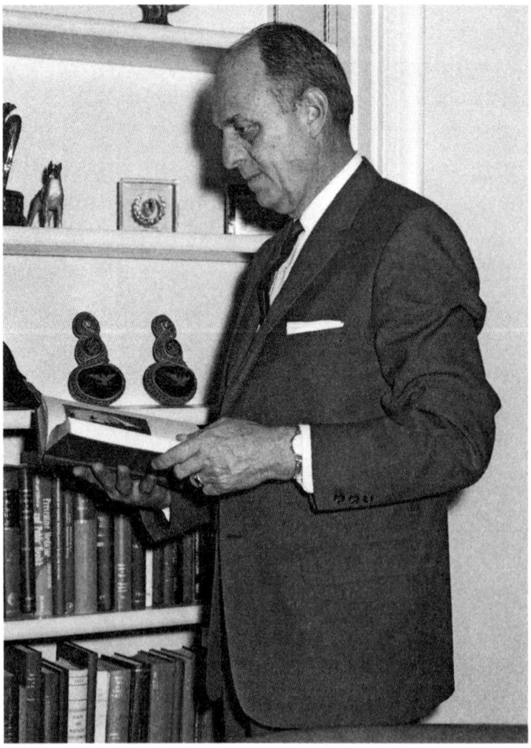

Luther Terry, MD, U.S. surgeon general from 1961 to 1965. Terry is best known for his groundbreaking work warning the public about the dangers of tobacco use. (National Library of Medicine)

After his tenure as surgeon general, Dr. Terry spent the rest of his career focusing on the dangers and prevention of diseases related to cigarette smoking. From 1967 to 1968, he was the chairman of the National Interagency Council on Smoking and Health. He later became vice president for medical affairs and a professor at the University of Pennsylvania, where he remained until retiring in 1982.

Later in his life, Dr. Terry spoke extensively on smoking in the workplace, emphasizing the dangers of secondhand smoke. He urged companies to take steps to ensure nonsmoking employees are not exposed to cigarette smoke. As a result, many American businesses banned smoking or allowed it only in designated areas.

Throughout his career, Dr. Terry was recognized with many honors, including 17 honorary degrees. The American Cancer Society established the Luther L. Terry Awards in conjunction with the World Conference on Tobacco or Health to recognize outstanding worldwide achievements in the field of tobacco control. In 1985, Dr. Terry was honored with a burial in Arlington National Cemetery.

Susan J. Montgomery

See Also: Asthma; Cancer Risk from Environmental Exposure; Indoor Environment; Public Health Service; Respiratory Disease and Air Pollution; Tobacco Smoke, Secondhand and Thirdhand

Further Reading

Finkel, Ed. "2004 Health Care Hall of Fame: He Helped Clear the Air: Former Surgeon General Luther Terry Helped Lead Crusade against Smoking." *Modern Healthcare*, March 2004, http://www.modernhealthcare.com/article/20040301/INFO/403010315.

The National Cyclopedia of American Biography. New York: James T. White and Company, 1984.

U.S. National Library of Medicine. *Luther L. Terry Papers 1957–1995 (bulk 1965–1983)*. https://oculus.nlm.nih.gov/cgi/f/findaid/findaid-idx?c=nlmfindaid;idno=terry503 (accessed March 19, 2016).

TETANUS INFECTION

Tetanus (also called "lockjaw") is an infection caused by *Clostridium tetani*, a bacterium commonly found in soil, dust, and manure. Tetanus usually enters the body through cuts or puncture wounds caused by objects that carry the bacteria, and it has also been associated with burns, crush injuries, injuries with dead tissue, superficial wounds, surgical procedures, insect bites, dental infections, compound fractures, chronic sores and infections, and intravenous drug use. It does not spread from person to person, and tetanus infections are uncommon in the United States, with most cases occurring among unvaccinated people or adults who are not up to date on their 10-year booster shots.

A common symptom of tetanus is a tightening of the jaw muscles, making opening the mouth difficult (thus, the name "lockjaw"). Other symptoms include headache, sudden and involuntary muscle tightening (often in the stomach), painful muscle stiffness, difficulty swallowing, seizures, fever and sweating, high blood pressure, and fast heart rate. Complications may involve laryngospasm (contraction of the vocal cords), bone fracture, hospital-acquired infection, pulmonary embolism (blockage of the main artery of the lung or one of its branches), pneumonia, and breathing difficulty.

Tetanus has an incubation period that usually ranges from 3 to 21 days, with most infections occurring within 14 days. In some cases, depending on the type of wound, the incubation period may last several months. Because there are no laboratory tests to confirm the presence of tetanus, doctors must diagnose the disease based on symptoms. Tetanus is considered a medical emergency requiring hospitalization and immediate treatment.

The best way to prevent tetanus is to be fully immunized. The Centers for Disease Control and Prevention recommends tetanus vaccination for people of all ages and booster shots throughout life. People who have been infected do not develop immunity and can become infected again if not protected by vaccination. Often immediate care of wounds can help prevent an infection.

One early success of the tetanus vaccine was during World War II, when U.S. soldiers were at risk of infection because of wounds that could not be cleaned well on the battlefield. As a result of the military's vaccination program, only 12 soldiers were infected during the war, and half of them had not been vaccinated. In contrast, soldiers from other countries without vaccination programs were much more likely to develop tetanus. The vaccination of children began in the 1940s, and today only 40 to 60 cases of tetanus occur each year in the United States.

Richard Crume

See Also: Centers for Disease Control and Prevention; Communicable Diseases; Infectious Diseases

Further Reading

Bennett, John E., Raphael Dolin, and Martin J. Blaser. *Mandell, Douglas, and Bennett's Infectious Disease Essentials*. Philadelphia, PA: Elsevier, 2017.

Centers for Disease Control and Prevention. *About Tetanus*. http://www.cdc.gov/tetanus/about/index.html (accessed October 1, 2016).

Jonathan Cohen, William G. Powderly, and Steven M. Opal. *Infectious Diseases*. Amsterdam, the Netherlands: Elsevier, 2016.

Kasper, Dennis L., Anthony S. Fauci, and Tinsley R. Harrison. *Harrison's Infectious Diseases*. New York: McGraw-Hill Medical, 2010.

THERMAL POLLUTION

Thermal pollution, like noise and light pollution, does not consist of toxic chemicals or foreign substances, as we traditionally associate with the term "pollution." In a broader sense, pollution can be seen as anything nonnative that is introduced into the environment that has an undesirable effect. Thermal pollution, the waste heat introduced into a body of water, often from an industrial process, fits this definition. Thermal pollution can adversely affect the ecology, including causing injury or death to fish, aquatic plants, and other organisms. Thermal pollution indirectly affects human health by reducing the supply of healthy fish and diminishing water quality for recreation.

The most common form of thermal pollution is where an industrial operation disposes of process water into a nearby body of water, such as a stream, river, or lake. An example is water used as coolant for heavy machinery. Coal-fired and nuclear electric power plants produce large quantities of wastewater and heated water (thermal pollution) from the power cycle and water treatment and pollution control systems. The Mississippi River is an example of a heavily trafficked waterway that receives intense thermal pollution from power plants. Less frequent causes of thermal pollution include runoff in urban areas, where water can be heated by pavement, and deforestation along shorelines, where the loss of shade can result in heating of water along the shore.

Thermal pollution is a problem for fish, aquatic plants, and other organisms because they can be sensitive to temperature changes and only survive within a restricted temperature range. If the temperature changes slowly, such as that which naturally occurs between seasons, fish and other aquatic organisms can adapt, but if the change is rapid, they may suffer thermal shock and die. Other consequences of thermal pollution include reduced reproduction rates, unhealthy offspring, and sometimes a dramatic shift in aquatic populations.

A dangerous consequence of thermal pollution is a reduction in the dissolved oxygen content of a body of water, causing fish and other organisms to suffocate. Another problem occurs when certain types of surface algae, which thrive in warm water, rapidly multiply and block the sunlight that other organisms depend on, resulting in decaying organic matter that can further reduce dissolved oxygen. And some types of algae, when too abundant, can release dangerous toxins into the water. Additionally, warmer water harbors more bacteria and pathogens that can be lethal to fish.

Thermal pollution can be mitigated by cooling the water before it enters a stream, river, or lake. For example, this could be accomplished with cooling towers, cooling ponds, and artificial lakes. These and other approaches are designed to address thermal pollution without disrupting the natural habitat.

Aaron Dorman

See Also: Deforestation; Electric Power Generation, Health Implications of; Light Pollution; Noise Pollution; Stormwater Runoff

Further Reading

Benedini, Marcello, and George Tsakiris. *Water Quality Modelling for Rivers and Streams*. Dordrecht, the Netherlands: Springer, 2013.

Kalinowska, Monika B., and Paweł M. Rowiński. "Thermal Pollution in Rivers—Modelling of the Spread of Thermal Plumes." In *Rivers—Physical, Fluvial, and Environmental Processes*, edited by Paweł Rowiński and Artur Radecki-Pawlik, 591–613. Cham, Switzerland: Springer, 2015.

Raptis, Catherine E., Justin M. Boucher, and Stephan Pfister. "Assessing the Environmental Impacts of Freshwater Thermal Pollution from Global Power Generation in LCA." *Science of the Total Environment*, vol. 580 (February 2017): 1014–1026.

U.S. Environmental Protection Agency. *Effluent Guidelines: Steam Electric Power Generating Effluent Guidelines*. https://www.epa.gov/eg/steam-electric-power-generating-effluent-guidelines (accessed March 11, 2017).

Verones, F., et al. "Characterization Factors for Thermal Pollution in Freshwater Aquatic Environments." *Environmental Science and Technology*, vol. 44, no. 24 (December 2010): 9364–9369.

THREE MILE ISLAND INCIDENT

Three Mile Island, an island in the Susquehanna River of Pennsylvania, is home to the Three Mile Island nuclear power plant. On March 28, 1979, a cooling system malfunction in one of the plant's reactors led to 700,000 gallons (2.6 million liters) of radioactive water leaking into the facility. A smaller portion of this radioactive material was released into the atmosphere.

Public alarm was widespread in the days following the incident. The media reported the possibility of radioactive uranium melting from the base of the reactor into the earth's crust, a phenomenon referred to as the China syndrome, based on a fictional movie released earlier that month about a similar disaster. The media also reported that a hydrogen gas bubble was building inside the reactor that might cause it to explode, releasing radioactive waste into the atmosphere. Pregnant women and children within a five-mile radius were evacuated from their homes, and in surrounding communities, 140,000 people fled. About two weeks after the accident, once fears of further meltdowns were assuaged, people were encouraged to return to their homes.

President Jimmy Carter (1924–) created a 12-person commission to investigate the accident and its potential health effects. The report released by the commission noted that there were mechanical failures that led to the accident, but ultimately the operators of the reactor were to blame. However, the report also indicated that the operators were not sufficiently trained on standard operating procedures, and this was a fault of company leadership. Because of the lack of accountability, the commission recommended that the nuclear power industry create a way to maintain and regulate safety standards for its workers. In the year following the accident, the Institute of Nuclear Power Operations (INPO) was created to ensure proper training for operators working at nuclear power facilities. In 1985, INPO created the National Academy for Nuclear Training to oversee training programs at nuclear power plants.

The president's commission also found that the health effects from the incident were negligible due to speedy and effective containment of the radioactive material. Studies conducted from 1981 to 1991 by the Pennsylvania Department

The Debate over Nuclear Power

Although causing no deaths, the incident at Three Mile Island raised public skepticism in the United States about nuclear energy, and the Chernobyl and Fukushima Daiichi nuclear plant disasters added to the concern. Supporters of nuclear energy say it is the cleanest and most efficient way to transition away from fossil fuels because to generate electricity, no greenhouse gases are emitted. Opponents say the processes involved in creating nuclear energy are too dangerous, especially when plants are situated near communities, and the problem of long-term storage for spent fuel rods, which are highly radioactive, has not been resolved.

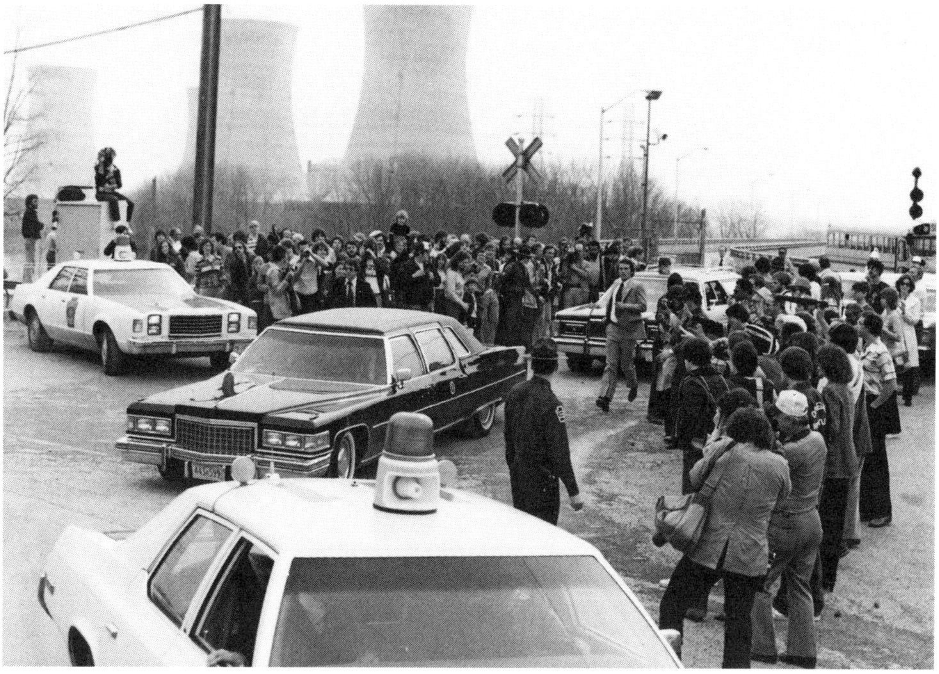

President Jimmy Carter visits the Three Mile Island nuclear plant after an accident in 1979. While there was no evidence of adverse health effects from the small release of radioactive material to the atmosphere, the incident caused the nation to reconsider the benefits and dangers of nuclear power. (National Archives)

of Health regarding infant mortality, hypothyroidism, cancer, and pregnancy also found no evidence of adverse health effects from the accident. In 1997, the Department of Health discontinued a study of 30,000 people living within 5 miles (8 kilometers) of Three Mile Island because they found no evidence of adverse health effects. More than a dozen independent studies have also found no evidence for negative health impacts. The average dose of radiation for people living within 10 miles (16 kilometers) of Three Mile Island is believed to be about the same as the radiation received during an X-ray.

Mallory L. Daily

See Also: Chernobyl Incident; Fukushima Daiichi Incident; Nuclear Regulatory Commission; Nuclear Safety; Radiation, Ionizing and Nonionizing; Radiation Sickness

Further Reading

Fact Sheet: Lessons from the 1979 Accident at Three Mile Island. Washington, DC: Nuclear Energy Institute, 2014.

Haberman, Clyde. "Three Mile Island, and Nuclear Hopes and Fears." *New York Times*, April 28, 2014, https://www.nytimes.com/2014/04/29/us/three-mile-island-and-nuclear-hopes-and-fears.html?.

The Need for Change, the Legacy of TMI: Report of the President's Commission on the Accident at Three Mile Island. New York: Pergamon Press, 1979.

Three Mile Island Accident. World Nuclear Association, London, 2012. http://www.world-nuclear.org/information-library/safety-and-security/safety-of-plants/three-mile-island-accident.aspx.

THREE Rs OF WASTE MANAGEMENT

The three Rs of waste management stand for "reduce," "reuse," and "recycle." All three are key to a sustainable future and to controlling the staggering amounts of garbage that have accumulated in the United States and other developed countries over the past century. Although there is no definitive origin for the "three Rs" as a slogan for environmentalism, its use coincides with the first Earth Day (April 22, 1970) and with the Resource Conservation and Recovery Act, which was enacted by the U.S. Congress that same year.

Reduce

Reducing consumption is necessary, not only to avoid the worst effects of climate change but also to maintain a healthy and sustainable biosphere. Every year, our society overshoots the biosphere's capacity for renewal. For example, in 2016, "earth overshoot day" was August 8, which means it took only 220 days to use up the quantity of resources that the biosphere could recover in one year. This calculation may actually underrepresent the amount of resources humanity is using because it does not account for nonrenewables, such as rare earth metals, which are used in many consumer products.

While waste management activities account for no more than 5 percent of greenhouse gas emissions in the United States, the entire life cycle of resource extraction through production of foods and consumer products accounts for a whopping 42 percent of greenhouse gases. Thus, the environmental benefits of recycling and other "green" waste management initiatives pale in comparison to what could be achieved if there was less consumption in the first place. Reducing consumption also helps address some of the health concerns associated with commercial and industrial operations that arise from air and water pollution. Additionally, there are other environmental benefits, such as reducing depletion of the earth's stratospheric ozone layer.

Reuse

Reusing products and materials reduces wastes and puts less strain on the global environment. One example is simply keeping products as long as possible before buying new ones. This approach is facilitated by companies that manufacture "quality" products lasting a long time. On the other hand, "planned obsolescence" causes products to be replaced sooner than necessary. (Planned obsolescence is a manufacturing and marketing strategy where products quickly become obsolete due to frequent design changes, unavailability of spare parts, and use of nondurable construction materials.) Unfortunately, raw material and labor costs are often such that it is cheaper to manufacture a new product than to fix an old one. This may change in the future as raw materials become scarcer and labor costs rise.

An emerging reuse success story involves reusable shopping bags (made of a durable fabric or plastic), which have become very popular with customers shopping at several large U.S. grocery store chains. This is an important step toward reducing waste in the United States, where over 1 billion disposable plastic grocery bags are discarded every week. Several large cities, such as Chicago and Los Angeles, have banned disposable plastic bags outright, while other cities (e.g., New York and Washington, D.C.) have resorted to regulatory measures, such as a bag fee, to encourage consumers to switch to reusable bags.

Recycle

Recycling helps keep valuable materials in circulation rather than discarded as waste. Most of what we consider recycling is actually "down-cycling," which means that the recycled materials lose their initial value but can still be used for other purposes. For example, many plastics can only be reprocessed into new plastics of lower quality, and the same is often true for certain metals and paper goods. Nevertheless, recycling helps extend the life cycle of raw materials and reduce the quantity of wastes going to landfills and incinerators.

Although recycling requires energy for collection, transportation to recycling centers, and reprocessing, the overall energy requirements are still often less than for extracting new raw materials. For example, the recycling of aluminum cans requires only 5 percent of the energy needed to mine new ore. It is sometimes less expensive to landfill certain renewable materials than to recycle them, although the long-term harm to the environment from the accumulation of garbage needs to be considered. According to the U.S. Environmental Protection Agency, the average person in the United States produces about 4.4 pounds (2.0 kilograms) of waste every day, and only about one-third of municipal waste is recycled.

The greatest gains to be made from recycling may involve packaging. Containers and packaging made from cardboard, paper, and plastic make up almost 30 percent of municipal solid waste, and often these materials are amenable to recycling programs. To reduce operational costs and promote sustainable operations, some manufacturers and online stores have switched to 100 percent recycled packaging for their products.

Aaron Dorman

See Also: Biosphere, Environmental Threats to; Earth Day; Environmental Protection Agency; Greenhouse Effect and Global Warming; Land Disposal of Waste Materials; Municipal Solid Waste Management; Recycling; Resource Conservation and Recovery Act; Stratospheric Ozone Depletion; Sustainable Development and Health

Further Reading

Advancing Sustainable Materials Management: 2014 Fact Sheet. Washington, DC: U.S. Environmental Protection Agency, 2016.

Global Footprint Network. *Earth Overshoot Day*. http://www.overshootday.org (accessed December 23, 2016).

Global Footprint Network. *Footprint for Nations.* http://www.footprintnetwork.org/en/index.php/GFN/page/footprint_for_nations (accessed December 23, 2016).
Humes, Edward. *Garbology: Our Dirty Love Affair with Trash.* New York: Avery, 2013.
McDonough, William, and Michael Braungart. *Cradle to Cradle: Remaking the Way We Make Things.* New York: North Point Press, 2002.
Rogers, Heather. *Gone Tomorrow: The Hidden Life of Garbage.* New York: New Press, 2006.
Scott, Nicky. *Reduce, Reuse, Recycle: An Easy Household Guide.* White River Junction, VT: Chelsea Green, 2007.
U.S. Environmental Protection Agency. *Reduce, Reuse, Recycle.* https://www.epa.gov/recycle (accessed December 23, 2016).

THRESHOLD DOSE

In the fields of environmental toxicology and risk assessment, there are two common measures of acceptable dose and adverse effect for noncarcinogens. The *no observed adverse effect level* (NOAEL) is the highest dose at which no deleterious effects of a toxic chemical have been observed in toxicological experiments or epidemiologic studies. A related concept is the *lowest observed adverse effect level* (LOAEL), which is the lowest dose at which a toxic effect has been observed in toxicological experiments (possibly including epidemiological studies). The NOAEL and LOAEL have been used in chemical risk assessments as a starting point for deriving an acceptable level of exposure for humans. However, there are limitations to the NOAEL/LOAEL approach to informing safety standards, including the following:

- The NOAEL and LOAEL are fully dependent on the design of toxicological experiments, which may involve granular, discrete doses (e.g., four treatments of 5 parts per million [ppm], 10 ppm, 100 ppm, and 500 ppm). For example, imagine a newly synthesized chemical for which only a single toxicology experiment is available. If a NOAEL is observed at one concentration (e.g., 10 ppm) and a LOAEL is observed at the next highest concentration (e.g., 100 ppm), then there is a wide range of possible concentrations between 10 and 100 ppm where toxicity might occur. Using a NOAEL may lead to an unnecessarily conservative exposure recommendation, whereas a LOAEL may lead to an inadequately protective recommendation.
- A NOAEL/LOAEL summary uses only two data points from the entire toxicological literature on a chemical, although data from other relevant studies, if any, are considered in the process of deriving the final NOAEL and LOAEL. The dose-response information from other doses is ignored.
- The NOAEL and LOAEL are often defined using a toxicological model organism (e.g., a rodent) that is different from humans. Although a risk assessment uncertainty factor (e.g., dividing the NOAEL/LOAEL by a default value of 10 to account for interspecies differences in toxicokinetics and toxicodynamics) may be applied as a buffer, this uncertainty factor can be arbitrary and may be insufficient to protect human health.

The U.S. Environmental Protection Agency, the California Environmental Protection Agency, and other government health agencies have begun moving away from the NOAEL/LOAEL model to alternative approaches, such as the *benchmark dose* method, which estimates a defined biological response at a given dose by fitting a dose-response curve to toxicity data and drawing predictions from the curve. The benchmark dose method explicitly addresses the granularity limitation of the NOAEL and LOAEL and uses more of the information available from toxicological experiments. Nevertheless, it is still limited by interspecies extrapolations if the evidence being used to inform the risk assessment comes from nonhuman models. There also may be limitations to any model if the data it draws upon come from research that is undermined by reporting or study design biases. Another approach of policy interest is *physiologically based pharmacokinetic modeling*, which accounts for metabolic processes to estimate more human-relevant target-organ doses from external environmental exposures.

Matthew O. Gribble

See Also: Dose-Response Assessment; Environmental Epidemiology; Environmental Protection Agency; Environmental Toxicology; Integrated Risk Information System

Further Reading

Bois, F. Y., L. Zeise, and T. N. Tozer. "The Use of Pharmacokinetic Models in the Determination of Risks for Regulatory Purposes." In *Risk Assessment in Setting National Priorities*, edited by James J. Bonin and Donald E. Stevenson, 573–583. New York: Plenum Press, 1989.

Davis, J. A., J. S. Gift, and Q. J. Zhao. "Introduction to Benchmark Dose Methods and U.S. EPA's Benchmark Dose Software (BMDS) Version 2.1.1." *Toxicology and Applied Pharmacology*, vol. 254, no. 2 (July 2011): 181–191.

Science and Decisions: Advancing Risk Assessment. Washington, DC: National Academies Press, 2009.

Shanks, Niall, Ray Greek, and Jean Greek. "Are Animal Models Predictive for Humans?" *Philosophy, Ethics, and Humanities in Medicine*, vol. 4, no. 2 (January 2009).

Vork, Kathleen, Jim Carlisle, and Joseph P. Brown. *Workplace Air and Worker Blood Lead Concentrations Using an Updated Physiologically-Based Pharmacokinetic (PBPK) Model*. Sacramento: California Environmental Protection Agency, 2013.

Wignall, J. A., et al. "Standardizing Benchmark Dose Calculations to Improve Science-Based Decisions in Human Health Assessments." *Environmental Health Perspectives*, vol. 122, no. 5 (May 2014): 499–505.

TOBACCO SMOKE, SECONDHAND AND THIRDHAND

Breathing someone else's tobacco smoke, referred to as involuntary or passive smoking, can be hazardous. This happens when tobacco smoke permeates an environment (e.g., at home or work) such that it is breathed by individuals other than the actual smoker. For nonsmokers, there is no safe level of exposure to tobacco smoke, which can cause various cancers and heart disease, aggravate asthmatic conditions, decrease pulmonary function, and impair blood circulation.

Secondhand Smoke and Cardiovascular Disease

Secondhand tobacco smoke increases the risk of coronary heart disease by about 30 percent. This noxious mixture of over 7,000 chemical compounds, including about 70 known carcinogens, has been recognized for some time as a cause of lung and other cancers. While the role of secondhand tobacco smoke as a cause of heart disease has been less well understood, the health effects of secondhand smoke are acknowledged to be greater than would be expected based solely on the risks associated with tobacco smoking and the relative amounts of smoke delivered to nonsmokers compared with smokers. Secondhand tobacco smoke is estimated to account for at least 35,000 deaths each year in the United States.

Secondhand tobacco smoke is a combination of smoke that comes from the burning end of a cigarette, cigar, or pipe (referred to as sidestream smoke) and the smoke that is exhaled from the lungs of a smoker (referred to as mainstream smoke). Sidestream smoke has higher concentrations of carcinogens, consists of smaller particulates, and is more toxic than mainstream smoke, which was partially filtered through its passage into the lungs of the smoker. The smaller particle size of sidestream smoke makes it easier for the harmful substances it contains, such as ammonia, arsenic, benzene, butane, cadmium, chromium, cyanide, formaldehyde, lead, nickel, and polonium, to make their way into the lungs and other body tissues of those exposed. The U.S. Environmental Protection Agency, National Toxicology Program, and International Agency for Research on Cancer (a branch of the World Health Organization) have all classified secondhand smoke as a known human carcinogen.

Thirdhand smoke consists of the residue that accumulates on surfaces exposed to tobacco smoke. This residual matter interacts with other common indoor pollutants, such as those routinely included in cleaning products, yielding a hazardous mixture that sticks to bedding, clothing, curtains, furniture, hair, skin, and other surfaces. When people interact with these surfaces, the toxic conglomeration can be inhaled, swallowed, or absorbed through contact with mucosal tissue, including the anus, eyelids, genitals, lips, and nostrils.

Individuals exposed to secondhand or thirdhand smoke are at greater risk for numerous health consequences compared to those who are not. If a pregnant woman is exposed to secondhand or thirdhand smoke, her baby is also exposed to the dangerous substances in these mixtures. Parents who smoked before or during pregnancy are more likely to have a child with hepatoblastoma (a rare liver cancer). Exposure causes lower respiratory tract infections in 150,000 to 300,000 children annually under 18 months of age, resulting in 7,500 to 15,000 hospitalizations every year. Other conditions linked to secondhand and thirdhand smoke exposure in children include asthma, cancers like leukemia, chronic obstructive pulmonary disease, sinus and nasal problems, and sudden infant death syndrome.

Furthermore, it is estimated that this exposure kills about 42,000 people from heart disease and 7,300 from lung cancer each year in the United States, where the added expenses associated with illnesses, medical care, and deaths are estimated at over $10 billion annually.

Considerable efforts have been directed at reducing or eliminating exposure to secondhand and thirdhand tobacco smoke. The U.S. surgeon general first addressed the harmful effects of environmental smoke in 1972, and numerous reports since have issued even stronger warnings. Community advocacy groups, such as the Group Against Smoking Pollution, have been organized to combat smoking in public. In contrast, beginning in the early 1990s, the tobacco industry has attempted to discredit the scientific research indicating that secondhand and thirdhand tobacco smoke exposure was harmful. In 1993, Vermont became the first state to ban smoking in restaurants. Currently, over 4,000 American municipalities have enacted similar laws restricting where individuals can smoke, and over 90 countries have passed laws and ordinances that limit smoking in public and work environments.

Victor B. Stolberg

See Also: Asthma; Cancer Risk from Environmental Exposure; Environmental Protection Agency; Indoor Environment; Particulate Matter and Bioaerosols Pollution; Respiratory Disease and Air Pollution; World Health Organization

Further Reading

Barnoya, Joaquin, and Stanton A. Glantz. "Cardiovascular Effects of Secondhand Smoke: Nearly as Large as Smoking." *Circulation*, vol. 24, no. 111 (May 2005): 2684–2698.

The Health Consequences of Involuntary Exposure to Tobacco Smoke: A Report of the Surgeon General. Atlanta, GA: Centers for Disease Control and Prevention, U.S. Department of Health and Human Services, 2006.

Hong, Mi-Kyung, and Lisa A. Bero. "How the Tobacco Industry Responded to an Influential Study of the Health Effects of Secondhand Smoke." *British Medical Journal*, vol. 325, no. 7377 (December 2002): 1413–1416.

Prickle, James L., et al. "Trends in the Exposure of Nonsmokers in the U.S. Population to Secondhand Smoke: 1988–2002." *Environmental Health Perspectives*, vol. 114, no. 6 (June 2006): 853–858.

TORREY CANYON INCIDENT

The *Torrey Canyon*, a supertanker filled with crude oil, ran aground along the Cornish Peninsula of Great Britain on March 18, 1967. The resulting spill of nearly 100,000 tons (90,700 metric tons) of crude oil remains one of the largest oil spills in history, causing widespread ecologic damage that occurred as far away as Normandy, France, and presenting a health hazard for both marine life and humans that continues today.

The incident occurred because the captain of the *Torrey Canyon* decided to go through the Scilly Islands instead of around them to save time. The ship struck Pollard Rock in the Seven Stones reef, running aground and bursting 6 of its

18 tanks filled with crude oil, spilling 30,000 tons (27,200 metric tons) of oil into the sea. Eight days later, weather patterns and rough seas caused the release of another 30,000 tons (27,200 metric tons) of oil.

The government waited to take action on cleanup for 10 days while experts considered whether to syphon off the remaining oil. However, this was judged too dangerous because of explosion hazards. Attempts were then made to refloat the ship, which failed and resulted in the ship further breaking apart, spilling the remaining crude oil. The government then decided to address the issue by setting fire to the spilled oil. Subsequently, the Royal Air Force reportedly dropped 62,000 pounds (28,100 kilograms) of bombs, 5,200 gallons (19,700 liters) of petroleum, 11 high-powered rockets, and an undisclosed amount of napalm on the wreck and surrounding waters. This approach failed because rough seas quickly put out the fire.

The government was pressured to take immediate action by the Cornish coastal communities, whose beaches were a large source of tourist revenue. In response, the government arranged for the beaches and oil spill to be sprayed with 2 million gallons (7.6 million liters) of highly toxic oil dispersants. The dispersants turned out to be the worst possible choice, as not only did they contain toxic aromatic hydrocarbons, but the dispersants also converted the oil to a water-soluble form that

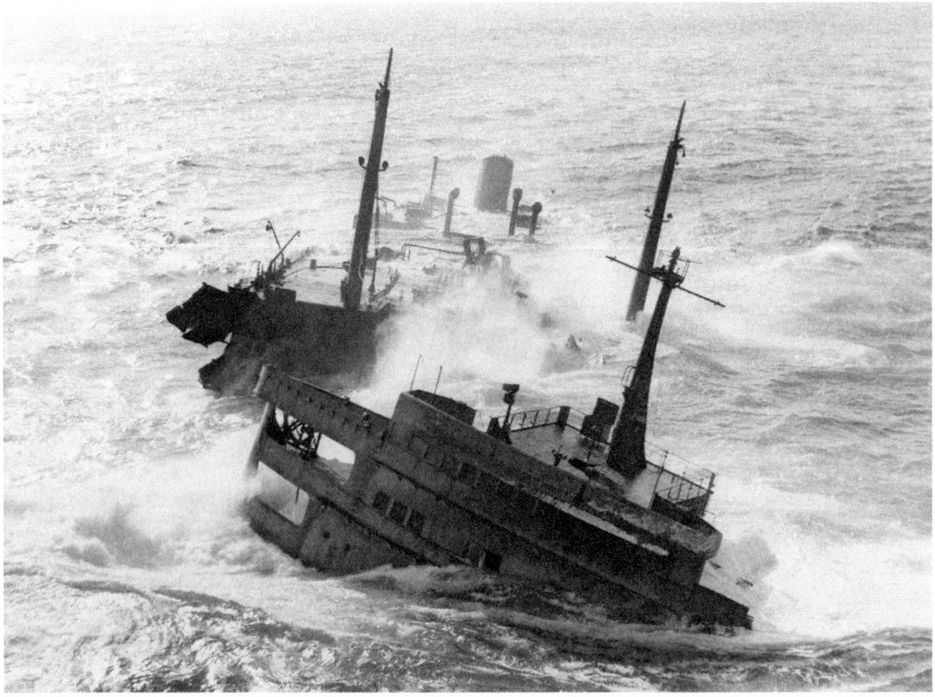

The oil tanker *Torrey Canyon* breaks apart after running aground on a reef off Land's End, England, in 1967. The subsequent oil spill contaminated vast areas of coastline and caused widespread ecological damage. (AP Photo)

was readily taken up by marine life. This toxic combination was responsible for the deaths of 15,000 seabirds, thousands of sea lions, innumerable fish, and other aquatic plant and animal life in open ocean. On shore, the dispersants destroyed lichens and other beach life, leaving the land toxic. Rapid recovery was recorded for the untreated shores, but ecological damage is still being reported 50 years later for the treated coastal areas.

The effects on the human population are more difficult to quantify, as little research has covered this aspect of the disaster. It is theorized by some researchers that the oil and contaminated plankton and other small marine organisms were eaten by successively larger predators, thereby concentrating the effects of the toxins. These predators were caught in large numbers by local fishermen and served to residents of the Cornish coastal communities. Research continues to identifying the health effects on the local population from this disastrous oil spill and equally disastrous cleanup.

Timothy J. Sutton

See Also: Deepwater Horizon Incident; *Exxon Valdez* Incident; International Environmental Law and Policy; Oil Spills, Health Consequences of; Persistent, Bioaccumulating, and Toxic Chemicals; Polycyclic Aromatic Hydrocarbons

Further Reading

Barkham, Patrick. "Oil Spills: Legacy of the *Torrey Canyon*." *Guardian*, June 24, 2010, https://www.theguardian.com/environment/2010/jun/24/*torrey-canyon*-oil-spill-deepwater-bp.

Hall, Grey. "*Torrey Canyon* Alerted the World to the Dangers That Lay Ahead." *Professional Mariner*, March 2007), http://www.professionalmariner.com/March-2007/*Torrey-Canyon*-alerted-the-world-to-the-dangers-that-lay-ahead/.

Hawkins, S.J., and A.J. Southward. "The *Torrey Canyon* Oil Spill: Recovery of Rocky Shore Communities." In *Restoring the Nation's Marine Environment*, edited by G. Taylor. College Park, MD: Maryland Sea Grant College, 1994.

Pillay, Anand, and J. Wang. *Technology and Safety of Marine Systems*. Amsterdam, the Netherlands: Elsevier Science, 2003.

Weintrit, Adam, and Tomasz Neumann. *Marine Navigation and Safety of Sea Transportation: Maritime Transport and Shipping*. Boca Raton, FL: CRC Press, 2013.

TOXIC SUBSTANCES AND DISEASE REGISTRY, AGENCY FOR

The Agency for Toxic Substances and Disease Registry (ATSDR) is a federal agency of the U.S. government housed within the U.S. Department of Health and Human Services. It was authorized by the Comprehensive Environmental Response, Compensation, and Liability Act of 1980 and formally established in 1983. While the ATSDR is an independent agency, it works in close association with the U.S. Centers for Disease Control and Prevention (also known as the CDC) and is administered by the CDC director, who appoints the director of the ATSDR. (The ATSDR has a joint Office of the Director with the National Center for Environmental

Health, also under the CDC.) The ATSDR's mission is to "serve the public through responsive public health actions to promote healthy and safe environments and prevent harmful exposures."

The ATSDR's primary role is to evaluate the potential health effects of hazardous chemicals and sites. It serves in an advisory capacity to communities and other federal and state agencies, but it does not regulate industry, and it is not involved in the cleanup of sites. The agency conducts public health assessments for sites on the U.S. government's National Priority List (otherwise known as Superfund sites), which allow the ATSDR to evaluate whether specific Superfund sites pose human health risks. The agency also provides public health consultations for other hazardous sites. The ATSDR, or states receiving funding from the agency, can initiate consultations when requested by the public or other government agencies. Both assessments and consultations provide stakeholders with information about hazards and health risks, including recommendations for ways to reduce community exposure.

The ATSDR staff members also investigate hazardous releases that have occurred during emergency events. Not only do they provide on-the-ground support during emergencies, but they also conduct surveillance to track emergency-related chemical releases, exposures, and health effects. The agency has developed several health registries to document and track human exposures and health impacts from emergency events. One such registry is the World Trade Center Health Registry, which commenced shortly after the terrorist attacks of September 11, 2001. The registry now contains information on over 70,000 people who were affected by the collapse of the World Trade Center buildings. This registry has been used to study both the mental and physical impacts of the disaster.

Finally, the ATSDR is charged with conducting research into the health effects of specific hazards and preparing toxicological profiles of hazardous chemicals. The agency's online Toxic Substances Portal contains information on over 250 toxic chemicals, including physical and chemical properties, sources, routes of exposure, health effects, and medical management guidelines.

Adrienne L. Katner

See Also: Disaster Preparedness and Response; National Center for Environmental Assessment; September 11 World Trade Center Attack; Superfund Act

Further Reading

Agency for Toxic Substances and Disease Registry. *Toxic Substances Portal.* http://www.atsdr.cdc.gov/toxprofiles/index.asp (accessed April 16, 2016).

Centers for Disease Control and Prevention. *Agency for Toxic Substances and Disease Registry.* http://www.atsdr.cdc.gov/about/index.html (accessed April 16, 2016).

Centers for Disease Control and Prevention. *National Center for Environmental Health.* http://www.cdc.gov/nceh/ (accessed April 16, 2016).

Centers for Disease Control and Prevention. *NCEA/ATSDR Organization Chart.* http://www.cdc.gov/nceh/information/org_chart.pdf (accessed April 16, 2016).

TOXIC SUBSTANCES CONTROL ACT

The Toxic Substances Control Act (TSCA) (15 USC (C. 53) 2601–2692) is a law passed by the U.S. Congress allowing the federal government to identify and control both existing chemicals and those entering U.S. markets. The TSCA was signed into law on October 11, 1976, by former president Gerald Ford and is administered by the U.S. Environmental Protection Agency (EPA).

In the 1970s, policymakers, scientists, and healthcare professionals began to express concern over the risks that toxic substances pose to human health and the environment. Reports observed a significant increase in the number of new chemicals that were entering commercial markets each year, many with little or no information about toxicity. Worker-related chemical exposure scares in the late 1960s, combined with the increasing number of new chemicals, prompted government action in the early 1970s. President Richard Nixon formed the Council on Environmental Quality in 1971, which published an influential report leading to the eventual drafting and passing of the TSCA.

The intent of the new law was to give the EPA power to evaluate the safety of raw materials and authority to control chemical risks that were not addressed under previous statutes. For example, Section 4 of the TSCA gives the EPA the authority to require testing of chemicals produced in substantial quantities that may pose a significant risk to human health or the environment. Section 5 requires companies planning to manufacture or import a previously unregulated chemical to submit to the EPA a premanufacture notice that includes information on the identity, use, anticipated volume, hazard, and disposal of the chemical. Under Section 6, the EPA may ban or control the production of any new or existing chemical due to excessive risk to the environment or human health.

Section 8 requires the EPA to compile and maintain a published list of every manufactured or processed chemical as part of the TSCA Inventory. Upon passage of the TSCA, it was declared that all existing chemicals should be considered safe, and nearly 62,000 existing chemicals were grandfathered in. The inventory, originally published in 1979, has grown to include roughly 85,000 chemicals. Substances that are generally excluded from TSCA oversight include food, drugs, cosmetics, and pesticides.

Title I of the original statute established the core of the law, which directed the EPA to control risks related to polychlorinated biphenyls. Subsequently, there have been five titles added to the law that address specific concerns. Title II, which was added in 1986, takes aim at asbestos. Title III (1988) addresses radon, Title IV (1992) seeks to control lead, Title V (2007) addresses energy and environmental issues in schools, and Title VI was added in 2008 to control formaldehyde emissions from composite wood products.

Most recently, attempts have been made by the U.S. Congress to modernize the act. In 2009, President Obama issued the "Essential Principles for Reform of Chemicals Management Legislation," which was designed to help inform ways that Congress could reauthorize and make the TSCA more effective. In 2015, competing reform bills were proposed in both U.S. congressional chambers. The House of

Representatives passed the "TSCA Modernization Act of 2015" (H.R. 2576), and the Senate drafted the "Frank R. Lautenberg Chemical Safety for the 21st Century Act" (S. 697).

Anthony C. Holderied

See Also: Asbestos; Formaldehyde; National Toxicology Program; Persistent, Bioaccumulating, and Toxic Chemicals; Polychlorinated Biphenyls; Toxic Substances and Disease Registry, Agency for; Toxics Release Inventory

Further Reading

Arbuckle, et al. *Environmental Law Handbook.* Rockville, MD: Government Institutes, 1993.

H.R. 2576—TSCA Modernization Act of 2015. As approved by the House on June 23, 2015. https://www.congress.gov/bill/114th-congress/house-bill/2576.

S. 697—Frank R. Lautenberg Chemical Safety for the 21st Century Act. As introduced by the Senate Environment and Public Works Committee on June 18, 2015. https://www.congress.gov/bill/114th-congress/senate-bill/697.

U.S. Environmental Protection Agency. *Essential Principles for Reform of Chemicals Management Legislation.* http://www.epa.gov/assessing-and-managing-chemicals-under-tsca/essential-principles-reform-chemicals-management-0 (accessed December 10, 2015).

U.S. Environmental Protection Agency. *Summary of the Toxic Substances Control Act, U.S.C. §2601 et seq. (1976).* http://www.epa.gov/laws-regulations/summary-toxic-substances-control-act (accessed January 2, 2016).

U.S. Environmental Protection Agency. *Toxic Substances Control Act and Federal Facilities.* http://www.epa.gov/enforcement/toxic-substances-control-act-tsca-and-federal-facilities (accessed December 10, 2015).

TOXICOGENOMICS

Sensitivity to chemicals differs between people. Many factors, including social and psychological influences and other environmental exposures, affect how people respond when exposed. In addition to external factors, some of the differences influencing susceptibility may be innate. Toxicogenomics is the name given to genomic investigations into the innate component of susceptibility to toxic chemicals.

There are two main ways that biology can affect a chemical's toxicity: toxicokinetics, defined as the movement and transformation of toxic chemicals within the body, and toxicodynamics, the biological response to a chemical at the dose in the organ where toxicity occurs. Toxicokinetic processes determine the dose of the chemical in the organ where toxicity occurs and may differ according to genetics. For instance, genetic differences may lead to distinct versions of relevant transporters or metabolic enzymes with different affinities for a particular chemical, or relevant proteins may be present in different concentrations across individuals. In some cases, a person may have no functional copies of a particular protein; for example, the enzyme glutathione-S-transferase mu 1 (GSTM1), which can help to eliminate certain toxic chemicals, is nonfunctional in many people. Sometimes genes can also influence the intake of a chemical; for example, nicotinic receptor genes influencing addiction are important for cumulative tobacco exposures.

Genetics can also play an important role in toxicodynamics. For example, a person may have a different form of a receptor with higher affinity for a toxic chemical, and therefore, a lower concentration of the chemical may elicit a similar response to a higher dose in a person with a lower-affinity receptor.

Some exposures have a few genes that are known to be particularly important. For example, the *PON1* (serum paraoxonase/arylesterase 1) gene is particularly important for sensitivity to organophosphate pesticides, and the *AS3MT* (arsenic III methyltransferase) gene is particularly important for the response to arsenic. However, for most exposures we do not have a clear picture of the human response genetics.

There are two main approaches to studying genetics. The first approach has the goal of identifying genetic regions that have similar inheritance patterns to the phenotype of interest. This similar inheritance is called linkage, and studies aimed at observing it are called linkage studies. The second approach, called association, compares how individuals' frequency of genomic variants (i.e., their genotype at a specific locus) is associated with the phenotype of interest. The linkage approach is concerned with transmission; the association approach is concerned with burden. There are epidemiological and animal model examples of both approaches. In general, linkage approaches are more powerful to detect large effects from genetic variants that may be rare overall in the population, while association studies are more powerful to detect modest effects from common variants.

Both linkage and association testing may be done on the scale of the whole genome. The late 1990s and early 2000s saw a large number of genome-wide association scans (GWAS) for myriad outcomes. GWAS results are generally available in the GWAS Catalogue, a partnership between the National Human Genome Research Institute in the United States and the European Molecular Biology Laboratory/European Bioinformatics Institute. When genome-wide association scans are used to test for interactions with environmental exposures, this may be called a gene-environment-wide interaction study (GEWIS). Testing a very large number of hypotheses in a genome-wide screen increases the risk of false positive findings, and thus, a more stringent criterion for statistical significance is used to limit the number of false positives. As a result, the minimum sample sizes required for GEWIS can be enormous (on the order of several thousand people).

A complementary approach is to focus on specific genetic pathways hypothesized to be involved in the biological response to specific compounds. Use of prior information on the biology of the chemical can be much more efficient than conducting an "agnostic" genome-wide screen and therefore may be feasible in smaller sample sizes. Furthermore, pathway hypotheses have the advantage of being amenable to representation in models that can explicitly incorporate toxicokinetic processes.

Recently, the scope of the field has expanded from a focus on sequence variation to how gene expression can affect toxic chemical responses. "Epigenetics" refers to potentially inherited features of the genome that may affect gene expression. Much of the epidemiological research considering epigenetics to date has focused on DNA methylation differences between people. This is of interest because more methylated DNA is harder for polymerases to bind to and therefore tends to have lower gene expression. There is also research looking at copy number variation (differences in the numbers of copies of a gene present in a person's genome) and RNA expression as key dimensions of toxicogenomics.

There is also growing interest in moving beyond studying nuclear genomic DNA. One emerging area is mitochondrial DNA, which may be particularly relevant for chemical exposures where toxicity is mediated by reactive oxygen species. Another emerging area is the effect of microbial communities living within people on how toxic chemicals are processed. Studying genomic features of resident microbial communities is called meta-genomics. In the future, these other kinds of DNA may become more prominent in toxicogenomic investigations.

Matthew O. Gribble

See Also: Dose-Response Assessment; Environmental Epidemiology; Environmental Toxicology

Further Reading

Adad, L. M., et al. "Occupational Exposure of Workers to Pesticides: Toxicogenetics and Susceptibility Gene Polymorphisms." *Genetics and Molecular Biology*, vol. 38, no. 3 (July–September 2015): 308–315.

Collins, Y., et al. "Mitochondrial Redox Signaling at a Glance." *Journal of Cell Science*, vol. 125, no. 4 (February 2012): 801–806.

Cortessis, V. C., and D. C. Thomas. *Toxicokinetic Genetics: An Approach to Gene-Environment and Gene-Gene Interactions in Complex Metabolic Pathways (IARC Scientific Publication)*. Lyon, France: International Agency for Research on Cancer, 2004.

Gao, J., et al. "The Genetic Architecture of Arsenic Metabolism Efficiency: A SNP-Based Heritability Study of Bangladeshi Adults." *Environmental Health Perspectives*, vol. 123, no. 10 (October 2015): 985–992.

Khoury, M., et al., eds. *Human Genome Epidemiology*. 2nd ed. Oxford, UK: Oxford University Press, 2009.

Khoury, M. J., and S. Wacholder. "Invited Commentary: From Genome-Wide Association Studies to Gene-Environment-Wide Interaction Studies—Challenges and Opportunities." *American Journal of Epidemiology*, vol. 169, no. 2 (January 2009): 227–230.

Klaassen, Curtis. *Cassarett and Doull's Toxicology: The Basic Sciences of Poisons*. 8th ed. New York: McGraw-Hill, 2013.

Loukola, A., et al. "Genetics and Smoking." *Current Addiction Reports*, vol. 1, no. 1 (March 2014): 75–82.

Murcray, C. E., et al. "Sample Size Requirements to Detect Gene-Environment Interactions in Genome-Wide Association Studies." *Genetic Epidemiology*, vol. 35, no. 3 (April 2011): 201–210.

Ott, J., Y. Kamatani, and M. Lathrop. "Family-Based Designs for Genome-Wide Association Studies." *Nature Reviews Genetics*, vol. 12, no. 7 (June 2011): 465–474.

Thomas, D. C., et al. "The Use of Pathway Information in Molecular Epidemiology." *Human Genomics*, vol. 4, no. 1 (October 2009): 21–42.

Welter, D., et al. "The NHGRI GWAS Catalog, a Curated Resource of SNP-Trait Associations." *Nucleic Acids Research*, vol. 42, Database Issue (January 2014): D1001–D1006.

TOXICS RELEASE INVENTORY

The Toxics Release Inventory (TRI) is a data repository consisting of toxic chemical releases as well as waste reduction and pollution prevention activities reported by industrial and federal facilities in the United States. This repository is maintained by the U.S. Environmental Protection Agency (EPA) and is updated annually with data provided by facilities subject to TRI reporting requirements. This program allows citizens to identify areas where toxic chemicals have been emitted into the environment as well as the waste reduction and prevention strategies used to minimize this activity.

The TRI reporting program originated from the Emergency Planning and Community Right-to-Know Act (EPCRA) enacted in 1986. The primary objectives of EPCRA were the following: (1) enhance the efforts of state and local emergency planning organizations with actions directed at chemical emergencies; (2) provide a mechanism for notifying relevant authorities about emergency releases of chemicals; and (3) increase the body of available data on toxic and hazardous chemicals, which will be used to address community concerns. Section 313 of EPCRA requires the EPA and the states to collect annual data on releases and transfers of certain toxic chemicals from applicable facilities and to make this data available through the TRI.

Facilities that meet the three applicability criteria below must report to the TRI program:

- Be classified as part of a specific industrial sector (note that federal facilities are required to report if they meet the employee and chemical use thresholds, regardless of their industry sector)
- Employ 10 or more full-time equivalent employees
- Manufacture or process greater than 25,000 pounds (11,340 kilograms) of a TRI-listed chemical or otherwise use greater than 10,000 pounds (4,536 kilograms) of a listed chemical in a given year (note that certain persistent, bioaccumulative, and toxic chemicals—PBTs—have lower reporting thresholds)

If a facility meets these criteria, it must submit a TRI Form R (known as the long form) for each TRI-listed chemical it manufactures, processes, or otherwise uses in quantities above the reporting threshold. Each TRI Form R must be submitted to both the EPA and the relevant division in the state in which the facility is located. Facilities may be eligible to submit a shorter version of a TRI form (Form A) if all of the following criteria are met:

- The chemical being reported is not considered a persistent, bioaccumulating, and toxic chemical
- The chemical has not been manufactured, processed, or otherwise used in excess of 1,000,000 pounds (453,592 kilograms)
- The total annual waste management (i.e., recycling, energy recovery, treatment, and disposal or other releases) of the chemical does not exceed 500 pounds (227 kilograms)

The deadline for submitting TRI forms for chemical releases and other related activity occurring in the previous calendar year is July 1.

The TRI program has improved the availability of data that can be accessed by the general public on sources of toxic releases in their communities. In recent years, the EPA and several other organizations have developed systems to enable users to understand the information in the TRI and use it for decision making. Examples include the following:

- TOXMAP: Available from the National Library of Medicine, this geographic information system helps users manipulate maps of the United States to analyze data from the EPA's TRI and Superfund programs.
- MapEcos.org: Developed by faculty and students at Dartmouth College, Duke University, and Harvard Business School, this system allows users to access an interactive map of the United States illustrating the most recent TRI data.
- RTKnet.org: Available from the Center for Effective Government, this system provides access to a variety of current EPA data, including data for the TRI. Queries allow users to download files with the raw data.
- Envirofacts: Available from the EPA website, this system allows queries to the underlying relational database produce downloadable text documents.

Richard F. Pandullo

See Also: Emergency Planning and Community Right-to-Know Act; Environmental Protection Agency; National Air Toxics Assessment; Pollution Prevention

Further Reading

Environmental Defense Fund. *Toxic Release Inventory Data*. https://www.edf.org/health/toxics-across-america/TRI-table (accessed March 16, 2017).

2015 TRI National Analysis: Executive Summary. Washington, DC: U.S. Environmental Protection Agency, 2017.

U.S. Environmental Protection Agency. *Toxics Release Inventory Program*. https://www.epa.gov/toxics-release-inventory-tri-program (accessed March 16, 2017).

TRACHOMA

Also known by the names granular conjunctivitis, Egyptian ophthalmia, and blinding trachoma, trachoma is the leading cause of infectious blindness. Blindness caused by trachoma is irreversible, and trachoma is the primary cause for the blindness or visual impairment of 1.9 million people. Trachoma is considered a public health problem in approximately 42 countries in Africa, Asia, Central America, and South America. While trachoma is not as prevalent in the United States as in to other countries, it is still present.

Chlamydia trachomatis is the organism responsible for causing trachoma as well as some genital tract infections. Serotypes A, B, Ba, and C are the primary causes of trachoma, while serotypes D through K cause urinary and genital tract infections. This disease is spread by direct contact with secretions from the eye, nose, and throat of infected individuals, but it can also be spread via fomites, such as handkerchiefs, towels, or washcloths contaminated with these secretions.

Trachoma appears to have two phases: an active, inflammatory trachoma and a cicatricial portion of the disease, in which scarring from the active phase causes the eyelid to turn inward, resulting in light sensitivity and ocular damage. Active trachoma is most commonly seen in young children up to nine years old, whereas the cicatricial disease and blindness are most often observed in adults.

The World Health Organization (WHO) has developed another categorization system for trachoma, termed the simplified WHO trachoma grading system. This classification helps determine the intervention required for the disease (see Table 18). The WHO and its partners in world health medicine endorse the surgery, antibiotics, facial cleanliness, and environmental improvement ("SAFE") strategy for trachoma control.

It is recommended that a good light and at least 2.5-times magnification be used to examine the eye when looking for inflammation, discharge, loss of eyelashes, rubbing on the cornea, and corneal opacity. The upper lid should also be everted to visualize the upper tarsal conjunctiva for evidence of follicles, inflammation, or scarring. If an eye has a grade of TT or CO in the WHO grading system, then there is a high propensity for blindness, and this observation should prompt ophthalmologic evaluation and surgical intervention.

If the cause of eye inflammation and discharge is in question, then there are laboratory tests available to test for *C. trachomatis*, such as immunofluorescent cytology, polymerase chain reaction, Giemsa cytology, and bacterial culture. Trachoma is often confused with eye irritation from viruses, chemicals, allergies, hypersensitivity to makeup, or infection by another bacterial organism, like *Streptococcus pneumoniae*, *Staphylococcus aureus*, and *Bartonella henselae*.

Table 18. Simplified trachoma grading system.

Classification	Description	Treatment
Trachomatous inflammation, follicular (TF)	Five or more follicles of > 0.5 mm on the upper tarsal conjunctiva	Antibiotic therapy and ocular hygiene
Trachomatous inflammation, intense (TI)	Papillary hypertrophy and inflammatory thickening of the upper tarsal conjunctiva, obscuring more than half the deep tarsal vessels	Antibiotic therapy and ocular hygiene
Trachomatous conjunctival scarring (TS)	Grossly visible scars on the tarsal conjunctiva	Ophthalmologic evaluation, antibiotic therapy, and ocular hygiene
Trachomatous trichiasis (TT)	At least one ingrown eyelash touching the globe, or evidence of epilation (eyelash removal)	Surgical intervention
Corneal opacity (CO)	Corneal opacity blurring part of the pupil margin	Surgical intervention and lifetime antibiotics

Trachoma is typically treated with a single high dose of azithromycin by mouth or topical forms of tetracyclines or azithromycin directly on the eyelid. Oral tetracycline cannot be used on pregnant women due to risk of harm to the unborn child, but the topical medicine is safe during pregnancy. If the severity of the illness has surpassed antibiotic intervention, then surgical methods are necessary.

Howard W. MacLennan Jr.

See Also: Communicable Diseases; Infectious Diseases; World Health Organization

Further Reading

Burton, M. J., et al. "A Randomised Controlled Trial of Azithromycin Following Surgery for Trachomatous Trichiasis in the Gambia." *British Journal of Ophthalmology*, vol. 89, no. 10 (October 2005): 1282–1288.

Evans, J. R., and A. W. Solomon. "Antibiotics for Trachoma." *Cochrane Database of Systematic Reviews*, vol. 16, no. 3 (March 2011): CD001860.

Negrel, A. D., H. R. Taylor, and S. West. *Guidelines for the Rapid Assessment for Blinding Trachoma*. Geneva, Switzerland: World Health Organization, 2001.

Solomon, Anthony W., et al. *Trachoma Control: A Guide for Program Managers*. Geneva, Switzerland: World Health Organization, 2006.

Trachoma. World Health Organization, Geneva, Switzerland, 2017. http://www.who.int/mediacentre/factsheets/fs382/en.

U

ULTRAVIOLET RADIATION AND THE UV INDEX

The sun emits radiation over a wide range of wavelengths, including wavelengths corresponding to radio waves, microwaves, infrared radiation, visible light, X-rays, gamma rays, and ultraviolet (UV) radiation. UV radiation is a particular concern because overexposure can cause reddening of the skin (erythema), reduced vitamin D synthesis, skin cancer, cataracts, and suppression of the immune system. We become overexposed to UV radiation when we spend too much time outdoors and neglect to take appropriate precautions to protect ourselves from the sun. Additionally, air pollution can worsen our exposure by weakening the UV radiation shielding provided by the stratospheric ozone layer.

Protecting Yourself from Too Much UV Radiation

In addition to causing a sunburn, too much UV radiation can cause skin cancer and other serious problems. Here are some simple steps you can follow to avoid overexposure while outdoors:

- Limit the time you spend in the midday sun, especially during the hours from 10:00 A.M. to 4:00 P.M.
- Avoid getting a sunburn, which can significantly increase the risk of developing skin cancer. (You can get a sunburn even on a cloudy day!)
- Try to stay in the shade as much as possible while outside.
- Be careful near water, snow, and sand, which can reflect sunlight and increase the risk of sunburn.
- Only buy sunglasses that provide 100 percent UV protection against both UVA and UVB radiation.
- Wear wide-brimmed hats and tightly woven, loose-fitting clothing.
- Stay away from suntanning salons and tanning beds, which increase the risk of skin cancer and wrinkling.
- Always apply a broad spectrum sunscreen before going outside, and reapply frequently.

Additionally, it is a good idea to check the National Weather Service's UV Index before planning outdoor activities to be sure you are adequately protected. And examine your skin at least monthly, looking for abnormalities, such as moles that have changed size, color, or shape and sores that have not healed.

Our health depends on sunlight. In particular, sunlight helps our bodies produce vitamin D, which is essential for healthy bones and for regulating the immune and neuromuscular systems. However, sunlight can sometimes be too much of a good thing when it affects our health. Many of us grew up thinking there is nothing wrong with a nice tan after a weekend at the beach. In fact, tanning is how your body protects itself from harmful UV radiation, and if you are developing a tan or, worse, a sunburn, you have probably been out in the sun too long.

Among the serious health consequences of overexposure to UV radiation, skin cancer is perhaps the best known. Here are the facts about skin cancer:

- The most common cancer in the United States is skin cancer.
- One in five Americans will develop skin cancer in their lifetime, and one American dies from skin cancer every hour.
- Among several risk factors for skin cancer, exposure to UV radiation is the most preventable. (Genetic factors and immune system deficiencies also increase the risk of developing skin cancer.)
- Overexposure to UV radiation and frequent sunburns, especially during childhood, enhance the likelihood of developing melanoma, the most serious type of skin cancer. (Melanoma represents only about 3 percent of skin cancer cases, but it accounts for over 75 percent of deaths attributable to skin cancer.)

Excessive UV radiation exposure can also cause actinic keratoses, which are growths of skin on overexposed areas of the body (especially the face, hands, neck, and forearms) that are risk factors for later development of cancer. Premature aging of the skin can also occur, making the skin look old and wrinkled. As people get older, up to 90 percent of the skin changes, often attributed to the aging process, are actually caused by the sun and are preventable if precautions are taken to reduce UV radiation exposure.

There are three types of UV radiation: UVA (having a wavelength of 315 to 400 nanometers), UVB (280 to 315 nanometers), and UVC (100 to 280 nanometers). While most UVA radiation reaches the surface of the earth, the earth's stratospheric ozone layer can block much of the UVB radiation from reaching the earth's surface, especially where the layer is thicker. However, when air pollution causes a thinning of the stratospheric ozone layer, more UVB can pass through. The atmosphere is very effective in blocking UVC radiation, with little ever reaching the earth's surface. Of all of the UV radiation reaching the earth's surface, about 90 to 95 percent is UVA, and the remainder is UVB. Overexposure to both UVA and UVB can adversely affect human health.

The UV Index is a daily forecast by the U.S. National Weather Service of the amount of UV radiation expected to reach the earth's surface, based the sun's elevation, the amount of stratospheric ozone, and cloud cover. The higher the index value, the more likely skin and eye damage will occur over a shorter period of time (see Table 19). Thus, it is a useful tool for planning outdoor activities. In addition to the UV Index, the National Environmental Education Foundation's SunWise program provides resources for teaching children about sun safety, UV radiation, and stratospheric ozone.

Richard Crume

Table 19. UV Index scale.

UV Index	Category	Precautions
0 to 2	Low (Green)	A UV Index reading of 0 to 2 means low danger from the sun's UV rays for the average person. Wear sunglasses on bright days. If you burn easily, cover up and use broad spectrum SPF 30+ sunscreen. Watch out for bright surfaces, like sand, water, and snow, which reflect UV and increase exposure.
3 to 5	Moderate (Yellow)	A UV Index reading of 3 to 5 means moderate risk of harm from unprotected sun exposure. Stay in shade near midday when the sun is strongest. If outdoors, wear protective clothing, a wide-brimmed hat, and UV-blocking sunglasses. Generously apply broad spectrum SPF 30+ sunscreen every two hours, even on cloudy days, and after swimming or sweating. Watch out for bright surfaces, like sand, water, and snow, which reflect UV and increase exposure.
6 to 7	High (Orange)	A UV Index reading of 6 to 7 means high risk of harm from unprotected sun exposure. Protection against skin and eye damage is needed. Reduce time in the sun between 10 A.M. and 4 P.M. If outdoors, seek shade and wear protective clothing, a wide-brimmed hat, and UV-blocking sunglasses. Generously apply broad spectrum SPF 30+ sunscreen every two hours, even on cloudy days, and after swimming or sweating. Watch out for bright surfaces, like sand, water, and snow, which reflect UV and increase exposure.
8 to 10	Very High (Red)	A UV Index reading of 8 to 10 means very high risk of harm from unprotected sun exposure. Take extra precautions because unprotected skin and eyes will be damaged and can burn quickly. Minimize sun exposure between 10 A.M. and 4 P.M. If outdoors, seek shade and wear protective clothing, a wide-brimmed hat, and UV-blocking sunglasses. Generously apply broad spectrum SPF 30+ sunscreen every two hours, even on cloudy days, and after swimming or sweating. Watch out for bright surfaces, like sand, water, and snow, which reflect UV and increase exposure.
11 or More	Extreme (Purple)	A UV Index reading of 11 or more means extreme risk of harm from unprotected sun exposure. Take all precautions because unprotected skin and eyes can burn in minutes. Try to avoid sun exposure between 10 A.M. and 4 P.M. If outdoors, seek shade and wear protective clothing, a wide-brimmed hat, and UV-blocking sunglasses. Generously apply broad spectrum SPF 30+ sunscreen every two hours, even on cloudy days, and after swimming or sweating. Watch out for bright surfaces, like sand, water, and snow, which reflect UV and increase exposure.

Source: U.S. Environmental Protection Agency.

See Also: Air Pollution; Cancer Risk from Environmental Exposure; Environmental Protection Agency; Stratospheric Ozone Depletion

Further Reading

Barrow, Mary M., and John F. Barrow. *Sun Protection for Life: Your Guide to a Lifetime of Healthy and Beautiful Skin*. Oakland, CA: New Harbinger Publications, 2005.

Consumer Reports. *Sunscreen Buying Guide*. http://www.consumerreports.org/cro/sunscreens/buying-guide.htm (accessed August 15, 2016).

Consumer Reports. *What Does SPF Stand For? Understanding How a Sunscreen Works Helps You Get the Best Protection*. http://www.consumerreports.org/cro/magazine/2015/05/what-does-spf-stand-for/index.htm (accessed August 27, 2016).

Hitchcock, R. Timothy. *Ultraviolet Radiation*. Fairfax, VA: American Industrial Hygiene Association, 2001.

National Environmental Education Foundation. *Home Page*. https://www.neefusa.org/sunwise (accessed August 15, 2016).

National Weather Service. *UV Index: Information*. http://www.cpc.ncep.noaa.gov/products/stratosphere/uv_index/uv_information.shtml (accessed August 15, 2016).

U.S. Environmental Protection Agency. *UV Index: What Is the UV Index for My Area of Interest Today?* https://www.epa.gov/sunsafety/uv-index-1 (accessed August 15, 2016).

U.S. Environmental Protection Agency. *UV Index Scale*. https://www.epa.gov/sunsafety/uv-index-scale-1 (accessed August 15, 2016).

U.S. Environmental Protection Agency. *Welcome to Radtown USA*. https://www3.epa.gov/radtown (accessed August 15, 2016).

UNDERGROUND STORAGE TANKS, HEALTH CONCERNS WITH

Underground storage tanks (USTs) exist throughout the country and contain a variety of materials (primarily liquids), such as gasoline, diesel, oils, other petroleum products, solvents, additives, cleaners, water, and used oil. Finely ground metals may also be present, particularly when storing used oil. Health effects related to USTs are caused both by the unique ways relatively common materials with known health effects can enter the environment and by human exposure to these materials through both air and water (respiration and ingestion).

When Underground Storage Tanks Leak

Virtually any liquid chemical can be stored within a UST. When chemicals leak from a UST system, they can migrate in the subsurface soil, groundwater, and air in many ways, leading to complex exposure pathways. Chemical migration can be influenced by many factors, such as soil type, soil layering, the presence of underground features (including rock layers and caves), air pressure, rainfall, groundwater, tides, earthquake faults, subsurface utilities, and past excavations and backfill. Thus, determining the environmental effects of underground storage tank leaks can be very difficult, requiring expert knowledge and experience.

There are several ways that UST systems can discharge chemicals into the environment. These include leakage from the UST itself (including the piping and pumps) and spills around the tank. Spills are most likely during the process of adding and removing the contents. When contaminants are released from a UST, they are generally pulled downward by gravity and, in the gaseous phase, expand outward. This path is influenced by the soil and subsurface features, creating an impacted area called the contaminant plume, which may extend to the groundwater. Chemicals lighter than water will pool on top of the water, while those denser than water will sink. Most chemicals will dissolve in the groundwater to some extent. Variations in the conditions of the release result in a distinctive contaminant plume for each release.

The materials stored within the tanks can cause health concerns. Virtually any liquid material can be stored in a UST, as long as the material is not reactive with the UST material itself. In addition, liquids in the tanks (such as a used oil tank) may contain metals and other finely ground and dissolved materials that will travel with the liquid in the event of a discharge into the environment. In practice, USTs typically contain chemicals such as petroleum hydrocarbons (e.g., gasoline and diesel), cleaning agents (e.g., chlorinated solvents), and waste materials (e.g., used oil). Many of these are considered volatile organic compounds and can be readily detected by smell. Some of the chemicals, such as benzene and methyl tert-butyl ether, are potential human carcinogens. The health effects are the same as exposure to the materials through other channels; however, the exposure pathways are unique. While leakage from surface and above-ground tanks can be quickly identified and addressed, USTs may leak for some time until the leak is discovered.

One well-documented release pathway to exposure is the contamination of groundwater through releases from USTs. Contaminants leaked into the subsurface can travel with the water when it is pumped for human use. The contaminants are often very dilute and remain hidden until the water is tested. Gasoline consists of chemicals with a distinctive odor, and some initial contamination issues related to USTs for gasoline were identified by petroleum odors in well water.

Vapor migration in the subsurface can also lead to human exposure to the contents of USTs. While gravity tends to pull liquids downward, chemicals may also be present in the gaseous state (depending on the chemical and the environmental conditions). In addition to the overall downward movement of liquid chemicals, gases will move laterally and may even move upward. Human exposure through respiration can occur in many situations, such as basements and crawl spaces, where the gas would move from the soil into a space with limited air circulation, and in buildings where the gas could enter through foundations.

Exposure can also occur when contaminated groundwater exits subsurface flow to surface flow. Chemicals from the UST leakage may travel with the groundwater as it enters the surface stream. If contaminants in the groundwater are dilute, they may not be noticed over contaminants that enter the surface water from stormwater runoff. With higher concentrations of chemicals in the groundwater, a discoloration, surface sheen, or biological growth may be observed where the groundwater meets the surface water.

Workers may be exposed to UST releases as they construct trenches, such as for storm drains, sanitary sewers, and other buried utilities, as well as during excavations on construction sites. When encountering subsurface contaminants, workers at the site are typically alerted to the contamination when they notice odors from the volatile organic compounds and other chemicals, by which time their skin, clothes, and equipment may already be contaminated with soil and groundwater containing the chemicals. When found, work is usually suspended in the area of the subsurface contamination, pending investigation and cleanup of the released materials.

In Southern California in the 1990s, the gasoline additive named MTBE was found in drinking water wells in the Santa Monica area, where there was no other indication of significant contamination in the water. Although MTBE had been found in other locations, its identification in the Santa Monica water wells triggered more extensive testing of water wells throughout the country, and MTBE was found in additional wells. Further research determined that the MTBE traveled through the subsurface faster than other commonly tested chemicals, and MTBE actually became an early indicator of a UST leak.

Another health-related factor that was illustrated by the MTBE leakage is that some chemicals, including petroleum hydrocarbons, may be susceptible to biodegradation upon release into the environment. While biodegradation can be useful in that it removes the chemical from the environment, it can also cause the creation of new chemicals that were not originally present in the chemicals released from the UST. In the case of the MTBE leakage, some of the MTBE biodegrades into tert-butyl alcohol, a skin irritant that may then biodegrade into other compounds.

Thomas B. Lawrence

See Also: Biodegradable Materials, Health Benefits of; Cancer Risk from Environmental Exposure; Groundwater Pollution and Depletion; Respiratory Disease and Air Pollution; Volatile Organic Compound Pollution

Further Reading

Coffey, Chris. *Hundreds of Underground Tanks Leaking in Chicago*. WMAQ-TV NBC-5, Chicago, IL, 2013. http://www.nbcchicago.com/investigations/Underground-Storage-Tanks-Creating-Toxic-Soil-231846081.html.

Ground Water Report to the Nation: A Call to Action. Oklahoma City, OK: Ground Water Protection Council, 2007.

U.S. Environmental Protection Agency. *Underground Storage Tanks (USTs)*. https://www.epa.gov/ust (accessed March 16, 2017).

UST Program Facts: Data about the Underground Storage Tank (UST) Program. Washington, DC: U.S. Environmental Protection Agency, 2016.

UNEXPLODED ORDNANCE

Unexploded ordnance (often abbreviated UXO) is active military weaponry that did not detonate upon deployment. It includes aerial bombs, hand grenades, tank mines, artillery shells, and landmines. This type of military weaponry has been used since the American Civil War. Unexploded ordnance is found all over the world, and it is unknown how much unexploded ordnance remains. Every year, about 24,000 people die from unexploded ordnance and landmines.

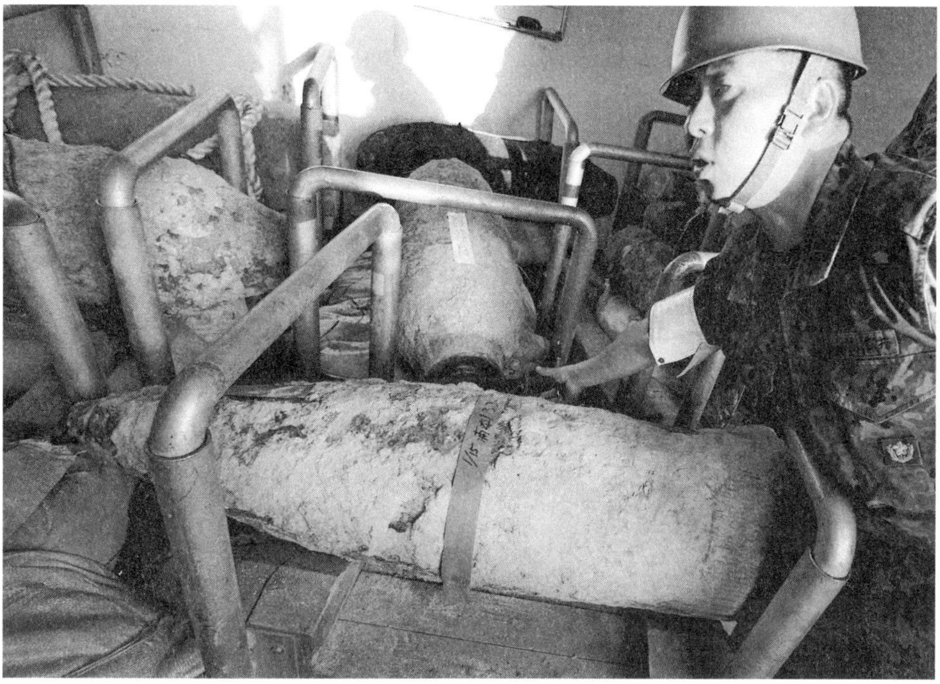

Unexploded World War II bombs at a warehouse in Okinawa, Japan. Every year many people throughout the world die from unexploded ordnance, including aerial bombs, hand grenades, tank mines, artillery shells, and landmines. (AP Photo/Itsuo Inouye)

A legacy of World War II, unexploded aerial bombs are commonly found in the United Kingdom, Germany, France, Japan, and the Pacific Islands. UXO is often discovered during construction projects. In France and Belgium, farmers plowing their fields turn up artillery in what they call the "iron harvest." Japan also regularly uncovers and defuses bombs left over from World War II. Since 1972, Japanese military forces have disposed of 5,500 tons (5,000 metric tons) of ordnance, and the discovery of bombs is almost a daily occurrence in Germany. This results in frequent evacuations while bomb-disposal teams do their work. Buried artillery becomes more unstable and therefore more dangerous over time, and in France alone, more than 630 demining workers have died while removing mines. This represents a fatality rate of one worker per every 5,000 defused mines.

Countries that have experienced recent or frequent conflict are most affected by unexploded ordnance. For instance, during the Vietnam War (1955–1975), the United States dropped more than 2 million tons (1.8 metric tons) of artillery on Laos, making it the world's most heavily bombed country per capita. In the four decades since this war, 8,000 people have been killed and 12,000 wounded from UXO, many of them children who did not know what they were playing with. The United States currently spends $12 million every year to remove UXO in Laos. In addition, Lebanon, Angola, and Afghanistan are each littered with millions of landmines and bomblets (cluster bombs) left over from military conflicts. This type of unexploded ordnance is considered more dangerous than large bombs because it is more difficult to detect. Mines and bomblets make agricultural land unusable until the land is cleared.

In the United States, over 10 million acres of land formerly used for military practice may contain unexploded ordnance, and restoring this land will cost at least $14 billion, according to the U.S. Environmental Protection Agency. The United States often uses sophisticated electronic or geophysical techniques to detect UXO, techniques that are effective but expensive.

Since 1980, international law has required countries to remove "explosive remnants of war" once the conflict has ended. Because civilians are victims of remaining mines, the United Nations believes that "antipersonnel" mines (mines designed to injure people) should not be used in warfare. Additionally, some people believe that antipersonnel mines accomplish only limited military goals. In 1997, UN efforts led to an international treaty, the Anti-Personnel Mine Ban Convention. The United States has not signed the treaty, criticizing it for allowing antivehicle mines and cluster bombs, which remain live for many years after deployment. The UN is currently working to find and remove UXO, assist victims, and educate people living in affected areas.

Alisha K. Newton

See Also: Chemical Weapons Elimination; Environmental Protection Agency; International Environmental Law and Policy

Further Reading

Convention on the Prohibition of the Use, Stockpiling, Production, and Transfer of Anti-Personnel Mines and on Their Destruction. Adopted September 18, 1997. http://www.apmineban convention.org.

Kaplan, Sarah, and Nick Kirkpatrick. "The Bombs Beneath Us: Unexploded Ordnance Lingers Long after Wars Are Over." *Washington Post*, August 13, 2015, https://www.washing tonpost.com/news/morning-mix/wp/2015/08/13/the-bombs-beneath-us-unexploded-ordnance-linger-long-after-wars-are-over.

UN Office for Disarmament Affairs. *Landmines.* http://www.un.org/disarmament/convarms/landmines/ (accessed December 21, 2015).

Walsh, Nicolas E., and Wendy S. Walsh. "Rehabilitation of Landmine Victims: The Ultimate Challenge." *Bulletin of the World Health Organization*, vol. 81, no. 9 (2003): 665–670.

UNITED NATIONS ENVIRONMENTAL PROGRAMME

The United Nations Environmental Programme (UNEP) oversees environmental progress and concerns around the world. As an agency of the United Nations, it works primarily with member states to identify, research, and mitigate environmental issues, such as air and water pollution, waste disposal, and climate change. The main functions of the UNEP are policy development and analysis, coordination among member nations and nongovernmental agencies, and resource mobilization and outreach.

Are You Too Lazy to Save the World?

If so, the United Nations has published a list of things you can do from the comfort of your couch, including the following:

- Save electricity by turning off electronic devices and appliances when not in use, such as your computer.
- Stop paper bank statements, and pay your bills online.
- Use social media to share interesting stories about, for example, climate change or women's rights.
- Speak up about important issues, like voicing your support for international climate agreements.
- Stop using your printer, and instead, jot down ideas in a notebook or a digital Post-it note on your computer.
- Order products from companies having sustainable practices.
- Stay informed about local and national issues by watching the TV news, reviewing online articles, and even the old-fashioned way—reading a newspaper.

And when you finally get up from the couch, turn off the lights, TV, and computer. Let's get with it!

The UNEP was established in December 1972 in direct response to concerns among people and governments around the world about rising pollution levels. It is headquartered in Nairobi, Kenya, and is organized around six regional offices located in Bahrain, Kenya, Panama, Switzerland, Thailand, and the United States. A number of other program offices are located throughout the world, giving the UNEP a strong international presence.

In many ways, the UNEP functions similarly to other UN agencies in that it seeks to provide key support by partnering with local groups. This focus is seen within each of the organization's seven divisions—Communication, Corporate Services, Economy, Ecosystems, Law, Policy and Programme, and Science.

A major UN concern is that current lifestyles and priorities may not be sustainable into the future. As a result, member states have adopted the following 17 sustainability goals, which include environmental health objectives supported by UNEP: no poverty; zero hunger; good health and well-being; quality education; gender equality; clean water and sanitation; affordable and clean energy; decent work and economic growth; industry innovation and infrastructure; reduced inequalities; sustainable cities and communities; responsible consumption and production; climate action; life below water; life on land; peace, justice, and strong institutions; and partnerships for the goals.

While achieving these goals is certainly a daunting task, partnerships with member states and local organizations have been making significant progress in each of these areas. One example is a project to bring clean water to a primary school in Sierra Leone for the first time in a decade. This and similar projects have increased access to safe drinking water from 37 to 63 percent of the Sierra Leone population in the past 25 years. Another project in Montenegro is helping the country develop a carbon-neutral, climate-friendly tourism industry by working with businesses to adopt sustainable practices. A third project in Georgia is addressing rural poverty and food security through sustainable agriculture development.

Charles Daniel

See Also: Earth Charter; International Environmental Law and Policy; Sustainable Development and Health; United Nations Framework Convention on Climate Change

Further Reading

Annual Report 2016. Nairobi, Kenya: UN Environment Programme, 2016. http://www.unep.org/annualreport/2016/index.php?page=0&lang=en.

Environmental Protection Agency. *International Cooperation: EPA's Role in the United Nations Environment Programme*. https://www.epa.gov/international-cooperation/epas-role-united-nations-environment-programme-unep (accessed May 5, 2017).

Hanhimaki, Jussi M. *The United Nations: A Very Short Introduction*. New York: Oxford University Press, 2015.

UN Environment Programme. *Home Page*. http://www.un.org (accessed May 5, 2017).

United Nations. *The Lazy Person's Guide to Saving the World*. http://www.un.org/sustainabledevelopment/takeaction (accessed May 5, 2017).

United Nations. *Sustainable Development Goals: 17 Goals to Transform Our World*. http://www.un.org/sustainabledevelopment/blog/2016/07/17goals17days-progress-made-on-sustainable-development-goals (accessed May 5, 2017).

UNITED NATIONS FRAMEWORK CONVENTION ON CLIMATE CHANGE

The United Nations Framework Convention on Climate Change (UNFCCC) is an international treaty that provides the foundation for coordinating national responses to both the causes and effects of climate change. This treaty has been instrumental in facilitating and encouraging nations to reduce their greenhouse gas emissions. Ultimately, this is enormously important from a public health perspective because global climate change will cause and contribute to phenomena that pose serious public health risks, such as floods, heat waves, water shortages, and food shortages. Actions taken to reduce greenhouse gas emissions will reduce the likelihood and/or magnitude of such phenomena.

The UNFCCC was negotiated in 1992 and entered into force in 1994. Today, it has near-universal membership, with 197 countries having ratified the agreement. The primary objective of the UNFCCC is to "stabilize greenhouse gas concentrations in the atmosphere at a level that would prevent dangerous anthropogenic interference with the climate system." While the original convention did not specify what this level would be or how that might translate to specific emissions limitations for particular countries or sectors, it did provide the basis for an ongoing international dialogue to reach consensus on these issues.

One of the key elements of the original convention is the formal recognition that all countries should implement measures to mitigate and adapt to climate change, in accordance with their common but differentiated responsibilities and respective capacities. This means that developed country parties should take the lead in combating climate change and its adverse effects, both because they are primarily responsible for the problem and because they have the resources to address it. Developing countries are also expected to implement mitigation and adaptation measures, but the convention recognizes that their ability to effectively implement their commitments is contingent on the provision of financial and technical support from developed country parties.

The convention also requires all parties to monitor anthropogenic sources and sinks of greenhouse gas emissions and to periodically submit national emission inventories to the UNFCCC secretariat. These reports provide a basis for determining the respective contributions of countries to global climate change and for evaluating the adequacy of national efforts to reduce greenhouse gas emissions.

Finally, the convention creates a framework for implementation and elaboration on commitments. It outlines a process whereby the Conference of the Parties can hold periodic meetings and negotiate subsidiary agreements, and it establishes a secretariat that is responsible for administrative matters, such as the collection and publication of national emissions inventories.

The Conference of the Parties has convened every year since 1995 to discuss implementation of the UNFCCC and has elaborated on many important issues in the decisional documents published for each annual meeting. For example, in the Cancun Agreements (the decision document for the 2010 conference), the parties agreed that they must limit global warming to 2°C (about 4°F) to meet the original objective of the UNFCCC. Commitments related to financial and technical assistance have also been laid out in these decisions. Unfortunately, the terms of these decisions are not legally binding. They can, however, can lead to the adoption of legally binding domestic laws in willing countries.

The Conference of the Parties has also promulgated two subsidiary agreements. The first was the Kyoto Protocol, which was adopted in 1997 but did not go into force until 2005. It established legally binding emissions targets for some developed country parties as well as flexibility mechanisms that permitted emissions trading and offsets. The success of the Kyoto Protocol is a subject of debate—most countries met their targets and the sum of emissions from those countries fell significantly. However, major emitters like the United States and China did not participate in the program, and emissions from developing and emerging economies increased substantially. One major concern regarding the effectiveness of the Kyoto Protocol is that the overall increase in global emissions is likely the result of emissions leakage (which occurs when there is an increase in greenhouse gas emissions in one country as a result of emission reductions in another country). Much of the emissions growth in China and other emerging economies was driven by the production of goods and services that were exported to developed countries, including the Kyoto parties.

The second subsidiary agreement is the Paris Agreement, adopted in 2015. The Paris Agreement takes a very different approach from Kyoto: it establishes a framework wherein parties develop and periodically revise national plans for reducing greenhouse gas emissions (known as "nationally determined contributions"). The adequacy and implementation of these plans is then assessed during a global assessment. The agreement also contains provisions related to adaptation and financial and technical assistance. Unlike the Kyoto Protocol, the Paris Agreement is on track to achieve universal participation, likely due to the lack of any quantitative emissions limitations on participating countries.

It is not possible to estimate the specific impacts of the UNFCCC and its subsidiary agreements in terms of emissions reductions or health benefits. However, it is safe to say that the framework established by the UNFCCC has played a significant role in motivating and facilitating national-level responses to climate change and that these responses have led to meaningful reductions in greenhouse gas emissions and other co-pollutants.

Jessica Wentz

See Also: Climate Change and Human Health; Greenhouse Effect and Global Warming; Intergovernmental Panel on Climate Change; International Environmental Law and Policy; Sea Ice, Global Warming Implications for

Further Reading

Adoption of the Paris Agreement. Paris, France: UN Framework Convention on Climate Change, 2015.

Kyoto Protocol to the United Nations Framework Convention on Climate Change. Kyoto, Japan: United Nations, 1998.

UN Framework Convention on Climate Change. *Paris Agreement—Status of Ratification*. http://unfccc.int/2860.php (accessed April 29, 2017).

World Health Organization. *Climate Change and Human Health*. http://www.who.int/globalchange/en/ (accessed April 29, 2017).

V

VOLATILE ORGANIC COMPOUND POLLUTION

Volatile organic compounds (VOCs) are carbon containing compounds (excluding carbon monoxide, carbon dioxide, carbonic acid, metallic carbides or carbonates, and ammonium carbonate) that participate in atmospheric photochemical reactions, such as the formation of smog. VOCs can be emitted from a variety of sources, including car exhausts, gas stations, paint and printing shops, and many types of industrial operations, such as chemical manufacturing plants and refineries. VOCs typically enter the body through respiration (breathing) and can have significant effects on both short-term and long-term health. VOCs can cause headaches, nausea, and irritation of the eyes, nose, and throat. Beyond these immediate health risks, some VOCs are also thought to be mutagens (DNA-altering agents), and some may cause cancer.

VOCs can react with nitrogen to form ozone. Ozone is naturally found high in the earth's atmosphere, 10 to 50 miles (16 to 80 kilometers) above the earth's surface. This is the "good" ozone that provides a shield against harmful ultraviolet radiation produced by the sun. However, ozone can also be formed at ground level, where VOCs react with nitrogen oxides in the presence of sunlight. This ozone is a major component of urban smog. Human exposure to ozone can cause respiratory problems, lung damage, and exacerbation of other diseases. Children and the elderly are at most risk from ozone exposures. Children are more sensitive to the effects of ozone exposure because their lungs are still developing and they typically spend more time outside. Elderly people may be more prone to the negative effects of ozone because of preexisting conditions and weakened immune systems.

VOCs can be found both outside and inside. Building materials, such as new carpets or furniture, can release VOCs slowly, and the "new car smell" is from VOCs. Dry cleaning solutions, nail polish and its remover, degreasers, deodorizers, air fresheners, colognes, perfumes, and household cleaning products are all examples of substances that may give off VOCs. Some VOCs, such as benzene, toluene, and xylene, are more harmful than others. These chemicals can be found in gasoline, kerosene fuel oil, and other petroleum-based products. Acetone, isopropyl alcohol, and ethyl alcohol are VOCs found in some personal care products, and various adhesives emit the VOCs toluene, cyclohexane, and methyl ethyl ketone.

In workplaces where manufacturing occurs and the use of chemicals is commonplace, extra safeguards are needed to avoid exposure. Paint thinners, fabric cleaners, various adhesives, degreasers, plywood, and pesticides can all emit

VOCs. Frequency and time of exposure determine the effects of these compounds, some of which may cause debilitating diseases and even cancer. The Occupational Safety and Health Administration (OSHA) is responsible for rules addressing VOCs in the workplace.

Andrew P. Barefield

See Also: Air Pollution; Cancer Risk from Environmental Exposure; Indoor Environment; Occupational Safety and Health Administration; Ozone and Smog in the Urban Environment; Personal Care Products, Health Issues with

Further Reading

Moore, Julian P., ed. *Volatile Organic Compounds: Occurrence, Behavior, and Ecological Implications*. Hauppauge, NY: Nova Science Publishers, 2016.

Ozone and Your Health. Washington, DC: U.S. Environmental Protection Agency, 2009.

U.S. Environmental Protection Agency. *Technical Overview of Volatile Organic Compounds*. https://www.epa.gov/indoor-air-quality-iaq/technical-overview-volatile-organic-compounds (accessed May 8, 2017).

VULNERABLE POPULATIONS, ENVIRONMENTAL THREATS TO

It is well established that people living in close proximity to environmental pollution from power plants, factories, and motor vehicles are at greater risk of adverse health effects. The risk can be ameliorated by reducing the quantity of pollution, making it less toxic, or reducing exposure by moving to a less polluted area. However, in the United States and throughout the world, a new type of environmental health threat is emerging—climate change—that is harder to avoid, particular for the most vulnerable populations.

Climate change has the potential to affect the health of Americans by causing more extreme heat and other weather-related events, degrading ambient air quality, spreading waterborne and insect-borne diseases, threatening food safety and security, and inundating low-lying areas by sea level rise. The extent to which these environmental threats will occur depends on U.S. and global actions to reduce greenhouse gases, and in particular, on a willingness to replace power plants that burn fossil fuels with clean, renewable energy alternatives. Many scientists believe that significant climate change effects are already being observed in many regions of the world, and without urgent worldwide efforts to cut greenhouse gases, these effects will only worsen.

As you might imagine, the populations most vulnerable to climate change are those that are most sensitive to environmental change, least able to afford good medical care and other public services, and unable to relocate their homes to less affected areas. This includes low-income and minority people; children and pregnant women; older adults; recent immigrants experiencing a language barrier; people with disabilities; and those with underlying diseases such as asthma, diabetes, cardiovascular and kidney disease, and chronic obstructive pulmonary disease. Indigenous populations may also suffer from loss of cultural identity, as sacred lands are disrupted by drought, flooding, and thawing of permafrost, and as ceremonial practices are altered by loss of relevant plant and animal species.

To illustrate the potential for vulnerable populations to suffer disproportionately from climate change, consider the effects of extreme heat events. In the United States, low-income, minority, immigrant, and homeless people often inhabit our largest cities, where unusually hot weather is made worse by the heat island effect. These groups of people may be less likely to have well-insulated and air-conditioned homes, access to cooling centers and other public shelters, and adequate healthcare services, and these factors have undoubtedly contributed to an observed increase in heat-related illnesses and deaths during heat waves in some low-income and immigrant populations. Furthermore, air quality made worse by extreme heat has resulted in increased hospital and emergency room admissions for asthma attacks, shortness of breath, and cardiovascular and respiratory system distress. Cases of premature death have also been reported during these air pollution episodes.

Climate change effects can be even worse when environmental, socioeconomic, and demographic factors combine to threaten health while allowing for fewer healthcare options. Under these circumstances, populations may suffer not only from physical conditions but also from mental health problems. These challenges, already present today, will only worsen as climate change becomes more entrenched, with fewer options for halting and reversing the trend. It is not difficult to imagine that at some point in the future, a sense of desperation may set in among vulnerable populations as climate change accelerates, with fewer options for adapting to or avoiding its effects.

As demographics change, the number of most vulnerable people may also be altered. For example, minorities are expected to become a majority of the U.S. population by around 2043, and the number of older adults (age 65 and older) will nearly double between the years 2015 and 2050 as the baby boomer generation ages. At the same time, the effects of climate change are expected to become more apparent and disruptive over the next two to three decades, placing a greater strain on the nation's ability to cope its most vulnerable populations.

Of course, climate change is not limited to the United States, and the effects could be most severe in the poorest countries, where malnutrition and illness may become more prevalent and crops may fail. As people in sub-Saharan Africa and other impoverished areas are increasingly displaced by expanding deserts, more frequent floods, rising sea levels, and spreading diseases like malaria, they may have no option but to become environmental refugees—fleeing their homelands for places less affected by the changing climate, potentially leading to political unrest as their numbers swell. The irony is that those potentially most affected by climate change—poor people often living in the low latitudes who already suffer from malnutrition and disease—are least responsible for causing the problem, which largely originates with energy use and industrial operations in the developed nations.

Richard Crume

See Also: Climate Change and Human Health; Environmental Justice; Environmental Refugee; Greenhouse Effect and Global Warming; Heat Island Effect in Urban Areas; Heat Waves

Further Reading

Climate Change and Famine (Fact Sheet). Washington, DC: Physicians for Social Responsibility, 2017.

Communication Materials on Climate Change, Health, and Populations of Concern: Summary Points from the U.S. Climate and Health Assessment. Washington, DC: U.S. Environmental Protection Agency, 2016.

Gutierrez, Kristie S., and Catherine E. LePrevost. "Climate Justice in Rural Southeastern United States: A Review of Climate Change Impacts and Effects on Human Health." *International Journal of Environmental Research and Public Health*, vol. 13, no. 2 (February 2016): 189.

Health Implications of Global Warming: Impacts on Vulnerable Populations (Fact Sheet). Washington, DC: Physicians for Social Responsibility, 2013.

Human Rights Watch. *There Is No Time Left*. https://www.hrw.org/report/2015/10/15/there-no-time-left/climate-change-environmental-threats-and-human-rights-turkana (accessed March 24, 2017).

Levy, Barry S., and Jonathan A. Patz. "Climate Change, Human Rights, and Social Justice." *Annals of Global Health*, vol. 81, no. 3 (May–June 2015): 310–322.

UN Environmental Programme. *Our Planet: Empowering the Vulnerable*. http://web.unep.org/ourplanet/october-2016/articles/empowering-vulnerable (accessed March 24, 2017).

U.S. Global Change Research Program. *The Impacts of Climate Change on Human Health in the United States: A Scientific Assessment, Populations of Concern (Section 9)*. https://health2016.globalchange.gov/populations-concern (accessed March 24, 2017).

Wodon, Quentin. *Climate Change and Migration Evidence from the Middle East and North Africa*. Washington, DC: World Bank, 2014.

World Health Organization. *Environmental Health in Emergencies: Vulnerable Groups*. http://www.who.int/environmental_health_emergencies/vulnerable_groups/en (accessed March 24, 2017).

W

WASTE INCINERATION

Incinerators, where garbage is burned in a closed furnace, were created toward the end of the 19th century in England and were called "destructors." The first incinerator in the United States was built on New York's Governors Island in 1885. This method of garbage disposal was prevalent throughout the 1930s and 1940s, until environmental concerns and the cheaper cost of landfilling wastes outweighed the advantages of waste incineration. New York City and Los Angeles, in particular, had major problems with smog associated with incinerators and other air pollution sources, with bans on residential incinerators enacted in those cities in 1957 and 1971, respectively.

There were attempts in the 1980s to significantly increase the number of U.S. waste incinerators, with the intent of deriving energy from these units to generate steam or electricity. However, nationwide protests and environmental activism helped stall or kill many of these projects, with the slogan, "Not in My Backyard" (also known by its acronym, NIMBY), emerging. Today, NIMBY has become shorthand for a community's fight against undesirable infrastructure. Nevertheless, waste incineration survived, and today a number of waste incinerators are operating in the United States.

Incinerators can be harmful to the environment in several ways. The by-products of burning waste include air pollutants, such as dioxin and mercury, that are hazardous to human health. Other air pollutants contribute to urban smog and regional haze and are associated with lung and heart disease and other health problems. Expensive air pollution control equipment is required on waste incinerators to reduce the amount of air pollution to levels prescribed by state and federal regulations. Incinerators also create a toxic ash that needs to be managed carefully to avoid contaminating nearby water resources.

A mass-burn incinerator involves depositing the garbage in a large combustion chamber supplied with excess air to ensure good combustion. At many of these incinerators, garbage is unloaded by trucks into bunkers and then deposited into the furnace by crane, or alternatively, the garbage flows from the trucks along a conveyor belt. Two forms of ash are produced from incinerating garbage, "bottom ash" and "fly ash." The former is waste materials that is not completely burned, while the latter is particulate matter in the exhaust gas. Most of the bottom ash, as well as the fly ash collected by pollution control devices, is stored on-site or sent to landfills.

At a waste-to-energy incinerator, heat from burning the garbage is used to produce steam and to drive a turbine to produce electricity. For typical waste-to-energy incinerators, a ton of burned garbage produces about 550 kilowatt hours of electricity.

Nationwide, energy from U.S. incinerators powers the equivalent of 2 million homes. The U.S. Environmental Protection Agency considers waste-to-energy facilities to be a type of renewable energy source because of the continuous, never-ending flow of garbage. There are currently about 80 waste-to-energy incinerators in the United States.

Countries in northern Europe, such as Germany and Denmark, have relied on large incinerators to burn about one-third of their trash, and these incinerators are equipped with powerful pollution control devices to prevent most of the air pollution from entering the atmosphere. In contrast, Denmark has installed smaller incinerators, a strategy that helps reduce local impacts, and because the incinerators are located closer to communities, they are able to provide heat to homes and businesses. European countries also have efficient waste recycling programs, with some countries recycling up to two-thirds of their wastes.

Despite the availability of efficient pollution control technology, support for waste incineration in the United States remains low due to environmental concerns and construction costs, and the landfilling of wastes is usually less expensive. From an environmental health perspective, whether incineration versus the landfilling of waste is preferable is a complicated question requiring careful, case-by-case analysis of greenhouse gas emissions, toxic air emissions and controls, potential contamination of water resources, ash disposal alternatives, waste composition, availability of recycling programs, proximity to urban areas, and energy recovery options. Regardless of which disposal method is preferred, most experts agree that the best approach for waste management is to "reduce, reuse, and recycle."

Aaron Dorman

See Also: Dioxin Pollution; Environmental Protection Agency; Land Disposal of Waste Materials; Municipal Solid Waste Management; Ozone and Smog in the Urban Environment; Particulate Matter and Bioaerosols Pollution; Regional Haze Pollution; Respiratory Disease and Air Pollution; Three Rs of Waste Management

Further Reading

Humes, Edward. *Garbology: Our Dirty Love Affair with Trash.* New York: Avery, 2013.

Pyper, Julia. *Does Burning Garbage to Produce Electricity Make Sense? Scientific American*, New York, 2011. https://www.scientificamerican.com/article/does-burning-garbage-to-produce-energy-make-sense.

Rogers, Heather. *Gone Tomorrow: The Hidden Life of Garbage*. New York: New Press, 2006.

Suzuki, David, and Ian Hanington. *Incinerating Trash Is a Waste of Resources*. David Suzuki Foundation, Vancouver, Canada, 2013. http://www.davidsuzuki.org/blogs/science-matters/2013/09/incinerating-trash-is-a-waste-of-resources.

U.S. Environmental Protection Agency. *Energy Recovery from the Combustion of Municipal Solid Waste (MSW)*. https://www.epa.gov/smm/energy-recovery-combustion-municipal-solid-waste-msw (accessed December 23, 2016).

Williams, Timothy. "Garbage Incinerators Make Comeback, Kindling Both Garbage and Debate." *New York Times,* January 10, 2015, https://www.nytimes.com/2015/01/11/us/garbage-incinerators-make-comeback-kindling-both-garbage-and-debate.html.

Young, Gary C. *Municipal Solid Waste to Energy Conversion Processes: Economic, Technical, and Renewable Comparisons*. Hoboken, NJ: Wiley, 2010.

WATER CONSERVATION

Water conservation efforts aim to protect water resources for a sustainable future. In this context, water conservation refers specifically to freshwater resources. Water conservation includes how water resources are used and managed as well as how policies shape the use and management of water resources. Conservation of water resources is often closely associated with water-use efficiency, which is achieving the maximum productivity with minimal waste.

In a general sense, water conservation is related to environmental health because humans depend on clean water for various purposes, and many water conservation strategies change how humans use water. Using less water and creating less wastewater is usually considered an important water management strategy. However, some water conservation efforts have the potential to pose a public health threat if not carried out appropriately. For example, one method of water conservation is gray water recycling, which is the use of domestic wastewater (e.g., shower or laundry water) for a secondary purpose, such as watering a lawn. If the gray water used to water a lawn drains into a nearby creek, contamination of the creek with water used by humans could occur. Thus, we cannot take for granted that water conservation and water quality always go hand in hand.

Water supply is driven by what is referred to as water demand, which indicates how much water is needed. Water demand tends to increase with increasing population. While estimates vary, an average estimate of water use per person in the United States is about 100 gallons per day. As the population of a town or region increases, more water is required to satisfy the needs of more people. For example, the additional food consumed by an increasing population requires increased agricultural production, which tends to use large amounts of water. An increasing population also requires additional energy, which can also use water in large quantities, depending on the energy source. Because satisfying water demand depends on finite water resources, water conservation is one way to ensure that water is used efficiently and sustainably.

Water on the earth appears plentiful, covering about 70 percent of the earth's surface. However, almost all of the water on the earth is saltwater in the oceans, and only about 2.5 percent is freshwater suitable for humans use. Much of this freshwater is frozen in the icecaps of Greenland and Antarctica, and consequently, only about 1 percent of the water on the earth is easily accessible. This is why water is often referred to as a finite resource, which means the availability of water is limited and conservation may be needed to ensure an adequate supply.

This limited amount of the earth's freshwater is considered a vital resource that is essential for a variety of purposes, including human consumption, agricultural irrigation, energy production, sanitation and hygiene, and various industrial, commercial, and leisure activities. According to the U.S. Geological Survey, the top three uses of freshwater in the United States are thermoelectric power generation, irrigation, and public water supply. Realizing that water, a finite resource, has so many essential uses helps us put the importance of water conservation into perspective.

The top use of freshwater in the United States is for energy. This is often referred to as the water-energy nexus because water and energy are so intimately interconnected. It generally takes a large amount of water to produce energy, and a considerable amount of energy is needed to manage water resources. Water and wastewater utilities have programs in place to increase both energy and water efficiency.

Irrigation is the second most demanding sector for water. Several advances in irrigation practices have helped reduce the amount of water needed to achieve the same crop yield on farms. For example, converting from high-pressure to low-pressure irrigation systems has made a significant difference in water use. Additionally, watering at the appropriate time of day can reduce water that is lost to evaporation. There are many other good examples of how water has been conserved in agricultural irrigation practices.

At the residential level, water-efficient appliances, such as washing machines that use less water and low-flow toilets, can conserve water. Behavioral changes can aid in water conservation too, such as taking shorter showers or turning off water flow while lathering the soap in your hands or brushing your teeth. While estimates vary, research suggests that outdoor water use accounts for over half of residential water use. Effective outdoor water conservation measures include limiting lawn watering and planting native crops that are adapted to a region's natural precipitation patterns.

Urban areas are increasingly optimistic about implementing water conservation strategies. As urban populations increase, water demands are growing, and the supply infrastructure may not always be adequate. Consequently, most major cities in the United States have launched water conservation programs. For example, New York City has implemented several programs, including a Water Demand Management Plan, Municipal Water Efficiency Program, Residential Water Efficiency Program, and Upstate Water Conservation Program. Urban water conservation plans are often targeted to save water and energy, with the added advantage that consumers may spend less on their water bills.

One important uncertainty in planning for future water demands and the potential impact of water conservation involves the growing threat of climate change. There is overwhelming consensus in the scientific community that global warming will affect future climate patterns, including more severe droughts and flooding, which will ultimately impact water supplies. Many cities are incorporating water conservation into their water management plans to counter the potential effects of climate change.

A large number of city, state, and federal programs exist to achieve water conservation goals. Two notable examples are the WaterSense program, run by the U.S. Environmental Protection Agency (EPA), and the Energy Star program, which is a joint venture between the EPA and the U.S. Department of Energy. A number of organizations have formed to advocate for water efficiency, conservation, and education, such as the Alliance for Water Efficiency. Additionally, ongoing academic research aims to evaluate and improve water conservation efforts.

Elise C. Hunter

See Also: Drinking Water Quality and Regulation; Drought and Desertification, Health Consequences of; Energy Star; Environmental Protection Agency; Intensive Farming Practices and Health; Municipal Solid Waste Management; Safe Drinking Water Act; Water Reuse and Recycling

Further Reading

Department of Environmental Protection Commits $350,000 to Help Largest Upstate Wholesale Water Customers Develop Conservation Plans. New York City Department of Environmental Protection, New York, November 26, 2014. http://www.nyc.gov/html/dep/html/press_releases/14-095pr.shtml#.WaW8rNQjHcd.

Gies, Erica. "Turning to Water Conservation to Save Energy." *New York Times*, May 17, 2010, http://www.nytimes.com/2010/05/18/business/energy-environment/18iht-renwat.html.

Nagourney, Adam. "California Imposes First Mandatory Water Restrictions to Deal with Drought." *New York Times*, April 1, 2015, https://www.nytimes.com/2015/04/02/us/california-imposes-first-ever-water-restrictions-to-deal-with-drought.html.

Perrone, Debra, Jennifer Murphy, and George M. Hornberger. "Gaining Perspective on the Water-Energy Nexus at the Community Scale." *Environmental Science and Toxicology*, vol. 45, no. 10 (April 2011): 4228–4234.

U.S. Environmental Protection Agency. *Energy Star*. https://www.energystar.gov (accessed December 30, 2015).

U.S. Environmental Protection Agency. *WaterSense*. https://www.epa.gov/watersense/ (accessed December 30, 2015).

WATER POLLUTION

Safe and clean water is essential to human and environmental health. Water pollution is the contamination of waterbodies by chemical, physical, or disease-causing substances. According to World Health Organization (WHO), water pollution is considered a leading cause of death and disease worldwide. Water pollution also impacts the health of aquatic organisms, disrupts food chains, and destroys ecosystems.

Water pollution comes from a variety of sources, although most instances are a result of human intervention. Point-source water pollution refers to contamination

Arsenic in Bangladesh

The geological composition of aquifers can cause leaching of toxic elements into drinking water supplies. The main elements of concern are arsenic, fluoride, selenium, chromium, and uranium. In Bangladesh, arsenic-contaminated groundwater affects between 35 and 77 million people. Arsenicosis, or arsenic poisoning, symptoms can include skin problems and lesions, high blood pressure, and cancers of the bladder, kidney, and lungs. Approximately 1 in 100 people who drink arsenic-contaminated water (0.05 milligrams of arsenic per liter or greater) for a long period may eventually die from arsenic-related cancers.

originating from a single, identifiable source, such as a pipe or oil spill. Point-source pollutants typically are found near business, industry, agricultural, or urban sources. About 30 percent of the globally accessible freshwater is used by industry and municipalities. After processing, factories and sewage treatment plants discharge point-source wastewater, or effluents, directly into streams and rivers. In many parts of the world, these wastewaters are still untreated or else undergo treatment that does not effectively remove the majority of the pollutants.

When water pollution comes from many sources, it is considered nonpoint-source pollution. These diffuse pollutants often are associated with runoff from agricultural or urban areas. As stormwater flows over surfaces like pastures, parking lots, and lawns, it picks up chemicals and pollutants. This untreated water then flows directly into waterbodies. Large amounts of stormwater runoff can make small concentrations of pollutants, like fertilizer, sediment, and trash, a serious problem. All types of waterbodies, including lakes, streams, oceans, and groundwater, are susceptible to point-source and nonpoint-source pollution. Management and prevention of pollution is highly dependent on source type as well as the type of pollution.

Pollutants can be classified according to their chemical, physical, or disease-causing contaminants. Regardless of whether chemicals are naturally occurring or introduced by human interference, their concentrations and toxicities determine the degree of contamination and health hazard. Some chemical pollutants cause acute illnesses, while others damage human health (and the health of other organisms) over long periods, and some man-made chemical pollutants can be dangerous to human health even at low concentrations.

Common chemical pollutants include nutrients (nitrogen and phosphorus) from agricultural runoff, heavy metals from mining activities, toxic synthetic organics from pesticides, and radioactive waste. The sources and impacts of these common pollutants are reasonably well understood, but designing sustainable treatment technologies for them remains a challenge. For example, nutrients enter the environment from a wide range of human activities (agriculture, stormwater, wastewater, and residential runoff) that are difficult to pinpoint and reduce. High nutrient concentrations can lead to increased production of biomass, oxygen depletion, and toxic algal blooms.

Another source of chemical pollutants is gold mining by chemical extraction using mercury amalgamation (the process of merging gold and mercury for easier recovery of the precious metal). About 13 million miners in 55 countries increasingly practice this mining approach. During the process, waste mercury is discharged into the environment, including surface water, where it biomagnifies and then presents a health risk to indigenous populations. (Biomagnification is the increasing concentration of a substance in the tissues of organisms at successively higher levels in a food chain.) People are exposed to mercury by eating contaminated fish and wildlife that are at the top of aquatic food chains. When concentrations in humans are high enough, the mercury may act as a neurotoxin, causing harm to the brain and nervous system. Mercury exposure is especially dangerous to pregnant women and young children.

Persistent organic pollutants (POPs) are chemicals that are of great environmental concern. These chemicals persist for long periods and can bioaccumulate, passing from one species to the next through the food chain. Many of these toxic chemicals have proved beneficial in pest and disease control, crop production, and industrial manufacturing. These same chemicals, however, are believed to effect human health and the environment. For example, some of these chemicals are very similar to human hormones and are called endocrine disruptors, which may cause human developmental problems, deformations, and cancers. Well-known POPs, such as PCBs, DDT, and dioxins, are now highly regulated and are no longer produced in the United States.

Radioactive substances represent a small portion of chemical pollutants, although the associated health hazards could be significant. The degree of health concern is determined by the concentration of the contaminants, energy of the radiation being emitted, type of radiation, duration of exposure, and proximity of the contamination to the human body. Ingestion of radioactive contamination can cause cell death, genetic mutations, cancers, birth defects, and reproductive, immune, and endocrine system disorders. Radioactive contamination sources include nuclear power plants and research facilities, phosphate fertilizer, and naturally occurring nuclides in rocks and soil.

Unlike chemicals, physical pollutants alter the physical properties of the water, such as temperature and turbidity (water clarity or cloudiness). Thermal pollution changes the ambient water temperature and can be caused by the release coolant water by industrial facilities or by urban stormwater runoff. Elevated temperatures reduce dissolved oxygen concentrations, which can harm aquatic organism. As a result, food chains can be disrupted and biodiversity decreased. Excessive sediment, resulting from overintensive land-use practices, is considered the leading cause of pollution in rivers and streams in the United States, where sediment pollution causes approximately $16 billion in environmental damage annually. Sediment blocks sunlight, destroys habitat, and clogs fish gills, ultimately disrupting the natural food chain and altering water flow.

Disease-causing microorganisms, or pathogens, are often found in waters contaminated with human or animal feces. According to the WHO, 3.4 million people, mostly children, die from water-related diseases each year. High levels of pathogens may result from inadequate treatment of sewage discharge or poorly managed livestock. This is a common problem in developing countries, where many areas lack sanitation systems altogether. In Africa and Southeast Asia, cholera and typhoid fever are the primary causes of infant mortality. Although water-associated diseases are more prevalent in areas with inadequate sanitation, they are also a serious challenge in developed countries. Compiled data of disease outbreaks in the United States (1986–2000) indicate nearly 6,000 cases and 100 outbreaks associated with contaminated recreational water and over 400,000 cases and approximately 50 outbreaks caused by contaminated drinking water. Two common disease agents are *giardia lamblia* and *cryptosporidium*, both of which are parasitic, single-celled organisms common in the fecal material of many mammals.

The main cause of water pollution is improper management of water resources. The WHO as well as individual national governments have adopted strategies to manage water quality, with the goal of protecting and promoting human health. These agencies work to improve access to safe drinking water and sanitation and to encourage behavioral changes. It is estimated that over the years, better water management has provided 2.6 billion people access to an improved drinking-water source, although improved sources are not necessarily safe.

In the United States, water pollution reached crisis proportions by the early 1970s. This resulted in Congress passing the 1972 Clean Water Act, with the main objective "to restore and maintain the chemical, physical and biological integrity of the Nation's waters." The act requires regulation of point-source pollution through limitations set by the U.S. Environmental Protection Agency. Industrial, municipal, and other facilities must obtain a National Pollutant Discharge Elimination System permit to legally discharge pollutants into a waterbody. Additionally, under Section 303(d) of the act, states, territories, and authorized tribes are required to develop lists of impaired waters that are too polluted or degraded to provide acceptable water quality. The law requires jurisdictions to establish priority rankings for waters on these lists and develop Total Maximum Daily Loads (TMDL). A TMDL is a calculation of the maximum amount of a pollutant that a waterbody can receive and still safely meet water quality standards. The act was later expanded to include section 319, which aids jurisdictions in reducing non-point source pollution by granting money to support a wide range of nonpoint source management programs. To tackle drinking water quality, the Safe Drinking Water Act was passed in 1974 and stands as the principal federal law to ensure safe drinking water for the public by setting national health-based standards for both naturally occurring and man-made contaminants.

Remediating global water pollution requires an effective set of policies, technologies, and scientific advances. Water, unlike many other natural resources, does not have a substitute. Restoring and protecting the quality of water, therefore, is of highest priority. With more than one-third of the earth's accessible renewable freshwater used for agricultural, industrial, and domestic purposes, and with most of these activities leading to water contamination, water pollution will continue to be a major societal concern.

Chelsea N. Peters

See Also: Arsenic Pollution; Bioaccumulation of Environmental Contaminants; Clean Water Act; Combined Sewer Overflow; DDT Exposure; Deepwater Horizon Incident; Drinking Water Quality and Regulation; Great Lakes Pollution; Groundwater Pollution and Depletion; Mercury Pollution; National Estuary Program; National Pollution Discharge Elimination System; Oil Spills, Health Consequences of; Persistent, Bioaccumulating, and Toxic Chemicals; Pesticides and Herbicides; Polychlorinated Biphenyls; Radiation, Ionizing and Nonionizing; Radiation Sickness; Radioactive Wastes; Safe Drinking Water Act; Sewage Treatment and Disposal; Stormwater Runoff; Thermal Pollution; Waterborne Diseases; Watershed Management, Health Implications of; Wetlands and Healthy Waterways; World Health Organization

Further Reading

Schwarzenbach, Rene P., et al. "Global Water Pollution and Human Health." *Annual Review of Environment and Resources*, vol. 35 (2010): 109–136.

Singh, Prati P., and Vinod Sharma. *Water and Health.* New Delhi, India: Springer India, 2014.

U.S. Environmental Protection Agency. *Federal Water Pollution Control Act, 33 U.S.C. §1251 et seq. (1972).* (Also known as the Clean Water Act.) http://www.epa.gov/laws-regulations/summary-clean-water-act (accessed January 1, 2016).

U.S. Environmental Protection Agency. *National Pollutant Discharge Elimination System (NPDES).* http://www.epa.gov/npdes (accessed January 1, 2016).

U.S. Environmental Protection Agency. *Pollution Prevention and Control.* http://water.epa.gov/polwaste/ (accessed August 31, 2015)

Vigil, Kenneth M. *Clean Water: An Introduction to Water Quality and Water Pollution Control.* Corvallis, WA: Oregon State University Press, 2003.

World Health Organization. *Health Topics: Water.* http://www.who.int/topics/water/en/ (accessed August 31, 2015).

WATER REUSE AND RECYCLING

Water is fundamental to life. Not only do humans need it to survive, but virtually every human activity requires water. For example, manufacturing facilities, power plants, oil and gas refineries, and agricultural operations all rely on water to produce the food we eat, the energy we rely on, and the products we buy. Agriculture alone accounts for approximately 80 percent of daily U.S. water consumption. Water reuse and recycling is essential to having a healthful and plentiful supply of water, particularly as water uses continue to grow. ("Recycling" and "reuse" are generally considered synonymous terms.)

Increasing population, especially in arid regions, and growing threats of severe drought due to climate change have boosted the demand for freshwater and made water conservation efforts more urgent. Finding ways to safely and effectively reuse wastewater increases the supply of freshwater and may also improve water quality, protecting the environment and human health and providing economic benefits.

Ensuring Future Clean Water Supplies

With worldwide population growth, particularly in urban areas, and climate change threatening more severe and prolonged droughts, public water supplies are becoming increasingly stressed. One solution to this problem involves the concept of direct potable reuse (DPR), where treated municipal wastewater meeting drinking water standards is introduced to a water treatment plant or channeled directly into a water distribution system. The technology is currently available, and many communities in the United States are beginning to explore the possibilities. (In 2013, Big Springs, Texas, became the first U.S. town to implement DPR.) Although overcoming the "yuck" factor may be a challenge, DPR could become commonplace in the future as water supplies become increasingly threatened.

Virtually any water that flows into a sewer or is discharged from an industrial facility can be reused. One example is sewage from our toilets that is channeled to a wastewater treatment plant, representing a potential source of reusable water for many cities. We already practice a form of wastewater reuse when upstream wastewater treatment plants discharge treated water to a river while downstream populations draw drinking water from that river. However, this type of unplanned reuse is not as efficient as planned projects to reuse water.

Currently, most planned water reuse projects involve using domestic wastewater for purposes other than drinking water. This includes water for irrigation, landscaping, and industrial uses. Because domestic wastewater typically contains only about 0.1 percent solid waste, the remaining 99.9 percent can be treated and safely reused. Recycled water often is treated only enough to satisfy the needs of its intended use, avoiding end users the cost of unnecessary further treatment.

One example of domestic wastewater reuse comes from Honolulu, Hawaii. The city has constructed a water reuse facility that filters and further treats effluent (the polluted discharge) from its wastewater treatment plant and then uses that water for golf course, agriculture, and landscaping irrigation and for industrial purposes. This results in decreased reliance on fresh drinking water supplies. Additionally, the treatment plant discharges less wastewater into the Pacific Ocean, resulting in a cleaner ocean environment.

Reuse of gray water has also become more popular and can have substantial environmental benefits. Gray water refers to water in offices or homes that has not come in contact with human or animal waste, for example, water from kitchen sinks, washing machines, and showers. This water can be safely reused on-site, with little or no additional treatment, for irrigating lawns and landscaping and flushing toilets, thereby reducing the amount of fresh drinking water typically used for these purposes.

Some areas are now considering direct potable reuse (DPR), where wastewater is treated with advanced technologies and then pumped directly into a drinking water treatment plant or supply system. Of course, the water must meet all drinking water quality standards before it is distributed to the drinking water system. DPR has been used successfully both internationally and in the United States. Although some people are concerned about drinking wastewater, it can be entirely safe to drink if properly treated and handled. The technologies associated with water reuse are sufficiently advanced such that regulatory authorities have recognized that safe, reliable drinking water can be produced from wastewater. However, cost can be a limiting factor for DPR.

Recycled water is also used to recharge underground aquifers (sources of underground drinking water) in a process known as indirect potable reuse. When underground sources of drinking water become depleted, injecting clean water into them can replenish the supply. In coastal areas, this can be especially important because saltwater can migrate into aquifers if there is insufficient freshwater to keep it out. For these purposes, recycled water is treated, typically to drinking water standards, and then injected into wells or placed in recharge ponds, where the treated water filters through soil before moving into the aquifer. This injected water can later be recovered from the aquifer for human consumption.

Many states, tribes, and other authorities have regulations addressing recycled water use and treatment, and the U.S. Environmental Protection Agency has developed comprehensive water reuse guidelines to support these regulations and facilitate further development of water reuse practices.

Leah A. Dundon and Richard S. Davis

See Also: Drinking Water Quality and Regulation; Drought and Desertification, Health Consequences of; Environmental Protection Agency; Groundwater Pollution and Depletion; Industrial Effluents; Recycling; Sewage Treatment and Disposal; Water Conservation

Further Reading

Guidelines for Water Reuse (EPA/600/R-12/618). Washington, DC: U.S. Environmental Protection Agency, 2012.

Idelovitch, Emanuel. *SAT (Soil Aquifer Treatment)—The Long-Term Performance of the Dan Region Reclamation Project (Presentation)*. Washington, DC: The World Bank, 2003.

Johnson, Ted. "Using Recycled Water for Groundwater Recharge in the Central and West Coast Basins—A Successful History." *Water Replenish District (Southern California) Technical Bulletin*, vol. 16 (Spring 2008).

Raucher, Bob. *The Opportunities and Economics of Direct Potable Reuse (White Paper)*. Alexandria, VA: WateReuse, 2014.

U.S. Department of Agriculture. *Irrigation and Water Use*. http://www.ers.usda.gov/topics/farm-practices-management/irrigation-water-use.aspx (accessed October 1, 2015).

U.S. Environmental Protection Agency. *Water Recycling and Reuse: The Environmental Benefits*. http://www3.epa.gov/region09/water/recycling/ (accessed October 1, 2015).

WATERBORNE DISEASES

Water is essential for life on the earth. However, water can also be a source of illness when contaminated with pathogenic (disease-causing) organisms or toxic elements. A wide variety of waterborne diseases are caused when certain bacteria, protozoa, viruses, parasites, and metabolic toxins are present in water. These agents cause disease when they are ingested as contaminated water or food, come in contact with skin, or are inhaled as water vapor. The most common type of illness they cause is gastrointestinal diarrhea disorders. However, some waterborne agents may cause skin disease, ear, nose, and throat problems, respiratory disease, or neurological disorders. The severity of waterborne disease can range from mild to potentially fatal, depending on the particular disease agent, the level of exposure, and the ability of the person or animal to respond to the infection or toxin. The World Health Organization estimates that waterborne disease globally accounts for 1.5 million human deaths annually, with 58 percent of those due to unsafe water supply and lack of sanitation and hygiene. The importance of waterborne disease has grown in recent years due to several factors: more people are susceptible to

Sensitivity to Waterborne Pathogens

It is estimated that 20 to 25 percent of Americans are more susceptible to illness, including waterborne diseases, than the average population. This includes the elderly, the very young, those with chronic illness, and those with compromised immune systems from diseases (e.g., AIDS) or medical therapy (e.g., chemotherapy or organ transplants). These sensitive subpopulations are more likely to experience illness from exposure to low levels of waterborne pathogens that would not otherwise cause illness. This manifests in higher rates of disease, medical treatment, hospitalizations, and deaths among sensitive populations.

illnesses, diseases are spread more easily with rapid global commerce, the increasing virulence of microbes, and changing environmental conditions that favor more waterborne disease outbreaks.

People and animals can be exposed to different waterborne pathogens through a variety of contaminated water sources. These sources include contaminated treated drinking water; treated swimming pool or bathing water; untreated ambient waters in lakes, streams, and oceans; and exposure to contaminated industrial waters (e.g., cooling systems in buildings). The most common exposures occur from drinking water that is contaminated due to either the failure or absence of effective water treatment practices. In spite of strict water treatment requirements, there are still millions of cases of waterborne diseases each year of various etiologies (causes). The actual disease burden is not known since so many cases go unreported. However, U.S. federal agencies have been tracking significant waterborne disease outbreaks for several decades. Between 1971 and 2002, they reported on 764 waterborne disease outbreaks associated with drinking water. Of those outbreaks, 12 percent were caused by chemicals, 14 percent by bacteria, 19 percent by protozoa, and 8 percent by viruses. However, in nearly half of the outbreaks since 1971, they were not able to identify the cause and were simply labeled as unknown acute gastrointestinal illness. The undiagnosed cases are often thought to be viral in origin, but that is difficult to verify. Those 764 outbreaks resulted in over 575,000 cases of illness and 79 deaths. However, the actual incidence of waterborne disease is likely much higher due to lack of medical care and nonreporting. One study estimated that as many as 7 million people may fall ill each year from waterborne microbial infections, with up to 1,000 deaths per year in the United States.

Recreational water use is another significant source of waterborne illness. This can occur both in treated waterbodies, such as swimming pools and hot tubs, and in open ambient water in rivers, lakes, and oceans. Exposures in treated water are generally caused by inadequate water treatment or unsafe behaviors by users, such as fecal contamination of the pool. Exposures in natural water bodies are often associated with heavy rainfall events that raise the level of pathogen load in the water body through polluted stormwater runoff or failure of sewer lines or septic systems. In 2010, a rare natural event allowed researchers to study the rate of waterborne disease in triathlon swimmers in the oceans off Denmark and Norway. They compared the disease incidence in swimmers for the same triathlon race on two separate dates: one race following a major rainfall event and the other following a normal dry period. The rate of disease was 42 percent in the group that swam following the heavy rain and only 8 percent in the control group, for which rainfall did not precede the race. Infections in this study included *Campylobacter, Giardia lamblia*, and diarrhea-causing *Escherichia coli*. This and other studies have confirmed that there is risk to swimmers in contaminated freshwater or seawater.

Currently, more than 140 microorganisms have been recognized as waterborne pathogens able to cause disease from contaminated water sources. A variety of types of microorganisms, parasites, and toxins are capable of causing disease. The most common agents are protozoa, bacteria, and viruses. In addition, there are helminth parasites (worms), toxic algae, and other biotoxins that may also cause waterborne disease.

Protozoan parasites are single-celled organism that are frequently associated with diarrheal disease. They live in the intestinal tract of people and animals and are spread by fecal contamination. Their reproductive oocysts are resistant to conventional disinfectants used in water treatment and thus can persist in treated drinking water supplies. The two most common protozoa diagnosed are *Giardia* and *Cryptosporidium*, both of which have caused significant disease outbreaks in the United States.

- *Giardia* is a protozoan parasite and is the most common pathogen diagnosed in waterborne outbreaks. It can be found in water, soil, and food.
- *Cryptosporidium* (Crypto) is a single-celled protozoan parasite that infects people and animals. It can cause infection by ingestion or skin contact with water or soil.

Bacteria are the second most common cause of waterborne disease. As a group, they are more sensitive to water treatment practices and most often cause disease through direct fecal contamination or failure of a treatment system. Examples of these single-celled organisms and the illnesses they can cause include *Salmonella* (diarrhea and typhoid), *Shigella* (diarrhea), *Campylobacter* (diarrhea and nervous system disorders), *Vibrio cholera* (diarrhea and skin infections), *Escherichia coli* (pathogenic strains: diarrhea and hemorrhagic colitis), and *Legionella* (pneumonia and respiratory infections).

- *Escherichia coli* is a normal part of healthy intestinal bacterial flora. However, there are a number of pathogenic strains of *E. coli* that cause illnesses ranging from mild diarrhea to serious disease. The most virulent strain is *E. coli O157:H7*, which causes hemorrhagic colitis in its most severe form. The typical exposure is through contaminated food or water, especially from cattle, deer, sheep, and goats. It can be life-threatening in children and other susceptible individuals.
- *Salmonella* can cause serious, sometimes chronic diarrheal disease in people and animals, also known as typhoid fever.

- *Shigella* causes a disease called shigellosis, primarily in humans and other primates.
- *Campylobacter* causes a diarrheal illness and is mostly found in poultry, other animals, and people.
- *Vibrio cholera* is commonly associated with coastal marine waters and shellfish. It can also be transported in ship ballast water. Exposure occurs from ingesting contaminated water, eating raw shellfish, especially oysters, or entry through a wound in the skin. It causes cholera, which is resistant to antibiotics and can cause fever, chills, skin infections, and life-threatening septicemia.
- *Legionella* is associated with inhalation of contaminated water vapor from industrial sources, such as cooling systems in buildings. It causes two types of respiratory disease: Legionnaire's disease (severe pneumonia) and Pontiac disease (influenza-like disease).

Viral pathogens also frequently cause waterborne illnesses. Most of these viruses are in the enterovirus family (intestinal viruses), which colonize the intestinal tract and damage cells, causing inflammation, vomiting, and diarrhea. Some viruses can survive weeks or months in water and still cause disease. Viral infections in people are often self-limiting and of short duration, but they can be serious in sensitive individuals. More virulent viruses can also cause meningitis, myocarditis, respiratory disease, and nervous system disorders. Examples of the more common waterborne viral agents are hepatitis A (inflammation of the liver), Norovirus (diarrhea), Rotavirus (diarrhea, especially in children), plus astroviruses, adenoviruses, and other enteroviruses.

Biotoxins are another type of waterborne pathogen. They are most often associated with harmful algal blooms that occur with excessive nutrient water pollution and warmer, stagnant waters. Harmful algal blooms are becoming more frequent and disruptive, especially in the Great Lakes region and along the Florida coastlines. The biotoxins released from the thick algal mats pose a serious risk to people and aquatic life. They also disrupt use of source waters for drinking water treatment and have caused water shortages until eliminated from the area.

Helminth parasites are worms, such as trematodes (tapeworms) and cestodes (flukes), that infect people and animals. In many cases, these helminths have life cycle stages that involve an intermediate host animal, such as an aquatic snail or copepods, before they reach their final host in either people or other animals. They may exist free in the water for part of their life cycle and tend to be resistant to water treatment techniques. The diseases they cause vary with each agent, ranging from intestinal colonization to skin infections to invasion of nasal passages or eyes.

Many of these waterborne diseases are zoonotic disease agents, meaning that the disease can be transmitted between (or shared by) both animals and humans. The transmission potentially goes both ways for many bacteria, protozoa, viruses, and parasites. This means that wildlife, livestock, companion animals, and people share many of the same waterborne diseases. Examples of zoonotic waterborne parasites includes *Giardia, Cryptosporidium, Blastocystis, microsporidia, toxoplasma, Cyclospora*, amoeba, trematodes, cestodes, and others.

In rural communities, where open fields may be used to spread untreated livestock waste or biosolids from treated municipal sewage, this becomes a ready source for fecal contamination downstream during heavy rainfall events. Some outbreaks have occurred in cities where a major rainfall or spill from a manure lagoon has occurred in an upstream rural location. The largest outbreak in U.S. history occurred in the city of Milwaukee when an epidemic of *Cryptosporidium* protozoan parasites sickened over 400,000 people in the spring of 1993. The Milwaukee water source is Lake Michigan, and it was speculated that the water source in Milwaukee harbor was polluted by upstream cattle, slaughterhouses, or possibly human sewage. The waters of the Great Lakes continue to be at risk from various waterborne microorganisms and toxins, especially in light of increasingly warm waters and extreme rains sending excessive contamination of nutrients and fecal material into the lake ecosystem. Harmful algal blooms with exposure to algal toxins is another ongoing risk in the Great Lakes and other lakes around the country.

The factors that cause a waterborne disease outbreak involve much more than just the pathogen. When considering any waterborne disease, it is important to understand their full life cycle and the interrelationships with the ecosystem and organisms that are susceptible to their pathogenic effects. An outbreak happens as a result of complex interactions between weather conditions, water quality and quantity, presence or absence of treatment practices, occurrence of a pathogen, the immune competence of the patient, and the ultimate incidence of disease. Water quality is very closely associated with a variety of environmental conditions, including air and water temperature, extreme precipitation patterns (flood or drought), the land use of the watershed that drains to the source water, and the nature of contaminants carried by rainfall into streams, lakes, and reservoirs. Water temperature is a sensitive parameter, and many pathogens or toxic algae thrive in warmer waters while native aquatic species are often harmed by warmer waters with lower oxygen levels.

The strongest environmental influences on disease outbreaks are heavy rainfall events that result in large volumes of stormwater runoff flowing into lakes and streams. This runoff often carries heavy loads of pathogens and chemicals picked up across the landscape on its way to the body of water. A number of studies have shown a consistent correlation between heavy rainfall and outbreaks of waterborne disease. Intense rain and flooding reduces water quality in three main ways: direct contamination with fecal material from stormwater runoff into surface and groundwater sources, infiltration of contaminated runoff into drinking water lines due to aging infrastructure, and combined sewer overflow events that overwhelm the drainage system and send raw sewage directly into nearby rivers and streams. The high volumes of water and pathogens can temporarily overwhelm water treatment facilities and lead to contaminated finished drinking water.

Many studies have also documented an association between increased turbidity (cloudiness) of water sources and increased rates of pediatric illness. Higher turbidity levels can decrease the effectiveness of water purification methods and increase the pathogen load in the water supply. These associations with heavy rainfall and increased turbidity are of increasing importance with changing climate conditions. More frequent intense precipitation and flooding events are already occurring in every region, and that pattern is projected to increase in future decades. The combination of heavy rainfall, warmer waters, and increasing rates of land disturbance from farming or development is causing more erosion and turbidity. This, along with greater pathogen contamination, is setting the stage for higher rates of disease on a regular basis in the future. Understanding the environmental factors contributing to disease outbreaks is important for developing methods to predict and mitigate increased risks in the future.

The variety and complexity of different waterborne diseases make it difficult to identify simple prevention measures that benefit most of the causes of illness. General prevention methods primarily hinge on vigilant surveillance of bodies of water and disease incidence in the population. Beyond surveillance, it is important to take a system-wide approach to understanding the multifactorial nature of these disease outbreaks. These outbreaks take a serious toll on social and economic resources of society. A multidisciplinary "one health" approach may be beneficial to reducing adverse effects. Outbreaks occur when the conditions are right for ecological systems, weather conditions, water quality and quantity, animal health, human health, water treatment systems, and watershed conditions. Prevention efforts could be improved with a collaborative structure involving ecologists, public health agencies, veterinary health professionals, water utilities, agricultural agencies, stormwater managers, recreational leaders, and facility operators to work together to educate water users and optimize systems to protect human, animal, and ecological health.

Gwen Griffith

See Also: Cholera; Climate Change and Human Health; Drinking Water Quality and Regulation; *Escherichia coli (E. coli)* Infection; Infectious Diseases; Legionnaires' Disease; Norovirus Infection; Stormwater Runoff; Water Pollution; World Health Organization; Zoonotic Diseases

Further Reading

Collier, S.A., et al. "Direct Healthcare Costs of Selected Diseases Primarily or Partially Transmitted by Water." *Epidemiology and Infection*, vol. 140, no. 11 (November 2012): 2003–2013.

Harder-Lauridsen, Nina M., et al. "Gastrointestinal Illness among Triathletes Swimming in Non-Polluted versus Polluted Seawater Affected by Heavy Rainfall." *PLOS ONE*, vol. 8, no. 11 (November 2013): e78371.

Healthy Swimming. Centers for Disease Control and Prevention, Atlanta, GA, 2017. https://www.cdc.gov/healthywater/swimming/index.html.

Portier, C.J., et al. "Chapter 10: Waterborne Diseases." In *A Human Health Perspective on Climate Change: A Report Outlining the Research Needs on the Human Health Effects of Climate Change*, edited by Kimberly Thigpen Tart, 51–55. Research Triangle Park, NC: National Institute of Environmental Health Sciences, 2010.

Ralston, E.P., H. Kite-Powell, and A. Beet. "An Estimate of the Cost of Acute Health Effects from Food- and Water-Borne Marine Pathogens and Toxins in the USA." *Journal of Water Health*, vol. 9, no. 4 (December 2011): 680–694.

Reynolds, K.A., K.D. Mena, and C.P. Gerba. "Risk of Waterborne Illness via Drinking Water in the United States." *Reviews of Environmental Contamination and Toxicology*, vol. 192 (2008): 117–158.

WATERSHED MANAGEMENT, HEALTH IMPLICATIONS OF

Watershed management is the process of creating and implementing plans to protect watershed functions within the watershed boundary itself. The objective of watershed management is to sustain and enhance a watershed's ability to provide goods and services to the communities that depend on it. Using watersheds as basic organizing units allows effective management of mutually dependent interactions in a dynamic system. Healthy watersheds provide ecosystem, economic, and physical and mental health benefits, and the goods and services made possible by healthy watersheds are essential to social, environmental, and economic well-being.

Most natural resource problems are transboundary in nature, that is, they are intermunicipal, interstate, or international. Thus, there is rarely a single institution with legal jurisdiction over a natural resource. Natural resources, especially water, can cross recognized political boundaries, thereby creating situations where one jurisdiction's approach to resource management may not consider effects on neighboring jurisdictions. Watershed management addresses this problem by promoting a holistic, problem-solving approach that includes engagement with a variety of community stakeholders.

The U.S. Environmental Protection Agency (EPA) defines a watershed as a geographic area in which water drains to a common outlet, typically a point on a stream, lake, aquifer, estuary, or ocean. Watershed management is not limited to water supply, water quality, and water rights issues but extends to the overall planning and use of watersheds, including hydrological, geographical, geological, and biological aspects. Landowners, land-use agencies, stormwater management experts, environmental specialists, water-use surveyors, and communities all play an integral part in watershed management.

Watershed Management in New York City

New York City, the largest city in the United States, chose watershed protection over a more expensive filtration plant. The city was faced with an estimated $6 billion in capital costs and at least $300 million in annual operating and maintenance costs for the filtration plant. Instead, New York City opted to reduce its costs by negotiating a watershed protection program with state, federal, and environmental stakeholders, as well as with 70 watershed towns and villages. The program required a comprehensive watershed protection initiative in the Catskill-Delaware watershed, which supplies 90 percent of the New York City's drinking water.

Watershed management aims to regain healthy components of the landscape and ecosystem in disturbed watersheds. The health of a watershed can be defined by its landscape condition, biotic communities, ecological processes, water chemistry, and hydrologic and geomorphic processes. Together, these aspects support a healthy watershed.

There are many benefits to healthy watersheds. These benefits are called ecosystem services. Examples of these services include nutrient cycling, erosion control, increased biodiversity, soil formation, amelioration of air pollution, enhanced wildlife movement, water filtration, flood control, water storage, provisioning of food and timber, recreation, and finally, reduced vulnerability to invasive species, the effects of climate change, and other natural disasters. Watershed management seeks to sustainably protect and enhance these services in a sustainable manner within the watershed geographical boundary.

Healthy watersheds provide sufficient amounts of clean water required for aquatic ecosystems, habitat for fish and wildlife, drinking water, and recreation. This clean water has direct implications for the health and well-being of communities. For example, by preserving the ability of natural landscapes to filter pollutants, communities can reduce costs of drinking water treatment while ensuring a healthy drinking water supply. According to the National Resource Council, two-thirds of the U.S. population consumes water originating from forested lands. Precipitation in these areas infiltrates into the ground, where roots, soil, and sediments remove many of the impurities in the water. Through this process, toxins, excess nutrients, and sediments can be filtered before the water reaches a source of drinking water. A recent study found that about half of the variation in water treatment costs among municipalities could be explained by the area of forest cover in the water source area. Thus, a healthy watershed often means lower treatment costs as well as cleaner water.

Healthy watersheds can also help reduce vulnerability to climate change and natural disasters. Watersheds with sufficient natural land cover and soil resources can store significant amounts of carbon, helping to offset greenhouse gas emissions. Forest trees absorb carbon dioxide, ground-level ozone, carbon monoxide, and other greenhouse gases. It is estimated that the world's forests absorb as much as 30 percent of the annual global anthropogenic carbon dioxide emissions. Furthermore, intact floodplains and riparian zones are better adapted to changes in precipitation and floods. The EPA estimates that floods cause an average of $8 billion in damage every year in the Unites States. And according to the National Oceanic Atmospheric Administration, floods also cause an average of 70–80 U.S. fatalities annually. Healthy watersheds reduce the area and impact of floods by preventing runoff from moving rapidly across the landscape, often storing excess water.

There are social and health benefits to living in healthy environments. Proximity to green space and nature encourages physical exercise and provides mental stress relief. Evidence suggests that workplaces with views of green space have employees who report fewer incidences of illness, and the positive influences of green space may extend beyond general health by influencing the degree of social interaction, level of mental fatigue, and number of opportunities for reflection. It is even thought that urban green space users have greater longevity. The World Health Organization defines "health" as being a state of complete physical, mental, and social well-being, not only the absence of disease. This key public health concept of well-being encompasses a wide array of biological, sociological, economic, environmental, and cultural factors, some of which are addressed by watershed management.

The EPA implemented its Healthy Watersheds Initiative as an integrated, systems-based approach to watershed protection. The initiative aims to meet the Clean Water Act Section 101(a) objective of restoring and maintaining the chemical, physical, and biological integrity of U.S. waters. Because the rate at which new waters are being listed for water quality impairments exceeds the pace at which these waters can be remediated, the initiative provides support for state watershed programs, integrates watershed policies into national programs, and increases public awareness through outreach programs.

Chelsea N. Peters

See Also: Clean Water Act; Deforestation; Drinking Water Quality and Regulation; Environmental Protection Agency; Green Space in Urban Environments; National Oceanic and Atmospheric Administration; Natural Disasters; Safe Drinking Water Act; Stormwater Runoff

Further Reading

Davies, John-Mark, and Asit Mazumder. "Health and Environmental Policy Issues in Canada: The Role of Watershed Management in Sustaining Clean Drinking Water Quality at Surface Sources." *Journal of Environmental Management*, vol. 68, no. 3 (July 2003): 273–286.

Goldfarb, William. "Watershed Management: Slogan or Solution?" *Boston College Environmental Affairs Law Review*, vol. 21, no. 3 (1994): 483–509.

Hanson, Craig, John Talberth, and Logan Yonavjak. *Forests for Water: Exploring Payments for Watershed Services in the U.S. South (Issue Brief 2)*. Washington, DC: World Resources Institute, 2011.

Healthy Watersheds Initiative: National Framework and Action Plan. Washington, DC: U.S. Environmental Protection Agency, 2011.

Millennium Ecosystem Assessment. *Guide to the Millennium Assessment Reports*. http://www.millenniumassessment.org/en/index.aspx (accessed October 1, 2015).

Postel, Sandra L., and Barton H. Thompson Jr. "Watershed Protection: Capturing the Benefits of Nature's Water Supply Services." *Natural Resources Forum*, vol. 29, no. 2 (May 2005): 98–108.

U.S. Environmental Protection Agency. *Healthy Watersheds: Protecting Aquatic Systems through Landscape Approaches*. http://www.epa.gov/hwp (accessed October 1, 2015).

WEST NILE VIRUS

The West Nile virus (WNV) is a pathologic virus that is typically transmitted to people through the bites of mosquitoes. Mosquitoes also transmit WNV to, and cause illness in, other animals, most notably birds and horses. In addition to mosquito bites, the virus can be transmitted through blood transfusions, organ transplants, laboratory exposure, and mother-to-baby transmission during pregnancy, delivery, and breastfeeding.

Infection with WNV causes no symptoms in roughly 70 to 80 percent of people, according to the Centers for Disease Control and Prevention (CDC). However, one in five infected people will experience fever and other symptoms, such as headache, body ache, fatigue, vomiting, diarrhea, and rash. Most of those individuals fully recover within a few weeks. Such illness is known as nonneuroinvasive WNV disease.

In a small proportion of infected individuals—less than 1 percent—a severe and sometimes fatal neurologic illness can develop. Such illness is broadly classified as neuroinvasive WNV disease, though specific cases include such neurologic conditions as meningitis and encephalitis. Symptoms of these conditions may include disorientation, tremors, seizures, paralysis, and coma. Recovery from these conditions could require months, and some effects may be permanent. Death results in about 10 percent of cases of neuroinvasive WNV disease.

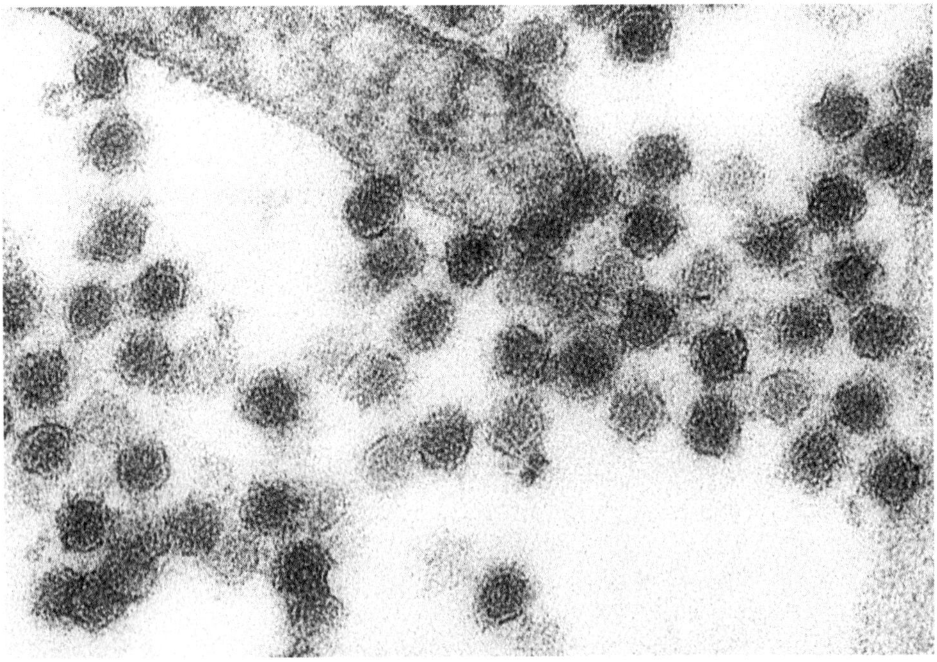

Image of the West Nile virus. The virus is most common throughout Africa, West Asia, and the Middle East, and it is typically transmitted by mosquito bites. (Centers for Disease Control and Prevention/Cynthia Goldsmith)

The prevalence of WNV disease varies from year to year. During 2016, the CDC received reports of 2,038 human cases of WNV disease throughout the United States. About 56 percent of those cases were neuroinvasive, and 44 percent were nonneuroinvasive. In the United States that year, 94 people died from WNV disease. From 1999 (the first year when WNV was detected in North America) to 2015, a total of 43,937 U.S. cases of WNV disease were reported to the CDC, including 1,911 deaths. Prevalence of the disease during that period was highest from:

- 2002 to 2008: ranging from a low of 1,356 cases with 44 deaths in 2008 to a high of 9,862 cases with 264 deaths in 2003.
- 2012 to 2015—ranging from a low of 2,175 cases with 146 deaths in 2015 to a high of 5,674 cases with 286 deaths in 2012.

Worldwide, WNV was first isolated in humans in 1937 in Uganda. Human cases of WNV disease continue to be most prevalent throughout Africa as well as in parts of the Middle East, West Asia, Europe, and Australia. Reliable global statistics on WNV disease prevalence are unavailable.

There are no effective medications to treat patients with WNV infection other than drugs to relieve the associated pain and reduce fever. Patients with severe WNV disease usually need to be hospitalized and receive such supportive treatment as intravenous fluids, prescription pain relievers, and nursing care.

A vaccine to prevent WNV infection is not yet available, although researchers around the world are working to develop one. The risk of contracting WNV can be minimized by covering the skin, including the arms and legs, with thick clothing to prevent mosquito bites and by spraying insect repellent over the skin. Windows and doors of homes should be kept closed or covered with screening to keep out mosquitoes during the warmer months.

A. J. Smuskiewicz

See Also: Centers for Disease Control and Prevention; Infectious Diseases; Insect-Borne Diseases; World Health Organization

Further Reading

Centers for Disease Control and Prevention. *West Nile Virus*. https://www.cdc.gov/westnile (accessed May 4, 2017).

Chancey, C., et al. "The Global Ecology and Epidemiology of West Nile Virus." *BioMed Research International*, vol. 2015, no. 11 (March 2015): 1–20.

Suthar, M. S., M. Gale Jr., and M. S. Diamond. "West Nile Virus Infection and Immunity." *Nature Reviews Microbiology*, vol. 11, no. 2 (February 2013): 115–128.

World Health Organization. *West Nile Virus*. http://www.who.int/mediacentre/factsheets/fs354/en (accessed April 30, 2017).

WETLANDS AND HEALTHY WATERWAYS

Wetland refers to an area of land that is frequently saturated with water. It is a unique ecosystem inundated by water where soils are dominated by anaerobic processes and plants are adapted to flooding or water-saturated soils. "Waterway" is a term used to describe a navigable body of water, such as a river, a canal, or another channel used by ships, boats, and small water vessels. Since wetlands and waterways provide habitat for wildlife, irrigation and drinking water, food, and other ecosystem services for humans, it is very important to ensure they remain productive and healthy.

Wetlands occur naturally in all countries and climatic zones, from the polar regions to the tropics. The largest wetlands include the Amazon River basin, the West Siberian Plain, and the Pantanal in South America. Wetlands can be either natural or artificial (constructed) and either permanent or temporary. The total area of wetlands in the world is about 33 percent larger than the United States, but massive losses of wetlands have occurred over the past decades worldwide, and the majority of remaining wetlands are degraded or under threat of degradation.

While the rate of wetland loss in North America is significant, the rate has slowed since the 1980s and remains low. However, a serious wetland loss problem exists in Asia. For example, the natural wetlands in China (3.8 percent of the terrestrial area) have suffered great losses and degradation, mainly due to severe population pressure and misguided policies over the past 50 years. In contrast, passage of the Clean Water Act of 1972 in the United States brought many improvements to surface water and removed much of the toxic and organic pollution going into wetlands and waterways.

There are four main kinds of wetlands: marsh, swamp, bog, and fen. The water in wetlands can be freshwater or saltwater. One unique characteristic of wetlands is the vegetation of aquatic plants that have adapted to the hydric soil (i.e., soil subject to saturation, flooding, or ponding such that anaerobic conditions have formed in the upper part of the soil.) Aquatic plants are essential for healthy wetland ecosystems because they reduce the amount of sediment in the water, remove nutrients, enhance pollutant breakdown, and provide food and shelter for invertebrates, frogs, reptiles, fish, and waterbirds.

Wetlands and waterways play an important role in the environment. Wetlands provide a wide variety of ecosystem services, such as (1) improving water quality by filtering sediment, nutrients, and pollutants; (2) reducing flood damage; (3) preventing shoreline erosion; (4) providing habitat for fish and wildlife; and (5) producing food, forest, and fuel products. Wetlands are considered one of the most biologically diverse and productive ecosystems, serving as home to a wide range of plant and animal life. Waterways provide resources for drinking, transportation, agricultural production, fisheries, flood control, and other services, including recreational and scenic values.

The multiple uses of wetlands and waterways have often led to significant changes in their structure and function, including alterations to catchment hydrology and sediment delivery, declining water quality, and loss of aquatic biodiversity. Pollution in the form of nutrients, such as nitrogen and phosphorus, and fine sediments can cause significant environmental problems. For example, nitrogen and phosphorus enhance the growth of algae and aquatic plants and, above certain levels, cause algae to grow very fast. Large algal blooms can eliminate the oxygen in a body of water, eventually killing most of the aquatic organisms, and the toxins produced by algal blooms can circumvent water treatment systems and directly threaten human health. If ingested or contacted, these toxins can cause skin irritation, stomach cramps, diarrhea, and even liver damage. Drinking water contaminated with bacteria may also lead to disease. This problem is greater in underdeveloped countries without water treatment systems but still sometimes occurs in developed countries.

Constructed wetlands have been widely used to improve water quality. These are artificial wetlands built to remove various types of pollutants, such as bacteria, nutrients (predominantly nitrogen and phosphorus), and metals present in wastewater and stormwater runoff. Constructed wetlands are designed to recreate the structure and function of natural wetlands that use natural processes involving wetland vegetation and soil and their associated microbial assemblages to improve water quality.

There are two types of constructed wetlands: surface-flow and subsurface-flow. Surface-flow constructed wetlands mimic natural environments and often have permanent standing water. In subsurface-flow wetlands, water passes laterally through a porous medium (usually sand and gravel) with a limited number of macrophyte species (i.e., plants visible to the naked eye). These systems often have no standing water. Constructed wetlands treat wastewater by filtration, settling, and bacterial decomposition, and the planted vegetation in constructed wetlands also plays a significant role in contaminant removal. In some cases, artificial wetlands provide additional benefits, such as groundwater recharge or habitat for waterfowl.

Assessing wetland health through monitoring is vital to their protection. This requires a strategic adaptive management plan that provides regular monitoring of a range of water quality parameters and other ecosystem attributes. Aspects of wetland and waterway health to be monitored include water quality and quantity (e.g., the concentrations of nutrients and pollutants in water), physical habitat (e.g., protective cover for fish, including woody debris), vegetation (e.g., types and productivity of species), physical parameters (e.g., the extent of erosion and sedimentation), and aquatic biology (e.g., the type and abundance of fish, invertebrates, phytoplankton macrophytes, exotic species, and algae). Effective management involves conservation and restoration of wetlands and their functions, including methods and approaches to protect wetland and aquatic resources, limit the pollution sources affecting waterways, and select and prioritize wetlands for restoration.

Dafeng Hui and Thomas D. Byl

See Also: Clean Water Act; Drinking Water Quality and Regulation; Ecosystems, Importance of; Stormwater Runoff; Water Pollution; Watershed Management, Health Implications of

Further Reading

An, Shuqing, et al. "China's Natural Wetlands: Past Problems, Current Status, and Future Challenges." *Ambio*, vol. 36, no. 4 (June 2007): 335–342.

Burton, Thomas M., et al., eds. *Great Lakes Coastal Wetlands Monitoring Plan*. Ann Arbor, MI: Great Lakes Commission, 2008.

Davidson, Nick C. "How Much Wetland Has the World Lost? Long-Term and Recent Trends in Global Wetland Area." *Marine and Freshwater Research*, vol. 65, no.10 (September 2014): 934–941.

Haag, Kim H., and Terrie M. Lee. *Hydrology and Ecology of Freshwater Wetlands in Central Florida—A Primer (Circular 1342)*. Reston, VA: U.S. Geological Survey, 2010.

Manuel, John. "Nutrient Pollution: A Persistent Threat to Waterways." *Environmental Health Perspectives*, vol. 122, no. 11 (November 2014): A304–A323.

Palmer, Margaret A. "Reforming Watershed Restoration: Science in Need of Application and Applications in Need of Science" *Estuaries and Coasts*, vol. 32, no. 1 (January 2009): 1–17.

U.S. Environmental Protection Agency (EPA). *Wetlands Protection and Restoration*. www.epa.gov/wetlands/wetlands-monitoring-and-assessment (accessed May 29, 2016).

WOODSTOVE AIR POLLUTION

Emissions from residential wood heaters are an important air pollution problem and human health issue. Wood burning, even under ideal conditions, results in incomplete combustion during which the volatilized wood fuel condenses to form hazardous air pollution. Exposure to woodstove air pollution is widespread. Emissions from woodstoves and other wood heaters occur near ground level in residential communities across the country.

Unlike industrial stacks with sophisticated air pollution control devices and elevated emission release heights, millions of residential chimneys emit largely uncontrolled wood smoke relatively close to the ground and ultimately into homes and breathing spaces. Wintertime atmospheric inversions (dense cold air captured under warmer air) cause air pollution to be trapped close to the ground, where the fine (i.e., very small) wood smoke particles outdoors can readily enter homes and pollute indoor air. Consequently, even people living in homes without woodstoves or fireplaces are exposed to indoor air pollution from wood smoke if their neighbors burn wood. People in homes with woodstoves,

Wood Smoke: As American as Apple Pie?

For many people, wood smoke conjures up good memories and warm feelings of family time in front of the hearth and friends around a campfire. The truth is that the pleasant aroma of wood smoke belies its danger to human health and the environment. Wood smoke is a major contributor to particulate air pollution, especially in the winter. The serious health and environmental effects of particulate pollution are well studied and widely recognized. Wood smoke also contains carbon monoxide, nitrogen oxides, carcinogenic hazardous air pollutants, and climate change pollutants.

especially old, leaky woodstoves that emit some smoke into indoor air, are the most significantly exposed.

According to the U.S. Census Bureau's 2013 American Housing Survey, over 2 million U.S. residences burn wood as their primary heating fuel. However, it has been widely reported that there are approximately 12 million woodstoves being used in the United States as primary, secondary, or occasional heat sources. Moreover, the Hearth, Patio, and Barbecue Association estimates that more than half of all U.S. households have at least one fireplace or freestanding woodstove. The wood smoke emitted from these millions of chimneys across the country is a complex mixture of gases and fine particles composed largely of unburnt carbon and organic (carbon-containing) compounds. This mixture contains many different air pollutants that adversely affect human health and the environment, including fine particulate matter (PM), carbon monoxide, nitrogen oxides, toxic chemicals, and climate-change pollutants.

In the year 2011 alone, the U.S. Environmental Protection Agency (EPA) estimates that smoke from residential wood heaters and fireplaces contributed over 380,000 tons (345,000 metric tons) of fine PM throughout the country, mostly during the winter months. Wood smoke contains primarily $PM_{2.5}$, which is very small PM with an aerodynamic diameter of 2.5 microns or less. (A micron, also called a micrometer, is a unit of length equal to one-millionth of a meter.) These particles, which are less than 4 percent of the diameter of a human hair (much too small to be seen with the unaided human eye), are inhaled deeply into the smallest sections of human lungs. There they can remain lodged for long periods while contributing to respiratory diseases and structural damage. According to the EPA, exposure to PM, and in particular $PM_{2.5}$, has been linked by numerous scientific studies to health problems, including premature death in people with heart or lung disease, nonfatal heart attacks, irregular heartbeat, aggravated asthma, decreased lung function, and respiratory symptoms, such as irritation of the airways, coughing, and difficulty breathing.

Carbon monoxide in wood smoke decreases the blood's ability to carry oxygen to the brain, impairing thinking and reflexes and even leading to death. Carbon monoxide is also known to cause lower birth weights and increased deaths in newborns. Adverse health effects from nitrogen oxides include damage to the immune system by compromising the body's ability to fight respiratory infection. Those populations most susceptible to health effects resulting from inhaling wood smoke are infants and young children, the elderly, and anyone with existing heart or lung conditions or impairments, including smokers and ex-smokers.

The fine PM in wood smoke also carries into the lungs toxic chemicals classified by the EPA as hazardous air pollutants (HAPs). The EPA defines HAPs, also known as air toxics, as those pollutants that are known or suspected to cause cancer or other serious health effects, such as reproductive problems and birth defects. HAPs in wood smoke, including acetaldehyde, acrolein, benzene, formaldehyde, and numerous polycyclic aromatic hydrocarbons, damage the respiratory tract, and many are known to cause cancer. In fact, according to the EPA's National Air Toxics Assessment published in December 2015, residential wood combustion in the United States accounts for nearly 50 percent of cancer risk from HAPs emitted by area sources. (Area sources are small air pollution emission sources like dry cleaners and auto body shops that individually do not account for much pollution but taken all together can be very significant in urban areas).

Beyond damaging human health, wood smoke also harms the environment. Reduced visibility (haze) is smoke's most obvious impact. Less obviously, the fine PM in wood smoke can be carried over very long distances before settling on the ground and water, where it can cause adverse environmental impacts, including acidification of lakes and streams. According to the EPA and numerous studies, PM deposition also changes the nutrient balance in watersheds and large river basins, leading to similar problems in coastal waters and the oceans. Additionally, soil nutrients can be depleted and forests and crops damaged, and ultimately, PM deposition can adversely affect the diversity of entire ecosystems. Finally, some pollutants in wood smoke, such as methane and black carbon, contribute to climate change.

Given the hazards of wood smoke, it is important to minimize woodstove emissions. The EPA has recognized this and first regulated PM emissions from some newly manufactured residential wood heaters in 1988. In May 2015, the agency promulgated updated PM emission limits for all newly manufactured residential wood heaters, which are to be phased in over five years, and even more stringent PM emission limits must be met starting in May 2020. The law does not apply to existing wood heaters in people's homes, but all new residential wood heaters for sale in the United States (including woodstoves, central wood furnaces, and indoor and outdoor wood boilers) must be certified to meet these PM limits. Furthermore, the PM level emitted by each wood heater model and the heater's energy efficiency (as measured by an EPA-required certification test) must be made available to the consumer on both the manufacturer's and the EPA's websites. To minimize woodstove air pollution, people should shop for the lowest emitting and most efficient wood heater and always use proper burn techniques, as discussed on the EPA's Burn Wise website.

Jill Warnasch Mozier

See Also: Air Pollution; Ambient Air Quality; Carbon Dioxide and the Carbon Cycle; Climate Change and Human Health; Environmental Protection Agency; Formaldehyde; Hazardous Air Pollutants; National Air Toxics Assessment; Particulate Matter and Bioaerosols Pollution; Polycyclic Aromatic Hydrocarbons; Regional Haze Pollution; Respiratory Disease and Air Pollution

Further Reading

Brown, David, et al. "Outdoor Wood Furnaces Create Significant Indoor Particulate Pollution in Neighboring Homes." *Inhalation Toxicology*, vol. 26, no. 10 (August 2014): 628–635.

Hearth, Patio, and Barbecue Association. *Home Page.* http://www.hpba.org (accessed December 15, 2016).

How Wood Smoke Harms Your Health Publication (Publication #91-br-023). Olympia, WA: Department of Ecology, State of Washington, 2012.
Naeher, Luke P., et al. "Woodsmoke Health Effects: A Review." *Inhalation Toxicology*, vol. 19, no. 1 (January 2007): 67–106.
U.S. Census Bureau. *American Housing Survey (AHS)*. http://www.census.gov/programs-surveys/ahs.html (accessed December 15, 2016).
U.S. Environmental Protection Agency. *Burn Wise*. https://www.epa.gov/burnwise (accessed December 15, 2016).
U.S. Environmental Protection Agency. *Final New Source Performance Standards for Residential Wood Heaters*. https://www.epa.gov/residential-wood-heaters/final-new-source-performance-standards-residential-wood-heaters (accessed December 15, 2016).
U.S. Environmental Protection Agency. *List of EPA Certified Wood Stoves*. https://www.epa.gov/compliance/list-epa-certified-wood-stoves (accessed December 15, 2016).
U.S. Environmental Protection Agency. *National Air Toxics Assessment*. https://www.epa.gov/national-air-toxics-assessment (accessed December 15, 2016).

WORLD HEALTH ORGANIZATION

The World Health Organization (WHO) is an agency of the United Nations with a mission to advance international public health. Founded on April 7, 1948—now celebrated as World Health Day—the WHO provides leadership, surveillance, and technical support to countries around the world. This includes sharing expertise, logistical support, training, and directing research.

Headquartered in Geneva, Switzerland, the organization is made up of 194 member states. Representatives from these states form the World Health Assembly, which is the WHO's governing body. As an agency of the United Nations, it is administered through the Economic and Social Council. The member states are organized into six regions across the world, each with a regional office. These geographical groupings are the Americas, Africa, Southeast Asia, Europe, Eastern Mediterranean, and Western Pacific.

Using this global network, the WHO seeks to improve health among all people. It defines the concept of health broadly as a state of complete physical, mental, and social well-being and not just the absence of disease. Because many diseases and health conditions share environmental risk factors, the WHO's focus includes environmental health, which is prioritized to the needs of each region. According to WHO data, 23 percent of all deaths in the world (an estimated 13 million deaths) are attributed to unhealthy environments.

Current efforts include a focus on many environmental concerns, such as air quality, food and chemical safety, and vector control. The WHO is also a leader in water and sanitation, waste management, and climate change. For example, in response to the changing climate, the WHO provides information and technical support and advocates for science-informed public policy. While climate change affects all countries, it will be most severe for the poorest populations in developing nations. The WHO partners with groups in these nations to help raise awareness and build capacity for an effective response.

Water and sanitation remain key environmental concerns around the world. According to the WHO, almost 2 billion people worldwide get their drinking water from a contaminated source. Some diseases are directly linked to unsafe drinking water. In addition, scientists predict that in the future, half of the world's population will be living in areas where access to clean water is uncertain.

Further challenging the environment is unsustainable waste disposal. Sustainable waste management informed by science allows for safe disposal of a variety of waste materials, including chemical, solid, liquid, and hazardous wastes. As the global population increases, waste management is becoming a more pressing issue. The WHO works to find waste management solutions, especially in developing countries.

Charles Daniel

See Also: Climate Change and Human Health; Drinking Water Quality and Regulation; Hazardous Waste Disposal; Infectious Diseases; United Nations Environmental Programme; Waterborne Diseases

Further Reading

Hanhimäki, Jussi M. *The United Nations: A Very Short Introduction*. Oxford, UK: Oxford University Press, 2015.

Preventing Disease through Healthy Environments: A Global Assessment of the Burden of Disease from Environmental Risks. Geneva, Switzerland: World Health Organization, 2016.

Working for Health: An Introduction to the World Health Organization. Geneva, Switzerland: World Health Organization, 2007.

World Health Organization. *Home Page*. http://www.who.int/en (accessed May 5, 2017).

Y

YELLOW FEVER

Yellow fever is a well-known viral infection found throughout the tropical regions of the world, such as sub-Saharan Africa and South America, that is regularly monitored by the World Health Organization (WHO) and the Centers for Disease Control and Prevention. It is a virus of the *Flaviviridae* family that is typically spread by mosquitoes biting monkeys and, when transmitted to humans, leads to a mosquito-borne viral hemorrhagic fever having a high fatality rate. Yellow fever is transmitted by the same "day-biting" mosquito, *Aedes aegypti*, that transmits the chikungunya and Zika viruses.

Historical disasters often lead to major developments in medicine. For example, the 1918 influenza pandemic that killed approximately 1 million people in the United States and more than 50 million worldwide led to research creating the influenza vaccine in 1938. Similarly, the yellow fever epidemic between 1817 and 1905 led to research into generating the yellow fever vaccine in 1936. Today, the yellow fever vaccine is recognized as being highly effective, safe, and inexpensive.

There is no treatment or antiviral therapy available for yellow fever once it is acquired, and only supportive and comfort measures are available (e.g., treating associated dehydration, liver and kidney failure, and bacterial infection). The chance

Yellow Fever in the United States

It is a little known fact that the United States was hit by a major yellow fever epidemic—way back in 1793. The epidemic struck Philadelphia, which was then the young nation's capital and home to many Revolutionary War figures and free African Americans. At the time, Thomas Jefferson wrote to James Madison that everyone who could leave the city was doing so. Those left behind were mostly poor with no place to escape to, and it is estimated that 5,000 people out of a population of 45,000 died. African Americans, who were thought to be immune to yellow fever, were asked to care for the sick. However, after several months, when African Americans began falling ill and dying at the same rate as whites, this theory was proven wrong. Dr. Jean Devèze, a French doctor who took over treatments at the local Bush Hill hospital, would become recognized as a world authority on yellow fever. Later, between 1817 and 1905, over 40,000 people may have died in New Orleans, which was built in a swampy area ideal for mosquito breeding. The city tried unsuccessfully to eradicate the disease by burning tar to purify the air and by firing cannons.

of survival is improved with modern intensive care medicine, although this level of care is generally not available in the areas most affected by the virus. Thus, the best treatment for yellow fever is prevention with the yellow fever vaccination, which is particularly important for travelers departing to endemic areas.

Due to the severity of the yellow fever illness and its recurring resurgence, including the 2016–2017 outbreak in a region of South America frequented by tourists, the WHO established the Eliminate Yellow Fever Epidemics (EYE) program in 2016 to control, if not eliminate, the disease. The EYE initiative incorporates three pillars: (1) preventing yellow fever in at-risk populations, (2) stopping international spread of the disease, and (3) containing outbreaks rapidly. Along with vaccinations, the EYE yellow fever strategy promotes resilient urban centers, urban readiness, and stronger international health regulations. The program identifies 27 countries in Africa and 13 in the Americas that are at highest risk, requiring large-scale vaccinations to ensure high levels of immunity.

Howard W. MacLennan Jr.

See Also: Centers for Disease Control and Prevention; Environmental Epidemiology; Infectious Diseases; Insect-Borne Diseases; World Health Organization

Further Reading

Carrigan, Jo Ann. *The Saffron Scourge: A History of Yellow Fever in Louisiana, 1796–1905.* Lafayette, LA: University of Louisiana at Lafayette Press, 2015.

Centers for Disease Control and Prevention. *Yellow Fever*. https://www.cdc.gov/yellowfever (accessed March 12, 2017).

Control of Yellow Fever: Field Guide. Washington, DC: Pan American Health Organization, 2005.

Global Strategy to Eliminate Yellow Fever Epidemics (EYE). Geneva, Switzerland: World Health Organization, 2016.

New Orleans Public Library. *Yellow Fever Deaths in New Orleans, 1817–1905*. http://nutrias.org/facts/feverdeaths.htm (accessed March 12, 2017).

Paules, C. I., and A. S. Fauci. "Yellow Fever—Once Again on the Radar Screen in the Americas (Perspective)." *New England Journal of Medicine*, vol. 376, no. 15 (April 2017): 1397–99.

Sun, Lena H. "Yellow Fever Outbreak in Brazil Worries U.S. Officials." *Washington Post*, March 8, 2017, https://www.washingtonpost.com/news/to-your-health/wp/2017/03/08/yellow-fever-outbreak-in-brazil-worries-u-s-officials.

"The Yellow Fever Epidemic in Philadelphia, 1793." In *Contagion: Historical Views of Diseases and Epidemics*. Cambridge, MA: Harvard University, http://ocp.hul.harvard.edu/contagion/yellowfever.html.

Z

ZIKA VIRUS

Zika is a viral infection primarily spread by the bite of an infected *Aedes aegypti* mosquito. However, it can also be transmitted through sexual contact and blood transfusions. The main threat from Zika is that it can be passed from a pregnant woman to her fetus, causing an abnormal smallness of the child's brain at birth or developing within the first few years of life. Known as microcephaly, this condition can cause developmental delays, cognitive impairment, problems with coordination and balance, and seizures. Furthermore, doctors have observed other Zika-related problems among fetuses and in infants infected prior to birth, including eye defects, poor hearing, and impaired growth. And there is increasing evidence of a link between Zika and Guillain-Barré syndrome, a rare nervous system disorder.

Zika infections were initially reported for Americans returning to the United States after traveling to areas where Zika outbreaks have occurred. However, more recently there have been an increasing number of cases where the virus was acquired locally by individuals living in the United States who did not travel abroad. The virus was first discovered in 1947 at a virus research facility in Uganda's Zika forest. Since then, there may have been a number of Zika outbreaks that were not attributed to the Zika virus because its symptoms are similar to other viral diseases.

Many people infected with the Zika virus will have mild symptoms or no symptoms at all, and they may not be sick enough to be hospitalized. But for others, the symptoms may be more severe. Typical symptoms are fever, rash, joint pain, and conjunctivitis. Additionally, people may experience muscle pain and headache. These symptoms may last from several days to a week, and once infected, people may be protected from getting the infection again. Of course, if you believe you have an infection, you should see your doctor right away.

Zika infections can be diagnosed from a person's symptoms and travel history and confirmed with a blood or urine test. Because Zika symptoms are similar to other infectious diseases, a health professional may test for several different types of infections. Aside from treating the symptoms, there are no medicines or vaccines for the Zika virus, although several candidate vaccines are under development. Additionally, trials are under way for genetically modified *Aedes aegypti* mosquitoes whose offspring die before they can transmit the disease.

To avoid acquiring the Zika virus, the best approach is to prevent mosquito bites when in areas where the virus is believed to be present. Avoiding mosquitos is not always easy, but using insect repellent, wearing long-sleeve shirts and long pants, and eliminating standing water near your home can help. (When using an insect repellent, always follow the label instructions.) Use window and door screens to prevent mosquitoes from entering your home, and if you do not have air-conditioning and must open the windows to cool off at night, you can avoid mosquito bites by sleeping under a mosquito net. If you are pregnant, the Centers for Disease and Control and Prevention recommends that you do *not* travel to areas where ongoing Zika transmission by mosquito is occurring, and use condoms or do not have sexual contact if you are pregnant and your partner lives in or has traveled to a Zika-infected area.

Our understanding of the Zika virus is evolving, and it is important to stay informed about the latest research and developments. A good source of information for the latest updates is the CDC's Zika virus website.

Richard Crume

See Also: Centers for Disease Control and Prevention; Communicable Diseases; Infectious Diseases; Zoonotic Diseases

Further Reading

Bennett, John E., Raphael Dolin, and Martin J. Blaser. *Mandell, Douglas, and Bennett's Infectious Disease Essentials*. Philadelphia, PA: Elsevier, 2017.

Centers for Disease and Control and Prevention. *Zika Virus*. https://www.cdc.gov/zika (accessed October 6, 2016).

Cohen, Jonathan, William G. Powderly, and Steven M. Opal. *Infectious Diseases*. Amsterdam, the Netherlands: Elsevier, 2016.

Kasper, Dennis L., Anthony S. Fauci, and Tinsley R. Harrison. *Harrison's Infectious Diseases*. New York: McGraw-Hill Medical, 2010.

National Institute of Allergy and Infectious Diseases. *Zika Virus*. https://www.niaid.nih.gov/diseases-conditions/zika-virus (accessed November 21, 2016).

U.S. Department of State. *Zika Travel Information for Travelers*. https://travel.state.gov/content/passports/en/go/Zika.html (accessed October 6, 2016).

World Health Organization. *Zika Virus*. http://www.who.int/topics/zika/en (accessed October 6, 2016).

ZOONOTIC DISEASES

Zoonotic diseases, or zoonoses, are infectious diseases that are transmissible under natural conditions from vertebrate animals to humans (see Table 20). Zoonotic diseases can be caused by viruses, bacteria, parasites, and fungi. These diseases are common, and it is estimated that 6 out of every 10 known infectious diseases in people are spread from animals. In addition, 3 out of every 4 emerging infectious diseases in people are transmitted from animals. Emerging infectious diseases are defined as those that are caused by apparently new agents or by known agents that occur in regions or species that did not previously appear to be affected by these known agents. The rise of emerging zoonotic infections is due to ecological changes resulting from agricultural practices, such as deforestation. It is speculated that climate change and overpopulation will result in more zoonotic diseases as the habitats of animals change, and they come into more frequent contact with humans.

Table 20. Examples of zoonotic diseases and associated animals.

Animal Type	Zoonotic Disease
Cats	Rabies, toxoplasmosis
Cattle	*Escherichia coli* O157:H7, cryptosporidiosis, bovine spongiform encephalopathy (mad cow disease)
Dogs	Rabies, leptospirosis, campylobacteriosis
Poultry	Influenza, salmonellosis
Swine	Influenza, trichinosis
Bats	Rabies
Rodents	Hantavirus, plague, tularemia

The definition of a zoonotic disease is broad and includes disease-causing pathogens that operate in a variety of ways. Some diseases maintain an infection cycle in an animal host that is independent from the disease the pathogen causes in humans. Others cause disease in both the human and animal hosts. There are several possible routes of transmission between animals and humans, including skin contact, bites or scratches, and direct inhalation or ingestion. People who are immunocompromised, children under five years of age, and pregnant women may be at increased risk of infection from zoonotic diseases.

The bubonic plague is an example of a zoonotic infection in which the disease-causing pathogen maintains an infection cycle in a host that is independent from humans. This disease is caused by the bacterium *Yersinia pestis*, which is transmitted by the bite of infected fleas from rodents. One natural reservoir for the plague is the ground squirrel, which is common throughout the United States. The bubonic plague begins with nonspecific symptoms, such as fever and chills, and progresses to infect the lymph nodes. In very rare cases, it can be transmitted by coming into contact with infected tissue or exposure to the cough of an infected human.

Rabies is an example of a disease that can infect both humans and animals. It is an acute and highly fatal zoonotic disease that affects the central nervous system. This disease is caused by a virus that is most often transmitted through saliva from the bites of infected animals. Worldwide, dog bites are the principal source of transmission of rabies to humans. In mammals, this disease results in encephalopathy and paralysis of the respiratory system. Symptoms at the early stages of the disease are nonspecific and include fever, headache, and malaise. As the disease progresses, it leads to hallucinations and paralysis, and death ensues within days. Treatment typically consists of a vaccine that must be administered as quickly as possible. Without treatment, this disease almost universally results in death.

Jyotsna S. Jagai

See Also: Bubonic Plague; Deforestation; Ebola Virus; *Escherichia coli* (*E. coli*) Infection; Infectious Diseases

Further Reading

Armon, Robert, and Uta Cheruti. *Environmental Aspects of Zoonotic Diseases*. London: International Water Federation, 2012.

Centers for Disease Control and Prevention. *One Health: Zoonotic Diseases*. https://www.cdc.gov/onehealth/basics/zoonotic-diseases.html (accessed May 8, 2017).

Centers for Disease Control and Prevention. *Plague*. https://www.cdc.gov/plague (accessed May 8, 2017).

Centers for Disease Control and Prevention. *Rabies*. https://www.cdc.gov/rabies (accessed May 8, 2017).

Conover, Michael R., and Rosanna M. Vail. *Human Diseases from Wildlife*. Boca Raton, FL: CRC Press, 2015.

Romich, Janet A. *Understanding Zoonotic Diseases*. Clifton Park, NY: Thomson/Delmar Learning, 2008.

Appendix: Steps to Reducing Your Environmental Exposure

We are surrounded by toxic substances in the environment. They are in the air we breathe, in our drinking water and food, and even in consumer products like clothing. Fortunately, our exposure to most of these substances is so low that we have nothing to worry about. But for some toxic substances, particularly those having higher toxicities, exposure can sometimes cause illnesses and even death. We can never eliminate all toxic substances, but if we can reduce our exposure to those that are most egregious or avoid them all together, we stand a much better chance of living a long and healthy life.

The first step in reducing our environmental exposure is to know what substances we need to avoid. Unfortunately, this is not as simple as it sounds. While we have good information on many toxic chemicals and other substances in the environment, there are still many others we know little or nothing about. For example, an estimated 60,000 or more commercial chemicals on the market have never been safety tested, and roughly 2,000 new chemicals are introduced every year. Millions of Americans are exposed daily to these chemicals, many of which are contained in consumer products. Similarly, there are many other toxic substances in the environment we know little about. Often, we learn about these substances only after they have caused a problem.

This presents a dilemma: How do we reduce our exposure to toxic substances when we do not always know what substances to be concerned about? While we may never have certainty about what is toxic and what is not, there are some common-sense measures we can take to reduce our risk of injury and illness. Of course, everyone knows that eating healthy foods and exercising are essential to maintaining good health and building a strong immune system. And it goes without saying that smoking and substance abuse are bad ideas. But what more can we do?

The World Health Organization (WHO) estimates that environmental factors account for about a quarter of the global disease burden and about the same percentage of deaths from all causes. Many of these environmental factors are well understood, and we can take steps to reduce our exposure to these factors or avoid them all together. Here are some examples of the steps we can take:

- Air Quality: Over 120 million Americans live in areas where *air quality* does not meet federal health standards. Check the AirNow Air Quality Index in the morning, and if the air quality is poor, limit strenuous exercise and stay indoor as much as possible. (Visit airnow.gov for specific guidance.)

- Water Supply: If you are on a public *water supply* system, review the annual water quality testing report and consider filtering your water if any contaminant limits are exceeded. If you are on a private system, be sure to have your water tested regularly, particularly if there has been recent agricultural or industrial development in the neighborhood or if you live near a landfill or waste dump.
- Infectious Diseases: To prevent *infectious diseases* spread by ticks and mosquitos, use insect repellent and wear a long-sleeve shirt, long pants, and socks when in grassy and wooded areas. It is also a good idea to purchase flea and tick control products for your pets so that they stay healthy and do not bring fleas and ticks inside the house.
- Handwashing: Old-fashioned *handwashing* remains one of the best ways to keep you and others from getting sick, especially when preparing food, caring for someone who is sick, handling an animal, and using the toilet. It is easy to do it right: wet your hands, lather with soap, scrub your hands together for at least 20 seconds (as long as it takes to sing the "happy birthday" song twice), rinse with running water, and dry.
- Radon: *Radon* is the second leading cause of lung cancer in America (after smoking), resulting in an estimated 21,000 deaths annually. Have your home tested for radon, and if readings are high, hire a radon contractor to explore options for remediation.
- Shampoos, Detergents, and Cleaning Agents: It is a mistake to assume that the chemicals in our *shampoos, detergents*, and *cleaning agents* have been safety tested because often they have not. Consider using natural, nontoxic alternatives, which are better for your health and kinder to the environment too!
- Pesticides: When using commercial *pesticides* at home, be sure to carefully follow the directions to avoid exposure to you and your loved ones. Better yet, try pesticides made of natural, nontoxic substances, and seal any cracks in your floors, walls, and ceilings where the little critters can enter. Keeping the kitchen area clean also helps.
- Household Dust: Regular vacuuming of *household dust* can reduce indoor toxic substances and help prevent allergies and asthma attacks. Dusts have been found to include all sorts of dangerous substances, such as lead, pesticides, fire retardants, and various allergens. Because carpeting collects dust, consider replacing it with solid wood, cork, tile, or nonvinyl linoleum flooring.
- Home Heaters: Ensure your *fireplace, woodstove*, or *kerosene heater* meets safety codes and is well ventilated, and install several carbon monoxide monitors in your home. Do not burn treated lumber, which can give off toxic gases.
- Remodeling: If you are *remodeling an older home*, especially one built in the 1970s or earlier, it may contain asbestos in insulation, wiring, roof and siding shingles, and floor tile, and there could be lead in old plumbing and wall paint. Hire a qualified inspector or contractor to assess the hazards and discuss remediation options. Use paints and wood products that do not off-gas harmful chemicals.
- Contaminated Fish: Be cautious about eating *fish contaminated with mercury*, such as some kinds of tuna. This is especially important for young children and pregnant and breastfeeding women. Fish can be good for you, but consider eating lower on the food chain to avoid fish that have bioaccumulated high levels of heavy metals. (See seafood.edf.org for more information.)
- Bisphenol A: Consider using food packaging, beverage containers, and plastic dinnerware that are free of *Bisphenol A (BPA)*, watch out for the BPA-containing epoxy resins used in the protective linings of food cans, and never microwave polycarbonate

food containers. According to the Centers for Disease Control and Prevention (CDC) (cdc.gov/biomonitoring/bisphenola_factsheet.html), BPA is widespread in the human population, and while its human health effects at low environmental exposures are unknown, BPA has been shown to affect the reproductive systems of laboratory animals.

- Sunlight Exposure: If you spend time *out-of-doors* for work or recreation, apply a broad-spectrum sunscreen that protects against both UVA and UVB ultraviolet sunlight. Also, consider using an insect repellent and wearing a long-sleeve shirt, long pants, and socks when in grassy and wooded areas. (The Mayo Clinic presents additional sunscreen information here: mayoclinic.org/healthy-lifestyle/adult-health/in-depth/best-sunscreen/art-20045110.)
- Hearing Loss: *Hearing loss* is the third most common chronic health condition in the United States, where about 40 million Americans age 20 to 69 have noise-induced hearing loss. When mowing the lawn, using a noisy leaf blower, running a loud power saw, or attending a rock concert, be sure to wear ear protection.
- Exposures at Work: If you come into contact with *dust, fibers, chemical fumes, radiation, or biological agents* at work, wear the appropriate personal protective equipment, such as gloves, masks, coveralls, and respirators, and shower before leaving work so that you do not bring any contaminants home on your clothing.
- Medical Imaging: Avoid unnecessary *medical imaging tests* using ionizing radiation, such as X-rays, CT scans, and fluoroscopy. According to the CDC (cdc.gov/nceh/radiation/ionizing.htm), such tests can lead to a small increase in the likelihood of developing cancer later in life as well as skin reddening, hair loss, and possible allergic reactions associated with contrast dyes.
- Environmental Health History: Physicians are rarely trained on environmental exposures and how to take an *environmental health history*. If you are concerned about past environmental exposures, talk with your doctor about documenting your exposures and researching potential health implications.

Can cancer be prevented? Americans are especially concerned about cancer, and rightly so. Over 40 percent of Americans will be diagnosed with cancer during their lifetimes, and about 20 percent will die from cancer. The incidences of some cancers are decreasing as new treatments are discovered and people make lifestyle changes. On the other hand, some cancers, including cases among children, are increasing for unexplained reasons. Environmental factors do not cause all cancers, but they are definitely implicated in some.

According to the President's Cancer Panel (prescancerpanel.cancer.gov), a growing body of research finds that environmental factors linked to genetic, immune, and endocrine dysfunction can lead to cancer and other diseases, and the true burden of cancer caused by environmental factors has been grossly underestimated. Furthermore, the WHO reports that cancer is the leading cause of death worldwide, with about 20 percent of all cancers attributed to the environment, particularly air pollution (indoor and outdoor), ultraviolet radiation, radon, secondhand smoke, and occupational exposures, including asbestos. By taking precautions at home and work to avoid these and other cancer-causing environmental agents, you can go a long way in reducing your cancer risk.

The hazards of tobacco smoking are incontrovertible, and there are also health concerns about e-cigarettes. But what about smoking marijuana? Marijuana is growing in popularity for medical and recreation use, and the CDC reports over 22 million users in the United States. Additionally, an increasing number of states have legalized marijuana for medical use. On the other hand, recreational (non-medical) use is perhaps more controversial, in part, due to potential side effects. For example, the CDC indicates (cdc.gov/marijuana) there is "strong evidence" that marijuana use may lead to health effect such as addiction, breathing problems, short-term declines in memory, and increased risk for psychosis or schizophrenia, and there is "some evidence" for an increased risk of some types of cancer and for heart attack and stroke. School performance may suffer too, according to the CDC.

If you are concerned about environmental risks in your community, you can work with community members to build a safe community plan to reduce environmental exposures, particularly for children playing out-of-doors. Begin by identifying community concerns and vulnerabilities. For example, you may be concerned about standing water or ponds that breed mosquitoes, exposure to ticks from deer that wander into town, volatile organic compound fumes from shredded tires used as a base for playgrounds, or air pollution from a nearby manufacturing plant. Do your own research and get the facts. Organize teams of concerned citizens, and enlist the support of local city offices. If necessary, attend city council meetings and make your voice heard, loud and clear. Pollution in your specific community can be investigated with the My Environment tool (epa.gov/myenvironment) developed by the U.S. Environmental Protection Agency.

The widespread presence of toxic substances in the environment is a symptom of our modern lifestyle. As we drive and fly more, use more chemical pesticides and fertilizers, and manufacture more consumer goods, we also produce more toxic pollution. Fortunately, a number of technological innovations in recent years have helped pave the way toward a healthy, environment-friendly future. Getting there from here seems a daunting task, but by reducing our own environmental exposure, we are taking a stand for environmental health and helping drive the national conversation about this important topic.

Glossary

Acid rain Precipitation that is acidic due to sulfuric and nitric acids that form from pollution in the atmosphere, increasing the acidity of bodies of waters where the precipitation falls.

Action level A guideline used by environmental agencies to identify the concentration level of a substance that may present a health hazard when exceeded.

Acute illness An illness with rapid onset, as distinguished from a chronic disease that is long lasting.

Aerodynamic diameter When studying the behavior of an air pollution particle in a gas stream, the diameter of a spherical particle having a density of 1 gram per cubic centimeter and the same settling velocity as the particle under investigation.

Aerosol A solid or liquid particle that is suspended in the air.

Air toxics Air pollutants known to cause cancer or other serious health conditions. Also known as hazardous air pollutants.

Ambient air The outdoor air that people breathe and that can contain air pollutants.

Anthropogenic Referring to something originating with human activity, such as the creation of ground-level ozone pollution. (Stratospheric ozone would not be considered anthropogenic because it occurs naturally.)

Antigen A substance foreign to the human body that can evoke an immune response and bind with the product of the response. The substance can act alone or as a complex with a protein or other larger molecule.

Aquifer Underground water contained in a layer of rock, sand, gravel, or sediment that can be used for drinking water or irrigation.

Area sources A number of small air pollution sources, such as automobile body shops or dry cleaners, that taken together can represent a large amount of pollution.

Asbestosis A chronic lung disease caused by the inhalation of asbestos fibers, resulting in lung tissue scarring and shortness of breath.

Atopy A genetic disposition to develop an allergic reaction, including allergic rhinitis, asthma, and atopic dermatitis, when exposed to an environmental antigen.

Batesian mimicry The ability of an organism to gain extra protection by resembling or mimicking a more dangerous organism, for example, adopting the dangerous organism's coloration, thereby keeping predators away.

Bioaccumulation The concentration of a substance in an organism when the substance builds up faster than it is removed.

Bioavailability The degree to which a substance is absorbed into a living system or made available to a target tissue or organ.

Bioconcentration Bioaccumulation that occurs specifically by absorption directly from water.

Biodegradation The decomposition of a substance by microorganisms or natural processes like sunlight.

Biogenic emissions Acetaldehyde, formaldehyde, methanol, and other volatile organic compounds emitted from natural sources, such as plants and trees.

Biomagnification An increase in the concentration of a substance in organisms while moving up the food chain.

Biosphere The earth, including the crust, oceans, atmosphere, and living organisms that inhabit it.

BPA (bisphenol A) A chemical used in manufacturing polycarbonate plastics and epoxy resins that researchers believe may cause adverse health effects in humans.

Built environment The human-created buildings, parks, and spaces within a city where people live and work.

Carbon dioxide A colorless, odorless, and nontoxic gas formed by the combustion of carbon-containing fuels, such as coal, oil, and natural gas, and the principal gas contributing to climate change.

Carbon offset A credit for greenhouse gas emission reductions achieved by one party that can be sold to another party to compensate for (offset) that party's greenhouse gas emissions.

Carcinogenic Substances known or suspected to cause cancer.

Case-control study A study comparing exposures of people having a disease or condition with people not having the disease or condition for the purpose of identifying risk factors for the disease or condition.

Chronic disease A long-lasting disease, as distinguished from an acute illness having rapid onset.

Cohort study A study where a group of people previously exposed to some environmental factor are followed over time, and their health experience is compared with a control group not previously exposed to the environmental factor.

Colitis An inflammation of the large intestine that is often accompanied by abdominal pain, bloody stools, dehydration, diarrhea, and fever.

Communicable disease A disease spread from one person to another through, for example, contacting blood and bodily fluids, inhaling an airborne virus, or being bitten by an infected insect.

DDT (dichlorodiphenyltrichloroethane) An insecticide first developed in the 1940s that was highly effective against malaria, typhus, and other insect-borne diseases but was later associated with adverse environmental and toxicological effects, as described in Rachel Carson's seminal publication, *Silent Spring*.

Deforestation Logging or burning practices that result in a forested area being cleared of trees, often for harvesting timber for sale or for agricultural purposes.

Detection limit The lowest concentration of a chemical that can be measured with confidence such that the measurement can be reliably distinguished from zero.

Diesel particulate matter A mixture of particles in diesel engine exhaust that are associated with cancer and noncancer health effects.

Dioxin A group of chemical compounds with similar chemical and biological characteristics that bioaccumulate in the food chain, persist in the environment, and can be highly toxic. The most toxic form is 2,3,7,8-tetrachlorodibenzo-p-dioxin, also known as 2,3,7,8-TCDD.

DNA Deoxyribonucleic acid, the self-replicating material present in living organisms that carries genetic information.

Dose The amount of a substance taken or administered at one time, for example, a medicine, radiation for diagnosis or treatment, or an environmental agent tested in animals for toxicity.

Dose-response assessment A determination of the relationship between the magnitude of a dose and a specific biological response.

Dry deposition The sulfuric and nitric acids that form from pollution in the atmosphere and fall back to the earth in a dry form, potentially damaging automobile and building surfaces, injuring wildlife and vegetation, and increasing the acidity of bodies of water.

Endocrine disruptor Chemicals such as dioxin, PCB, DDT, and BPA that are believed to interfere with the body's endocrine system, resulting in adverse developmental, reproductive, neurological, and immune effects.

Enteritis An inflammation of the small intestine that is often accompanied by abdominal pain, diarrhea, fever, and vomiting.

Environmentalism A philosophy and social movement focused on protecting the natural environment from pollution and overuse.

Epidemiology Study of the frequencies, patterns, and causes of health and diseases in populations.

Epitope A location on the surface of an antigen that can both elicit an immune response and combine with the antibody produced by the response.

Erythema Reddening of the skin (i.e., sunburn) caused by overexposure to ultraviolet radiation.

Estuary The area at the end of a river where the current of the river meets the tide of the sea.

Exotoxin A toxic substance produced by a microorganism and released to the surroundings.

Exposure Inhalation, ingestion, or skin contact with a substance, which may be short term or long term.

Exposure pathway A route by which a substance in the environment can come into contact with humans, animals, and plants, for example, the inhalation of an airborne toxic chemical.

Fission The splitting of an atom, resulting in the release of heat that can be used to produce electricity.

Fly ash Particulate matter that does not completely burn up in the combustion process, for example, when coal is burned to generate electricity in an electric power plant.

Fugitive emissions Air pollution escaping from various points in a manufacturing process rather than through a stack, chimney, or vent, thereby making capture and removal difficult.

Fusion The bonding together of two light atoms, forming a heavier one and releasing a large amount of energy.

Genetic engineering The process of manually adding new DNA to an organism so as to add new traits not already present in the organism, for example, creating plants resistant to certain insects.

Genome An organism's complete set of DNA, containing all the information required to build and maintain the organism.

Greenhouse effect Warming of the earth's surface due to the accumulation of gases in the atmosphere that absorb heat and prevent it from escaping into outer space.

Greenhouse gas Atmospheric gases, for example, carbon dioxide, methane, nitrous oxide, and ozone, that contribute to climate change and often originate with electric power generation and other human activities.

Greenwashing Unsubstantiated or misleading labeling or marketing claims, making a product or practice appear better for the environment than it actually is.

Hazard index The sum of hazard quotients when multiple substances affect the same target organ or organ system.

Hazard quotient The ratio of the level of exposure of a substance to the level where no adverse health effects occur.

Hazardous air pollutants Air pollutants known to cause cancer or other serious health conditions. Also known as air toxics.

Heat island effect How urban areas, because of their dense materials (asphalt, brick, concrete, steel, and stone), heat up faster and hold their heat longer than rural area.

Heat wave A period of unusually hot weather lasting for a number of days and often resulting in an increase in heat-related illnesses.

Heavy metals A group of elements, such as chromium, copper, lead, and zinc, that are toxic at low concentrations and can accumulate in the food chain.

Hypoxia The condition where insufficient oxygen reaches the tissues of the human body.

Incidence The number of cases of a disease over a specified period.

Industrial hygiene A professional field concerned with protecting the safety and health of workers while on the job.

Industrial Revolution The growth of industrial manufacturing from roughly 1760 to 1840, when industry supplanted agriculture in many countries as the major driver of the economy.

Infectious disease A human disorder caused by bacteria, viruses, fungi, parasites, and other organisms that grow and multiply in the body. Some infectious diseases may be passed from person to person, while others are transmitted by insect or animal bites or by consuming contaminated food or water.

Latency period The period between exposure to an agent causing a disease and the onset of the disease.

Leaching The process by which water dissolves chemicals as it flows through contaminated soils or landfills and transfers the chemicals to groundwater or surface water.

Longitudinal study A study type that follows individuals over a prolonged period of time and is useful in evaluating the relationship between risk factors and the development of disease and in evaluating the outcome of treatments.

Low latitudes The part of the earth's surface that is located near the equator.

Melatonin A hormone that helps regulate other hormones and maintains the body's circadian rhythm.

Mesothelioma A form of cancer almost always attributed to asbestos exposure that most commonly affects the outer lining of the lungs or chest cavity, the lining of the abdominal cavity, or the sac surrounding the heart.

Methane A colorless, nontoxic, and flammable hydrocarbon gas created by the anaerobic decomposition of organic compounds, and a potent greenhouse gas.

Methyl isocyanate A highly toxic chemical used to produce pesticides that was accidentally released in 1984 from the Union Carbide plant in Bhopal, India, resulting in thousands of deaths and injuries.

Miasma Gases given off by putrid matter or marshy regions, once believed to cause diseases such as cholera and malaria.

Microbes Living organisms, such as bacteria, archaea, viruses, fungi, prions, protozoa, and algae, that are too small to be seen with the naked eye.

Microbiology The study of microbes, which are living organisms too small to be seen without a microscope.

Microbiome A community of bacteria, fungi, viruses, and other microorganisms that inhabits a particular environment; often referring to the microorganisms inhabiting the human body.

Micron A unit of length equal to one-millionth of a meter. Also called a micrometer.

Mutagen A substance that causes mutations, which are changes to DNA, genes, or chromosomes.

Mutagenic Substances having the potential to cause changes in genetic material, such as DNA.

Mutation A change to the DNA, genes, or chromosomes of a living organism.

Nanometer A unit of length equal to one-billionth of a meter.

Napalm A highly flammable and sticky substance containing gasoline and other chemicals that was used in bombs during the Vietnam War and unsuccessfully applied to the *Torrey Canyon* oil spill in an attempt to set fire to and disperse the oil.

Neonatal Referring to or affecting the newborn, particularly human infants in the first month following birth.

Nicotine The addictive substance found naturally in tobacco.

Nonpoint source pollution Pollution originating from multiple diffuse sources, such as drainage, land runoff, and atmospheric deposition.

Odor threshold The lowest concentration of a substance in the air that can be detected with the human nose. Substances have different odor thresholds, and people often have different sensitivities for detecting odors.

Organic compound A large class of chemical compounds containing carbon, where the carbon atoms are covalently bonded to other atoms, typically hydrogen, oxygen, and nitrogen.

Ozone A molecule comprising three oxygen atoms that is formed by a chemical reaction between nitrogen oxides and volatile organic compounds in the presence of sunlight. Ground-level ozone is a harmful air pollutant, whereas ozone in the stratosphere helps block the sun's harmful ultraviolet radiation.

Pandemic A disease outbreak that spreads quickly and affects a large segment of a population over a wide geographical area.

Parts per million (ppm) The number of molecules of a substance contained in a million parts of another substance.

PCB (polychlorinated biphenyl) A group of chemicals widely used in hundreds of industrial and commercial applications, such as electrical and hydraulic equipment, plasticizers, pigments, and dyes, until manufacturing was banned in 1979 due to concerns about adverse health effects.

Perinatal Pertaining to the period around the time of birth.

Permafrost A thick subsurface layer of soil in the polar regions that remains in a frozen state throughout the entire year.

Phthalates A group of chemicals used to make plastics, including polyvinyl chloride, and other materials found in a wide range of products. Phthalate exposure is widespread in the U.S. population, although the human health effects are unknown.

Point source pollution A single source of pollution, such as at an industrial or sewage treatment plant.

Premature mortality Death, due to an environmental exposure, that occurs sooner than would otherwise be expected.

Quality assurance/quality control (QA/QC) A system of checks and audits to control the quality of measurements or products. Quality assurance is often conducted by an independent consultant or organization.

Radiation, electromagnetic A form of energy produced by electric and magnetic fields oscillating at right angles to each other. It takes many forms and is all around us, such as TV signals, radio waves, sunlight, ultraviolet radiation, and X-rays.

Radiation, ionizing A form of radiation, such as alpha and beta particles, gamma rays, X-rays, and neutrons, that is powerful enough to produce ions by breaking molecular bonds and displacing electrons from atoms and molecules. Ionizing radiation has many medical applications, but it can be a threat to human health at high doses.

Radiation, nonionizing A form of radiation, such as radio waves, microwaves, infrared and ultraviolet radiation, and visible light, that is not powerful enough to produce ions. Nonionizing radiation is not considered as great a threat to human health as ionizing radiation at high doses.

Radioactivity The emission of alpha or beta particles or gamma rays from radioactive elements like uranium, polonium, and radium. Also known as radioactive decay.

Radon A radioactive, alpha particle–emitting gas that exists naturally in many regions of the world and can be a health hazard if it accumulates in the basements and crawl spaces of homes.

Record of decision A public document that records a federal agency's decision about a proposed action for which an environmental impact statement has been prepared.

Rickettsial infection An infection caused by a type of bacteria that can only live inside the cells of another organism and that spreads primarily by ticks, mites, fleas, and lice.

Risk assessment A determination of the likelihood of events, such as the probability of a disease following exposure to an infectious agent or toxic pollutant.

Secondhand smoke Tobacco smoke exhaled by a smoker or given off by a tobacco product and inhaled by someone nearby. Also called passive smoke.

Smog A mixture of ground-level pollutants consisting primarily of ozone.

Social capital The relationships among people that allow society to function effectively.

Solar insolation A measure of the solar radiation striking the earth's surface, which varies according to the angle of the sun, location, elevation, and atmospheric conditions, including cloud cover.

Soot A black substance composed of mainly small particles of carbon that is emitted during the combustion of fossil fuels.

Stationary source An air pollution emission source other than a motor vehicle, such as a power plant, refinery, dry cleaner, commercial cooking establishment, and woodstove.

Stratosphere The part of the atmosphere, ranging from about 6 miles (9.7 kilometers) to 30 miles (48 kilometers) above the earth's surface, where temperature is relatively steady and clouds rarely form.

Subarctic Region located just south of the Arctic Circle.

Surgeon general Often referred to as the nation's doctor, the surgeon general of the United States oversees the U.S. Public Health Service and is responsible for providing Americans information and guidance on how to improve health and reduce the risk of illness and injury.

Synergistic effect Exposure to multiple substances where one substance worsens the effect of another substance.

Temperance movement An effort organized mainly by women in the nineteenth and twentieth centuries to encourage moderation or complete abstinence in the consumption of alcohol, believing alcohol to be the source of health problems, destitution, and crime.

Thermal pollution Heated water from an industrial process that is discharged to a body of water and can adversely affect aquatic organisms.

Thirdhand smoke Tobacco smoke residue that settles on indoor surfaces and interacts with other indoor pollutants to create a toxic mix of chemicals that may or may not become airborne.

Toxicant A toxic substance created by human activity, for example, an air pollutant or pesticide.

Toxicology The study of how chemical, physical, and biological agents can adversely affect people, animals, and the environment.

Toxin A toxic substance that is found in nature, for example, a snake venom or poisonous mushroom.

Transuranic waste A material produced from the recycling of spent nuclear fuel or the fabrication of nuclear weapons that is contaminated with artificially made radioactive elements having atomic numbers higher than uranium.

Tropism The involuntary orientation of an organism or one of its parts in response to stimulation.

Troposphere The lowest part of the atmosphere, ranging from the earth's surface to the bottom of the stratosphere, where weather systems and most air pollution occur.

Tsunami A large ocean wave or series of waves that sometimes occur following strong offshore earthquakes.

Turbidity A basic water quality test that measures the degree of cloudiness or haziness.

Urban runoff Stormwater from city streets and properties that can pick up and carry pollutants present on the ground as the stormwater flows into sewers or bodies of water.

Valley fever A fungal infection, characterized by fever, chest pain, coughing, and other symptoms, that thrives in arid desert soils.

Vector An organism, such as an insect or rodent, that carries a disease.

Volatile organic compound An organic compound that participates in the formation of photochemical smog.

Wet deposition The sulfuric and nitric acids that form from pollution in the atmosphere and fall back to the earth with rain, snow, fog, or hail, potentially damaging automobile and building surfaces, injuring wildlife and vegetation, and increasing the acidity of bodies of water.

Wetland An area saturated with surface or groundwater, such as a swamp, marsh, or bog, that supports wetland vegetation and helps sustain many species of fish and wildlife.

WTC dust A highly alkaline mixture of crushed concrete, gypsum, fibers, and many other substances that descended upon New York City as a dense cloud following the September 11, 2001, terrorist attack and subsequent collapse of the World Trade Center twin towers.

Zoonoses Diseases and infections transmitted between vertebrate animals and humans, where the zoonotic agent may be a bacterium, virus, fungus, or other communicable agent.

Zoonotic Diseases and infections transmitted between vertebrate animals and humans.

Directory of Resources

Air and Waste Management Association

Pittsburgh, Pennsylvania
https://www.awma.org

The Air and Waste Management Association (AWMA) is a professional organization dedicated to enhancing knowledge and expertise in the areas of air quality and waste management by providing a neutral forum for exchanging information. The AWMA provides professional development opportunities to its members, promotes global environmental responsibility, and helps organizations make critical decisions that benefit society.

American Public Health Association

Washington, D.C.
https://apha.org

The American Public Health Association (APHA) is a professional association with over 25,000 members representing virtually every field of public health and medicine. The APHA's Environment Section (apha.org/apha-communities/member-sections/environment) sponsors initiatives to protect environmental health, promotes the work of environmental health professionals, and develops outreach programs to educate the public on environmental health issues.

Carter Center

Atlanta, Georgia
https://www.cartercenter.org

The Carter Center was founded by President Jimmy Carter and Rosalynn Carter as a nongovernmental organization to help advance peace and worldwide health by resolving global conflicts, advancing democracy and human rights, promoting economic opportunity, preventing diseases, improving mental health, and teaching farmers how to increase crop production. The center has been particularly effective in the environmental health field by reducing the incidence of infectious diseases.

Centers for Disease Control and Prevention

Atlanta, Georgia
https://www.cdc.gov

The mission of the Centers for Disease Control and Prevention (also known as the CDC) is to protect Americans from health, safety, and security threats originating both in the United States and overseas. The CDC conducts research, provides health information to health agencies and the public, issues health alerts, and coordinates response activities with state and local agencies. The National Center for Environmental Health (cdc.gov/nceh) and National Institute for Occupational Safety and Health (cdc.gov/niosh) are organizational components of the CDC.

Council on Environmental Quality

Washington, D.C.
https://www.whitehouse.gov/ceq

The Council on Environmental Quality (CEQ) is located in the White House and falls under the Executive Office of the President. The CEQ coordinates the federal government's environmental efforts by developing environmental policies and initiatives, overseeing implementation of the environmental impact assessment process, and working with agencies to select environmental actions consistent with the president's goals.

David Suzuki Foundation

Vancouver, British Columbia
http://www.davidsuzuki.org

The goal of the David Suzuki Foundation is to promote environmental conservation and sustainability through science-based research, education, and policy development. The foundation's priorities include protecting the climate, creating livable communities, establishing environmental rights and justice, transforming the economy through efficient resource use, helping youth connect with nature, and building community with earth-friendly infrastructure, smart energy choices, and efficient transportation.

Environmental Protection Agency

Washington, D.C.
https://www.epa.gov

The U.S. Environmental Protection Agency (EPA) is the nation's leading environmental agency for protecting human health and the environment. The EPA's priorities include developing and enforcing regulations, issuing research grants, studying environmental issues, sponsoring partnerships, teaching people about the environment, and protecting the rights of low-income and minority populations to a clean environment.

Federal Emergency Management Agency

Washington, D.C.
https://www.fema.gov

The Federal Emergency Management Agency (FEMA) provides support to citizens, first responders, and state and local governments to prepare for, protect against, respond to, and recover from all hazards. For example, FEMA routinely provides emergency supplies and assistance during natural disasters caused by severe storm outbreaks, hurricanes, forest fires, and earthquakes.

Food and Drug Administration

Silver Spring, Maryland
https://www.fda.gov

The Food and Drug Administration (FDA) has a variety of responsibilities for protecting the safety of food and drugs in the Unites States. Additionally, the FDA ensures that vaccines and medical devices are safe and effective, protects the public from electronic product radiation, assures cosmetics and dietary supplements are safe and properly labeled, regulates tobacco products, and helps speed up the pace of product innovation.

Intergovernmental Panel on Climate Change

Geneva, Switzerland
http://www.ipcc.ch

The Intergovernmental Panel on Climate Change (IPCC) is the world's leading international body for assessing the science related to climate change and providing the latest information to governments and policymakers. The IPCC conducts regular assessments of climate change science, impacts and future risks, and options for adaption and mitigation.

Land Institute

Salina, Kansas
https://landinstitute.org

The Land Institute is working to replace traditional agricultural practices, including the widespread use of pesticides, herbicides, and chemical fertilizers, with sustainable practices based on natural systems that preserve culture and ecology. The institute's goal is to develop an agricultural system featuring perennial plants that will have ecological stability and crop yield comparable to today's annual crops.

National Center for Environmental Health

Atlanta, Georgia
https://www.cdc.gov/nceh

The mission of the National Center for Environmental Health (NCEH) is to promote a healthy environment, prevent premature death, and help people avoid illness and disability caused by environmental factors other than infectious disease agents and occupational exposures. The NCEH focuses particularly on vulnerable populations, such as children, older adults, and people with disabilities.

National Institute for Environmental Health Sciences

Research Triangle Park, North Carolina
https://www.niehs.nih.gov

The goal of the National Institute for Environmental Health Sciences (NIEHS) is to promote healthier lives for Americans by conducting research on how the environment affects people and by disseminating information to the research community and the public. The NIEHS is world renowned as a leader in the field of environmental health sciences.

National Institute for Occupational Safety and Health

Atlanta, Georgia
https://www.cdc.gov/niosh

The National Institute for Occupational Safety and Health (NIOSH) conducts research on occupational safety and health issues and puts its research findings into practice in the workplace. NIOSH's goals are to reduce worker illness and injury and advance well-being, promote safe and healthy workers through interventions and capacity building, and sponsor and participate in global collaborations aimed at enhancing worker safety and health.

National Institutes of Health

Bethesda, Maryland
https://www.nih.gov

The National Institutes of Health (NIH) is the nation's leading medical research agency, with many research programs at the forefront of global health protection. The NIH is made up of 27 separate institutes and centers, each having specific research agenda concerning diseases, health challenge, and body systems. The National Institute of Environmental Health Sciences (niehs.nih.gov) is an organizational component of the NIH.

National Oceanic and Atmospheric Administration

Washington, D.C.
http://www.noaa.gov

The mission of the National Oceanic and Atmospheric Administration (NOAA) is to conduct research, collect data, and disseminate information on the nation's climate, weather, oceans, and coasts. NOAA studies the structure and behavior of the oceans and atmosphere, conserves and manages coastal and marine ecosystems and resources, and responds to environmental emergencies.

Occupational Safety and Health Administration

Washington, D.C.
https://www.osha.gov

The mission of the Occupational Safety and Health Administration (OSHA) is to ensure that working Americans experience safe and healthful working conditions by implementing the requirements of the Occupational Safety and Health Act. OSHA sets and enforces standards, delivers training to employers and workers, and provides technical assistance.

Ocean Alliance

Gloucester, Massachusetts
http://www.whale.org

The Ocean Alliance collects information on whales and other ocean life, with the goal of educating policymakers and the public on the wise stewardship of the oceans to prevent the collapse of marine mammal populations and promote ocean and human health. A project known as the Voyage of the Odyssey provided the world's first set of data on the widespread distribution of synthetic contaminants in the oceans and how they affect ocean life.

Water Environment Federation

Alexandria, Virginia
http://www.wef.org

The Water Environment Federation (WEF) is a professional organization representing over 33,000 individual members and 75 affiliated organizations around the world. The

WEF's goals are to protect public health and the environment by enriching the experience of water pollution professionals, increasing public awareness about the importance of water, and providing a platform for innovation.

Woods Hole Oceanographic Institution

Woods Hole, Massachusetts
http://www.whoi.edu

The Woods Hole Oceanographic Institution is one of the world's leading nonprofit organizations for ocean research, exploration, and education, including environmental threats to the oceans and coastal areas. The institution's research covers a range of topics related to ocean and earth science, marine policy, and climate change.

World Health Organization

Geneva, Switzerland
http://www.who.int

The World Health Organization (WHO) provides global leadership on matters critical to human health by shaping the global research agenda, setting norms and standards, articulating ethical and evidence-based policies, providing technical support, and monitoring health trends. The WHO employees over 7,000 people in its headquarters office and over 150 country offices.

About the Editor and Contributors

Editor

Richard Crume is an environmental engineer, educator, and journalist with over 40 years of experience in the environmental health field. He previously managed the program planning and budget staff for the U.S. Environmental Protection Agency's national air quality planning and standards office, where he received the agency's highest honor award, the Gold Medal for Exceptional Service, and the Suzanne E. Olive Award for outstanding service in promoting equal opportunity and diversity. Crume was also principal engineer at the Parson's Corporation, head of the Environmental Engineering Section at MRI Global, and adjunct associate professor at North Carolina A&T State University, where he taught classes for many years on air pollution, climate change, and renewable energy. Crume has written and lectured extensively on environmental health and renewable energy topics, with nearly 100 publications and seminars covering air pollution and climate change, waste management, environmental justice and leadership, and green building design. Additionally, he has published 19 feature stories in *Solar Today* magazine, and he has chaired sessions at eight national environmental conferences. As a member of the American Public Health Association, Crume recently authored their national policy on air pollution and the Clean Air Act, and he also belongs to the National Association of Science Writers and Society of Environmental Journalists. He is certified as a qualified environmental professional and hazard control manager.

Contributors

Talia E. Abbott Chalew is an adjunct faculty member at Johns Hopkins University, teaching and developing courses in environmental applications and implications of nanotechnology. Her previous research experience has focused on the fate and transport of nanomaterials in the environment and human health effects. Dr. Abbott Chalew is a member of the Society for Environmental Toxicology and Chemistry.

Ifeanyi Abuachi is a physician, medical researcher, and private consultant, and he previously served as medical director of the Jerry Hospital in Lagos Nigeria. Dr. Abuachi's research has included creating a medical diagnostic and communications system (patent pending) aimed at improving patient-doctor communications and outcomes. He is a member of the Inter-American College of Physicians and Surgeons, American Board of Surgical Assistants, and American Public Health Association.

Henry Babatunde Akinleye is a chemist and program leader in the Food Safety Department of *Consumer Reports*. Additionally, he is conducting research on dietary exposure to phthalates at the City University of New York's School of Public Health and Health Policy.

Andrew P. Barefield is a medical support assistant at the Veterans Administration clinic in Carrollton, Georgia, and he has been a registered radiographer for over 30 years. With two autistic adult children living at home, Barefield's passion for the environment is based on the epigenetic link to autism, how that relates to his children's futures, and his desire to leave the world a more ecologically friendly place.

Matthew W. Blair is a plant breeder and research associate professor at Tennessee State University, where he conducts breeding and genetics research on legumes and dicotyledonous C4 crop plants, such as cultivated amaranth. His plant genetics laboratory applies molecular biology research to cultivar and crop development using various agronomic and physiological testing techniques, with the goal of having a major impact on the productivity of small-holder agriculture in the United States and internationally.

Michael S. Bloom is an associate professor and associate chair in the Department of Environmental Health Sciences at the School of Public Health, University of Albany, State University of New York. Dr. Bloom's research is focused on elucidating the impacts of environmental pollutants on reproduction and endocrine function in human populations. He also teaches graduate-level introductory environmental health, reproductive environmental health, and reproductive and perinatal epidemiology.

John K. Borén is the founder of RÄV EHS Consulting. He has over 25 years of environmental health and safety experience covering areas such as compliance auditing, management systems design, hazardous waste and toxics substances control, storm water and wastewater management, climate change, and air permitting. Borén is a registered professional engineer, certified hazardous materials manager, certified industrial hygienist, and certified safety professional.

Georgiana Bostean is an assistant professor of environment, health, and policy at Chapman University. Her research is broadly in the area of social determinants of health, and she has examined the individual and ecological correlates of adolescent e-cigarette use. Dr. Bostean has published in various academic journals, including the *American Journal of Public Health, Health and Place*, and the *Journal of Immigrant and Minority Health*.

Jeanine Botta is a writer, editor, and consultant with particular interest in nonauditory effects of noise exposure and health benefits of access to quiet. As a member of the Right to Quiet Society for Soundscape Awareness and Protection, she provides educational programs at environmental trade shows. She is a cofounder of the Silence the Horns project and a founding member of the Quiet Coalition.

Ronda Bowen is an independent researcher covering subjects ranging from metaphysics and epistemology to the philosophy of technology. Her current research interests include environmental solutions, biomedical ethics, and corporate agriculture's responsibility to citizens. Additionally, Bowen has published or presented on why we need a green revolution, steps to sustainability, and focal practices in response to a hot, flat, and crowded world. She also contributed chapters to *Native America: A State by State History*.

Thomas D. Byl is a research biologist with the U.S. Geological Survey. He is stationed at Tennessee State University, where he oversees research on hydrology and water quality in natural systems having nonideal flow, such as wetlands and karst aquifers. Additionally, Dr. Byl teaches environmental chemistry, biogeochemistry, and water quality management courses. He is a member of the Society of Environmental Toxicology and Chemistry, American Water Resources Association, National Speleological Society, and Tennessee Academy of Science.

Philip A. Clifford is dean of math and science at Volunteer State Community College and has taught biology, ecology, research and statistics, and related courses for over 30 years. He has also worked in the environmental consulting business for a number of years as an ecotoxicologist. In that role, he studied many bioaccumulative substances, wrote numerous mathematical models for predicting their behavior in the environment, and authored a variety of articles describing relevant case studies.

Chatten Cowherd Jr. recently retired as principal advisor for environmental studies at MRIGlobal. He has more than 30 years of experience in field studies directed toward the characterization and control of fugitive dust, and he is a fellow member of the Air and Waste Management Association, having served on its board of directors. Dr. Cowherd is one of the world's foremost experts on fugitive dust.

Yoko S. Crume has over 30 years of work experience in the environmental and social work fields, most recently as a tenured professor at North Carolina A&T State University, where she started a community-based mental health service for the non-English-speaking population in Greensboro, North Carolina. Her latest activities include developing a senior transportation system in Nashville, Tennessee, and researching assistive technology innovations for older adults in Japan.

Mallory L. Daily is a freelance reporter with strong roots in the Midwest. She has worked for St. Louis public radio, reported on state politics in Missouri, and farmed organic vegetables in Iowa. Daily's latest project is to write environmental stories while helping small farmers in El Salvador incorporate sustainable, economically feasible growing practices.

Charles Daniel is an environmental health officer for the city of Melrose, Massachusetts, and a former infectious disease epidemiologist for the Massachusetts Department of Public Health. He teaches epidemiology and biostatistics at Kaplan University and is a health sciences lecturer at Northeastern University's College of Professional Studies. Daniel is a member of the American Public Health Association and National Environmental Health Association.

Richard S. Davis has been an environmental lawyer at Beveridge and Diamond PC in Washington, D.C., for over 30 years, specializing in the Clean Water Act and Safe Drinking Water Act. He works with industry and municipalities to help them ensure compliance with these important laws. Davis is chair of his firm's clean water practice group and helps direct one of the most innovative and dynamic clean water practices in the United States.

Qi Deng is a research associate at Tennessee State University. His research covers the broad area of plant ecology and global change ecology, including both laboratory and field experimentation. Dr. Deng is also interested in metadata analysis and applications of modeling approaches for processing experimental data.

Aaron Dorman is a freelance science writer and editorial assistant for *The American Gardener* magazine. Among his more recent projects, Dorman published articles on upstate New York environmental issues, such as electric vehicle charging stations and vermicompost, and he contributed fact sheet and curriculum materials for the Earth Day Network. Dorman's writing often concerns the human impact on ecosystems and the environment, particularly garbage and electronic waste. He is a member of the Society of Environmental Journalists.

Abhishek Dubey is an assistant professor in the Department of Computer Science at Vanderbilt University. Additionally, he is a senior research scientist in the university's Institute for Software Integrated Systems. Dr. Dubey oversees research into the problems of interoperability, scalability, and dependability of Internet of Things networks in the domain of smart transportation and smart grid. He is a senior member of the Institute of Electrical and Electronics Engineers.

Lawrence K. Duffy is a professor and director of the Resilience and Adaptation Program at the University of Alaska-Fairbanks, where he teaches biochemistry and environmental toxicology and conducts research on issues related to environmental biochemistry and health. Dr. Duffy previously held research positions at Boston University, the Roche Institute of Molecular Biology, the University of Texas Medical Branch, and Harvard Medical School. He is a fellow of the American Institute of Chemistry and the Arctic Institute of North America.

Leah A. Dundon is an environmental attorney with the Beveridge and Diamond PC law firm in Washington, D.C. She has over 15 years of experience in advising clients regarding major federal environmental statutes, such as the Clean Air Act and Clean Water Act, and their state counterparts. Dundon is a member of the Tennessee and DC Bars and the American Bar Association's Environment, Energy, and Resources section. She regularly speaks and publishes on environmental issues, including climate change, risk, environmental disclosures, and resiliency.

E. Kudjo Dzantor, an associate professor of soil microbiology/biochemistry at Tennessee State University, has over 30 years of experience involving bio/phytoremediation investigations and studies of soil contamination with pesticides, polychlorinated biphenyl, polyaromatic hydrocarbons, explosives, and coal fly ash. Dr. Dzantor's current research is focused on coupling bio/phytoremediation to bioenergy feedstock production on marginal and degraded lands.

Joe Elkins has worked for the federal government for over 30 years, managing monitoring and quality assurance programs over much of this time. Elkins has taught monitoring and quality assurance courses around the world for the World Health Organization, and he has also worked as a college professor. His professional memberships have included the American Chemical Society, the Air and Waste Management Association, and the American Society of Quality.

Hana Elliott is a senior business manager in the technology industry with a background in environmental studies. She currently resides in Nashville, Tennessee, in a platinum LEED-certified, passive solar home, built using reclaimed materials, including recycled drywall and exterior siding made from a combination of old tin roofing material and charred oak (a traditional Japanese technique to preserve wood). Her work has previously been published in *Solar Today* magazine.

Beth J. Feingold is an assistant professor in the Department of Environmental Health Sciences at the University at Albany School of Public Health, State University of New York. She teaches global environmental health policy, geographic information systems and public health, and introduction to environmental health sciences. Dr. Feingold conducts interdisciplinary research to understand the drivers of environmental health disparities.

Linda Forst is board-certified in the field of occupational and internal medicine, and she is a professor at the School of Public Health, University of Illinois at Chicago. Dr. Forst conducts research related to occupational safety and health, underserved working populations, worker compensation, and surveillance for occupational illnesses and injuries in Illinois. Additionally, she is the director of a World Health Organization Collaborating Center on Occupational and Environmental Health.

Elizabeth Ann Glass Geltman is an associate professor at the City University of New York's Graduate School of Public Health and Health Policy. Additionally, she serves as secretary and communications officer for the Environment Section of the American Public Health Association. Dr. Geltman is an attorney and author of 17 books on environmental health law and policy.

Matthew O. Gribble is an assistant professor of environmental health at Emory University. He is a genetic epidemiologist by training and has conducted research on arsenic toxicokinetic genetics using both linkage and association approaches, focusing on families recruited from Arizona, Oklahoma, North Dakota, and South Dakota. Dr. Gribble also has broader interests in exposure science, environmental epidemiology, marine ecosystems, and ecotoxicology, and he is a diplomate of the American Board of Toxicology.

Gwen Griffith is program director of the Cumberland River Compact in Nashville, Tennessee. Dr. Griffith is a veterinarian turned educator who applies her science and health background to promoting ecosystem health at the landscape scale, including watershed stewardship, low impact development, and water conservation. Her background includes veterinary practice and science fellowship positions, and she was previously executive director of the Tennessee Environmental Council.

Justin M. Gundlach is an associate research scholar at Columbia Law School and a fellow at the Sabin Center for Climate Change Law. His work at the Sabin Center focuses on using existing legal and regulatory tools to promote efforts on the part of government and the private sector to mitigate and adapt to climate change. He is a member of the New York bar.

Meredith Hale holds the position of Kress Fellow in art librarianship at Yale University. She formerly was a librarian at the U.S. Environmental Protection Agency, specializing in resources for environmental research and rule development and handling requests from the public for information on environmental issues. She is a member of the Art Libraries Society of North America.

Maryam Hatcher is an associate with Beveridge and Diamond PC in Washington, D.C., where she maintains an environmental regulatory and litigation practice. Hatcher advises clients on various environmental compliance, contamination, and liability matters and provides guidance on federal environmental and occupational safety laws. During law school, Hatcher served as editor-in-chief of the *Howard Law Journal* at Howard University.

Adam Hess is an environmental health and safety assistant in the Environmental Health and Safety Department of New York University's Langone Medical Center. He previously conducted research at the City University of New York's School of Public Health, where he coauthored a data set and articles for the LawAtlas, concerning mold remediation and certification laws in the United States.

Anthony C. Holderied is a librarian and current assistant director at the U.S. Environmental Protection Agency (EPA) library in Research Triangle Park, North Carolina. Under contract with the School of Information and Library Science at the University of North Carolina at Chapel Hill, the EPA Research Triangle Park Library is one of 24 libraries in the EPA National Library Network. Holderied oversees the areas of reference, literature searching, and user education, helping to support over 2,000 local EPA research scientists.

Melisa L. Holman is associate director of Donor Communications for the Nature Conservancy in Asheville, North Carolina. She focuses on the Asia Pacific region, raising funding and awareness for the Conservancy's work. Holman has a background in forest ecology and environmental science and has published on topics ranging from invasive species to forest conservation.

Marilyn Holt is a research assistant in the chemical and physical biology program at Vanderbilt University, where she is studying the effects of enzyme dynamics on DNA replication. Additionally, as an accomplished science writer, Dr. Holt assists students in the university's writing center. She is a member of the Biophysical Society and the American Medical Writers Association.

Dafeng Hui is an associate professor at Tennessee State University, where he teaches ecology and conducts research in the areas of plant, global change, and ecosystem ecology and modeling. He has authored or coauthored more than 80 papers and serves as editor and reviewer for scientific journals. Dr. Hui's research has been sponsored by the U.S. Department of Energy, U.S. Department of Agriculture, and the National Science Foundation.

Elise C. Hunter is a site design engineer specializing in urban water resources. Additionally, she is experienced with wastewater treatment, stormwater development plans, and regulatory compliance. Hunter previously conducted research at Vanderbilt University on multidisciplinary approaches to assessing urban water security, incorporating physical and social sciences, engineering, and policy.

Ans Irfan is an adjunct professor at George Washington University's Milken Institute School of Public Health, where he teaches environmental health science and public health biology. Dr. Irfan is a certified public health professional, and he is chair of the Environmental Health and Safety Committee of the Metropolitan Washington Public Health Association.

Jyotsna S. Jagai is a research assistant professor at the University of Illinois at Chicago's School of Public Health. She is an environmental epidemiologist whose broad research interest is characterizing the impact of changing water quality and land use on human health. Dr. Jagai is also interested in developing comprehensive indicators to characterize the cumulative environmental impact on human health. Her work includes time series analyses, meta-analysis methods, and development of environmental exposure measures.

Adrienne L. Katner is an assistant professor at Louisiana State University's Health Sciences Center in the School of Public Health. Dr. Katner's research involves evaluating human exposure to heavy metals. Formerly with the Louisiana Office of Public Health, she oversaw Louisiana's Environmental Public Health Tracking and Occupational Health programs. Dr. Katner teaches principles of occupational health and environmental policy, and she is a member of the Society of Toxicology and the American Public Health Association.

Alison K. Krajewski is research associate at the University of Illinois at Chicago's School of Public Health, where she specializes in environmental epidemiology and occupational surveillance research. Dr. Krajewski's primary research project involves assessing the relationship between cumulative environmental exposures and diabetes outcomes.

Emmanuel Kyeremateng-Amoah is a public health/occupational health physician with the Ghana Health Service, where he conducts research on the health impacts of extractive industries and associated air pollution. Dr. Kyeremateng-Amoah is currently conducting research on pesticide poisoning reporting and the Adult Blood Lead Registry at the Illinois Occupational Surveillance Program within the Department of Environmental and Occupational Health Sciences, University of Illinois at Chicago.

Rachel L. Lamb is a University of Maryland Flagship fellow and steering committee member for Young Evangelicals for Climate Action. Additionally, she teaches environmental law and policy at Au Sable Institute of Environmental Studies. Lamb previously worked as a fellow for the U.S. Environmental Protection Agency, where she produced a collection of tribal best practices for climate change adaptation. Her professional expertise is in cultivating interdisciplinary strategies to combat climate change that simultaneously address ecological, economic, and sociopolitical concerns.

Megan W. Latshaw is a member of the faculty at the Johns Hopkins Bloomberg School of Public Health and is past chair of the American Public Health Association's Environment Section, serving from 2015 through 2017. She created and formalized a national biomonitoring network at the Association of Public Health Laboratories, and she has published and presented on this topic both domestically and internationally. Dr. Latshaw's earlier research involved measuring biomarkers as part of a larger study focusing on memory in older Baltimore residents.

David A. Lawrence is a senior research scientist with the Wadsworth Center of the New York State Department of Health in Albany, New York. At the Wadsworth Center, Dr. Lawrence is laboratory chief of immunology. His research addresses the influences of environmental stressors on the multifunctionality of nervous, endocrine, and immune system interactions. Dr. Lawrence received the Vos Lifetime Career Achievement Award in Immunotoxicology from the Society of Toxicology.

Thomas B. Lawrence is a consulting engineer specializing in water quality protection and restoration, including projects as varied as underground storage tank remediation, construction site pollution prevention design and implementation, and municipal stormwater pollution prevention. He is an experienced speaker and instructor, having spoken at professional conferences throughout the country. Lawrence is a registered professional engineer, and he has worked in the civil engineering field for over 25 years.

Nichole LeClair is a research fellow at the City University of New York's Graduate School of Public Health and Health Policy. She is coauthor of data sets published by LawAtlas, involving technologically enhanced mapping of naturally occurring radioactive materials and radon laws in the United States.

Shao Lin is a professor of environmental health sciences and associate director for Global Health Research, University of Albany, State University of New York. As a principal investigator, she has directed multiple studies of the September 11 terrorist attacks as well as other research involving the health effects of extreme weather, natural disasters, air pollution and traffic, and the home/school environment. Additionally, Dr. Lin was a member of the advisory board of the World Trade Center Health Registry for many years.

Yi-Pin Lin is a research scientist at the Wadsworth Center, New York State Department of Health at Albany, New York. His research focuses on how Lyme disease–causing bacteria survive in two distinct host environments (ticks and vertebrate animals), causing transmission between these hosts and resulting in diseases. Dr. Lin also teaches immunology and medical entomology at the State University of New York at Albany.

Howard W. MacLennan Jr. is the lead physician in medical readiness standards for the North Carolina Army National Guard, where his specialties include genetics, molecular biology, and osteopathic medicine. Dr. MacLennan is a member of the American Academy of Family Physicians, American Board of Family Medicine, and American Osteopathic Association, and he has widely published in a variety of medical journals. (The views expressed by Dr. MacLennan are those of the author and do not reflect the official policy or position of the Department of the Army, Department of Defense, or U.S. government.)

Jessica M. Madrigal is a research specialist at the University of Illinois at Chicago, where she contributes to public health research related to diabetes and other chronic diseases. Her academic and research interests focus on environmental and occupational exposures and chronic disease outcomes. Madrigal is a member of

American Public Health Association, American College of Sports Medicine, and the Society for Epidemiologic Research.

Susan J. Montgomery has more than 40 years of experience as a professional journalist and teacher. For much of her career, her writing has focused on healthcare topics for major healthcare organizations, and she has an expertise in communicating technical, health-related topics to a lay audience. Montgomery has also published two artists' biographies and is currently managing an online magazine, Life-Uncorked .com, that includes articles on travel and cuisine throughout Southern California.

Jill Warnasch Mozier is an environmental engineer with SC&A, Inc., an environmental and energy consulting firm. Mozier is the project manager for technical support to the U.S. Environmental Protection Agency in developing its residential wood heater air emission standards. Additionally, she is the project manager for the inhalation risk modeling (cancer and noncancer) of emission source categories evaluated under the agency's Risk and Technology Review and National Air Toxics Assessment programs.

Alisha K. Newton is the environmental literacy coordinator for the Tennessee Department of Environment and Conservation, where she is responsible for implementing the Tennessee state environmental literacy plan. As a student at Vanderbilt University, Newton founded a publication about environmental issues. She previously worked for the National Park Service at Wrangell-St. Elias National Park and Preserve in Alaska.

Joanne O'Loughlin is an environmental scientist and registered nurse at SC&A, Inc., an environmental and energy consulting firm, where she analyzes air pollution emission sources, health effects from exposure to air pollutants, and emission mitigation options. O'Loughlin is currently supporting the development of a healthcare provider training course to educate providers on communicating with patients who are at high risk from air pollution exposure.

Mary V. O'Reilly, an industrial hygienist and ergonomist, is on the faculty of the State University of New York's School of Public Health and a member of the faculty advisory committee for the university's Institute for Health and the Environment. Dr. O'Reilly is board president for Workplace Health Without Borders (U.S. Branch), and she received the American Industrial Hygiene Association's 2016 Alice Hamilton Award. She also belongs to the American Conference of Governmental Industrial Hygienists and the Society for Risk Analysis.

Richard F. Pandullo has over 30 years of professional experience covering a broad range of environmental management issues, including air quality planning and permitting, climate change strategy, greenhouse gas emissions management, health and safety management systems, and various types of environmental auditing. Pandullo is currently director of Trinity Consultants' business line for environmental health and safety performance and risk management, overseeing client technical support work involving sustainability, management systems, and auditing.

Anthony G. Papetti is an environmental attorney at Beveridge and Diamond PC, a national environmental law firm of 100 lawyers, where he maintains a general environmental litigation and regulatory practice. He also has work experience with the United Nations and the U.S. Environmental Protection Agency. Prior to becoming an environmental attorney, Papetti worked as a chemical analyst in the elemental analysis section of a global company that provides testing and inspection services for the petroleum, refining, and petrochemical industries.

Chelsea N. Peters is a hydrologist specializing in drinking water resources. She is experienced with stream restoration planning and water quality modeling, and her recent research at Vanderbilt University focuses on groundwater-surface water interactions in southwest Bangladesh. Peters has taught a variety of K–12 hydrology and environmental stewardship courses across Tennessee.

R. Christopher Rustin is director of Environmental Health for the Georgia Department of Public Health, and he has 18 years of experience working in local and state environmental public health programs. He was previously an assistant professor at Georgia Southern University's Jiann-Ping Hsu College of Public Health, where he taught courses in environmental health science and conducted research on the application of environmental health programs, surveillance of mosquito vectors, and lead poisoning risk factors.

A.J. Smuskiewicz is a freelance writer and editor who specializes in science, medicine, and world events. Prior to entering the writing profession, Smuskiewicz worked as a laboratory and field biologist, including analyzing zooplankton species and water chemistry for the U.S. Environmental Protection Agency's Great Lakes Monitoring Project and conducting dose-response tests on National Institutes of Health projects at the Illinois Institute of Technology Research Institute.

Victor B. Stolberg is an assistant professor/counselor at Essex County College in Newark, New Jersey, where he previously directed the Office of Disability Support Services and Office of the Substance Abuse Coordinator. He has authored 49 scholarly articles, 87 encyclopedia articles, six chapters and contributed papers, and 63 other miscellaneous publications. Stolberg also has several publications in press, including the book *Painkillers: History, Science, and Issues*.

Kathy Stolley is a professor of sociology at Virginia Wesleyan College. Her emphasis is applied sociology, which involves using sociological tools and perspectives to bring about positive social change. A recipient of Virginia Wesleyan College's Samuel Nelson Gray Distinguished Teaching Award, Dr. Stolley formerly served as associate dean for Innovative Teaching and Engaged Learning. Her written work appears in a variety of professional journals, and she has published five books.

Timothy J. Sutton is a physician specializing in occupational and environmental medicine. Dr. Sutton's field of expertise lies in the evaluation and management of workplace injuries and toxic exposures, and he also focuses on evaluating environmental pollutants and their effects on the human population. Dr. Sutton is a member of the American College of Occupational and Environmental Medicine.

Ranjita Thapa is a plant breeding specialist experienced in the genotyping and phenotyping of *Amaranthus*, a highly nutritious and ancient pseudocereal. She is presently involved with a rice breeding project in the Department of Soil and Crop Sciences at Texas A&M University. The goal of this research is to improve rice through the deployment of genetics and genomics tools.

Leon D. Tillman Jr. is a resource conservationist with the Natural Resources Conservation Service, where he provides technical leadership, guidance, and assistance in developing and implementing Farm Bill conservation programs. His work contributes to increasing conservation implementation on private agriculture land and improving water quality through U.S. Department of Agriculture programs and initiatives.

Kelley Trahan is the environmental librarian at the San Francisco Public Library. She has worked previously as a librarian at the Oakland Public Library and as an archivist at the National Archives' San Francisco regional office. She is passionate about fostering the information literacy skills that patrons need to become critical information consumers and developing innovative programs to highlight collections.

Robert Ukeiley is a public interest environmental lawyer and consultant with his own practice based in Boulder, Colorado. He represents and supports nonprofit environmental and community organizations in their efforts to reduce air pollution and foster the transition to clean, renewable energy. Ukeiley has presented at numerous workshops and panels on air pollution and energy issues.

Simon Waldbaum has spent over a decade conducting biomedical science research, most recently at the University of Colorado Anschutz Medical Campus in a laboratory studying the contributing effects of environmental toxins on neurological disorders, such as Parkinson's disease and acquired epilepsy. Dr. Waldbaum's primary research focus and areas of publication have been in elucidating inhibitory synaptic signaling, studying neuronal control of respiration, and investigating the link between mitochondrial dysfunction and neurological disorders.

Jessica Wentz is a staff attorney at the Sabin Center for Climate Change Law at Columbia Law School. Her work at the center spans a variety of topics related to climate change mitigation, adaptation, sustainable development, and environmental justice. She is a member of the California Bar.

Xingbo Wu specializes in plant breeding in the Agricultural and Environmental Sciences program at Tennessee State University. He has a special interest in researching the plant genomics and genetics of cowpea, an important sub-Saharan African crop, with the goal of improving nutritional quality through molecular breeding. Dr. Wu is a member of the Crop Science Society of America.

Damba Yahaya is a plant biotechnologist and assistant lecturer at the University for Development Studies in Tamale, Ghana, where he conducts tissue culture and plant propagation on roots and tubers crops, such as cassava and yam. Additionally, he is conducting breeding and genetics research at Tennessee State University involving legumes and dicotyledonous C4 crop plants, such as cultivated amaranth.

Index

Note: page numbers in **bold** indicate main encyclopedia entries.